'Few people have contributed as much to the growth of mental health care in the United Kingdom as the late Dr. Malcolm Pines. Over more than sixty years he transformed the profession, not least the discipline of group analysis, increasing the number of patients in treatment by an unparalleled percentage. We extend our deep thanks to John Schlapobersky – an esteemed clinician and author in his own right – for having prepared these highly-readable, core papers with such meticulousness.'

Prof. Brett Kahr, *Senior Fellow, Tavistock Institute of Medical Psychology, London; Hon. Director of Research, Freud Museum London; Visiting Professor of Psychoanalysis and Mental Health, Regent's University*

'Malcolm Pines has piloted the ship of group analysis from its earliest days when Foulkes was at the helm, and he set its compass into the twenty first century with amazing prescience. In this enthralling compilation he revisits his journey from psychoanalysis to group analysis and brings together the social and biological worlds of discourse. His writing is coloured by reminiscences of the earlier pioneers. We find him admiring their ideas but refusing to be beholden to their monolithic schools. The result has been a liberating experience for practitioners all over the world whom he has inspired. He has not only chronicled the history of psychotherapy: he is an essential part of it and these papers represent the summation of his lifetime's work.'

Dr. Harold Behr, *Honorary Member and Training group analyst, Institute of Group Analysis, London; Consultant Psychiatrist; Former Editor, 'Group Analysis – The Journal'*

'I can almost hear Malcom speaking as I read the papers – some of which I knew but not all. He saw himself as a teacher and would talk softly, not at length, waiting for those he taught to add their own ideas to what he was bringing. These papers are often quite short but always stimulate the reader or the student to see their own ideas from a different perspective. Malcolm was a life-long clinician who had a very deep love of learning. These papers show his excitement at the drama of connecting new learning to our group analytic frame. An erudite, stimulating collection.'

Sue Einhorn, *Training group analyst, Institute of Group Analysis (UK)*

'Reading this book gave me great joy; it was like meeting Malcolm again still alive, with his spontaneity and freshness, clarity and depth. People who were lucky enough to know him will have the same joyful surprise on reading this book. Those who did not know him personally will have the opportunity to discover his great vitality and generosity. The enormous theoretical and organizational work done by Malcolm Pines throughout his life is impressive. Group Analysis is not only a healing discipline but an opportunity to expand the fields of linguistics, semiotics, communication and political science described here. The book is recommended not only for group therapists, psychoanalysts, and psychology students, but also for the general reader.'

Prof. Claudio Neri, *Professor in Psychology, la Sapienza University, Rome and la Università Statale, Turin; Training and supervising analyst, Italian Psychoanalytic Society; Member, International Psychoanalytic Association (IPA), Institute of Group Analysis (UK) and Confederation of Italian Organizations for Analytic Research on Groups (COIRAG)*

'Malcolm Pines develops group analysis on wonderfully coherent terms in this collection which gives 'an account of our lifelong and often unsuccessful struggle to become, and remain, relatively healthy human beings' – living on reasonably good, tolerant relations with ourselves – our inner society – and with others – our external society. John Schlapobersky has done a fine job selecting and editing the papers.'

Dr. Robi Friedman, *Past President, Group Analytic Society International; Co-Founder and Formerly Chair, Israel Institute for Group Analysis*

'Malcolm and I first met at the Maudsley Hospital in 1975, where I was a young psychiatrist specialising in psychotherapy. Working with and being supervised by him was a lesson in the art of perceptive but gentle enquiry, always respectful of the whole person while exploring the reaches of their inner world. The breadth and depth of his erudition was astounding, yet always offered in the spirit of a Socratic dialogue among equals. His contribution to the field of analytic psychotherapy has been immense, leaving a legacy of outstanding scholarship and clinical acumen. Those of us who counted Malcolm a friend, remember with lasting affection the gentle giant of group analysis. I strongly commend this volume of his papers so thoughtfully edited by John Schlapobersky.'

Dr. Andrew Powell, *Formerly Consultant Psychotherapist and Senior Lecturer in Psychiatry, St George's Hospital and University of London; Formerly Consultant Psychotherapist and Hon. Senior lecturer, Warneford Hospital and University of Oxford*

'Malcolm Pines is at his best in this fine collection, edited attentively by John Schlapobersky. The papers represent a distillation of 60 years embedded in group analysis and its culture of enquiry, from its very beginnings. He writes with beautiful clarity, a keen eye on the historical detail of the personalities and movements, and always with a gentle compassion. On reading him and integrating what he offers, you can easily discover his wisdom in your own work without realising its origins – something Oklander identifies in his Foreword. For those of us who trained with him, hearing his words again in these pages is like another immersion in the 'sound bath' he describes, and we are warmly reminded of the profound debt we owe to him. This book will be an essential, core text in our discipline. It is also a page turner!'

Dr. Jale Cilasun, *Formerly Consultant Medical Psychotherapist, South West London and St George's Mental Health; Member, Institute of Group Analysis (UK)*

'Beautifully written, these last papers of Malcolm Pines cover much of his wide-ranging thought in many of the fields in which he worked over a lifetime. He was a man I was glad to have known for over 60 years. Developments in Psychoanalysis, Group Psychoanalysis and Therapeutic Community are put in context, demonstrating how each one throws light upon the others. His quest was to promote the study and teaching of these endeavours and secure their future. He tells their story, and their success and spread are testaments to his work. There are also elegant papers using the myth of Narcissus and Echo to illustrate the to and fro of both auditory and visual communication from birth onwards, essential for the creation and maintenance of relationship throughout a lifetime. Malcolm envisaged this volume before he died and John Schlapobersky, his former pupil, colleague and friend, has completed and set it in its own context in an appropriate tribute.'

Dr. Jennifer Johns, *Psychoanalyst, British Psychoanalytical Society*

'This collection of Malcolm Pines's papers reflects changes in society and knowledge development over 30 years of practice. They illustrate Russian dialogism represented by Bahktin and Vygotsky to whom Pines returns, repeatedly. Their claims – that the personal and the social are indivisible, that the social precedes the psychological – demonstrate that we need the other to complete the task of becoming ourselves. Malcolm's contribution consequently evolves around concepts like dialogue, mirroring and resonance. I had not expected to find that these 'dated' texts would resonate so well with recent developments in relational psychology and social and affective neuroscience. He stands amongst contemporary theorists exploring the emotional drivers we are governed by, showing how the life of the mind is dialogue. I highly recommend this book to anyone with an interest in the life of groups. It will have an essential place in reading lists on group psychotherapy education.'

Dr. Christer Sandahl, *Professor Emeritus, Karolinska Institutet, Stockholm; Formerly President, International Association for Group Psychotherapy and Group Processes (IAGP)*

'No group analyst since Foulkes has done so much as Malcolm Pines to promote and shape the development of group analysis in theory and practice. He was also significantly involved in the return of group analysis to Germany. This book presents well-known central papers and many others previously unpublished, brought together through the excellent editorial work of a pupil of the next generation, John Schlapobersky. Providing deep insights into the history of psychotherapy, the papers include the intersubjective turn in psychoanalysis and the interdisciplinary orientation and philosophical tradition that Foulkes brought with him from his Frankfurt years, prior to his forced migration to England. Groundbreaking papers like *The coherency of group analysis*, and *From social mind to social brain*, bear witness to this. The further development of his own perspective is combined with an openness to other, sometimes strongly divergent schools of thought, as with *Building on Bion, following on Foulkes*. Contributions like *Dialogue and selfhood – Discovering connections; Listening and the sonorous self*; and *The 'in-between'*, will remain indispensable points of reference for group–analytic thinking. Everyone with a serious interest in the group analytic tradition and its comparison to other forms of group psychotherapy and to psychoanalysis, will need this book.'

Dr. Thomas Mies, *Director, Institute of Therapeutic and Applied Group Analysis Münster; Training group analyst, Deutsche Gesellschaft für Gruppenanalyse und Gruppenpsychotherapie (D3G); Co-editor, Gruppenpsychotherapie und Gruppendynamik*

'Malcolm Pines was one of the few remaining links to the great developments in dynamic individual and group psychotherapy – and social therapy – in the second half of the 20th century. He participated in all of it and passed on his accumulated knowledge through his practice, teaching, training and publications. As one of the founders of Group Analysis, he was close to Foulkes who was also his individual analyst. He was at the forefront in the development of new ideas, his own as well as other sometimes overlooked theories of man and society. He writes about complex topics with an ease that can only come from a man of great knowledge derived from a life in close and personal contact with other great minds of his time. This last book portrays and sums up an incredibly productive life representing the accumulated knowledge of 60 years of practice as a group analyst and psychoanalyst – a gift to everyone interested in Group Analysis, its foundations, history, contemporary context and practice.'

Svein Tjelta, *Training group analyst and Training psychoanalytical psychotherapist, Institute of Group Analysis, Norway. Formerly editor in chief, 'Matrix', The Nordic Journal for Psychotherapy*

'This book contains 20 of Malcolm Pines' key papers, edited by his good friend John Schlapobersky, the two working closely together before Pines died in July 2021. Several papers have been published previously others have been extended and many will be new to readers. They are ordered in six sections according to chronology and thematic category, presenting a rich selection of new themes and deepening group analytic theory. Pictures of Malcolm from numerous previous encounters and situations popped up as I read this book, as if I could hear him again. He has been a prolific writer, scholar, and mediator of knowledge as editor of the journal Group Analysis and as an eloquent speaker from the podium or with comments in large groups at international conferences – his influence and presence have been marked. He means something special to many of us trained outside the UK, as he originally effected contact between representatives of the Norwegian Psychiatric Association and IGA, London. There are two highly interesting introductions by the author and the editor respectively, and a Forword by Juan Tubert Oklander. Appendix 1 gives an excellent overview of all Malcolm's writing and Appendix 2 references all the books he edited in the International Library of Group Analysis. Congratulations to John Schlapobersky for his long years of work planning, preparing and integrating these papers. The book is a must for everyone who wants to understand the roots and history of Group Analysis!'

Steinar Lorentzen, *Professor Emeritus and Consultant Psychiatrist, Institute for Clinical Medicine, University of Oslo; Member, Institute of Group Analysis, Norway*

'Reading this selection of papers – some old, some new – takes you on a journey through the historical evolution of group analysis, a discipline in which Malcolm Pines has been a pioneer, narrator, historian, teacher, innovator and deep thinker – the creator of its main theoretical and technical principles. This new book confirms and sustains our conviction that group analysis is the basis of psychoanalysis in a bi-personal or a group setting and gives us the deepest insight into the human condition. This book is a must for anyone who studies, works with or has an interest in the human soul.'

Reyna Hernández-Tubert, *Member, Argentine Psychoanalytic Association, International Psychoanalytic Association; Professor and Researcher, Doctorate in Relational Psychoanalysis and Group Analysis, Marista University of Mérida, Yucatán, Mexico*

The Journey from Psychoanalysis to Group Analysis

The Journey from Psychoanalysis to Group Analysis presents a selection of papers from Malcolm Pines's long career, documenting his profound contribution to group analysis and its applications.

John Schlapobersky, editor, is a well-established author who organised the collection in History; Development of Method; Metapsychology/Neurology; Final Papers. The compilation distils the life's work of a pioneer in many fields – psychiatrist, psychoanalyst, group analyst, editor and author. Pines's writing encompasses psychoanalytic and group analytic theory, developmental psychology, neuroscience, ethology, social science, language theory and mythology. He seeks their integration in the crucible of group analysis.

The book will become an essential text in psychotherapy and therapeutic communities – of value to students and readers in psychoanalysis and psychotherapy, politics, social and neurological sciences, humanities and language theory.

Malcolm Pines trained in medicine at University College London and in psychoanalysis at the British Psychoanalytic Society. Founder member, Group Analytic Practice and Institute of Group Analysis; past president, Group Analytic Society, International Association of Group Psychotherapy and the Psychiatric Section of the Royal Society of Medicine; consultant psychotherapist, St. George's and Maudsley Hospitals and Tavistock Clinic; editor, *Group Analysis* and founder, *International Library of Group Analysis.*

John R. Schlapobersky graduated at University of Sussex, Institute of Education and London School of Economics. He qualified at the Institute of Group Analysis, where he serves as faculty. He was scientific secretary, Group Analytic Society; member, British Society for Couple Psychoanalytic Psychotherapy, American Group Psychotherapy Association; and founding trustee, Freedom from Torture. He practices at the Bloomsbury Psychotherapy Practice. Publications include *From the Couch to the Circle: Group-Analytic Psychotherapy in Practice.*

The Journey from Psychoanalysis to Group Analysis

Further Papers of Malcolm Pines

Malcolm Pines

Edited by
John R. Schlapobersky

Routledge
Taylor & Francis Group
LONDON AND NEW YORK

Designed cover image: © Simeon Pines

First published 2025
by Routledge
4 Park Square, Milton Park, Abingdon, Oxon OX14 4RN

and by Routledge
605 Third Avenue, New York, NY 10158

Routledge is an imprint of the Taylor & Francis Group, an informa business

British Library Cataloguing-in-Publication Data
A catalogue record for this book is available from the British Library.

Library of Congress Cataloging-in-Publication Data
Names: Pines, Malcolm, author. | Schlapobersky, John R., editor.
Title: The journey from psychoanalysis to group analysis : further papers of Malcolm Pines / Malcolm Pines ; edited by John R. Schlapobersky.
Identifiers: LCCN 2024037214 (print) | LCCN 2024037215 (ebook) |
Subjects: LCSH: Group psychoanalysis. | Group psychotherapy.
Classification: LCC RC510 .P56 2025 (print) | LCC RC510 (ebook) |
DDC 616.89/152–dc23/eng/20241112
LC record available at https://lccn.loc.gov/2024037214
LC ebook record available at https://lccn.loc.gov/2024037215

ISBN: 978-1-032-79953-7 (hbk)
ISBN: 978-1-032-79954-4 (pbk)
ISBN: 978-1-003-49471-3 (ebk)

DOI: 10.4324/9781003494713

Typeset in Optima
by Taylor & Francis Books

This collection of papers is dedicated first to the living members of my family – to our children Rosamond, Jonathon and Simeon, and our grandchildren, Jacob, Harry, Katie and Lizzie.

It is dedicated next to the memory of those members of my family who have passed away, to Iris, my beloved wife and life companion and the mother of our children; to my Russian Jewish medical parents, Noë and Marousia, and to my medical siblings, Dinora and Arnold, who are all sadly missed.

Contents

Previous publications

Malcolm Pines

Author

Circular Reflections: Selected Papers on Group Analysis and Psychoanalysis International Library of Group Analysis London, Routledge 1998.

Editor

The Evolution of Group Analysis International Library of Group Analysis London, Routledge 1984; reissued Jessica Kingsley Publishers 2000.

Bion and Group Psychotherapy International Library of Group Analysis London, Routledge 1985; reissued Jessica Kingsley Publishers 2000.

The Practice of Group Analysis (edited with J. Roberts) International Library of Group Analysis London, Routledge 1991.

Ring of Fire – Primitive Affects and Object Relations in Group Psychotherapy (edited with V. Schermer) International Library of Group Analysis London, Routledge 1994.

Self Experiences in Group: Intersubjective and Self Psychological Pathways to Human Understanding (edited with I. Harwood) International Library of Group Analysis London, Routledge 1998.

Group Psychotherapy of the Psychoses – Concepts, Interventions and Contexts (edited with V. Schermer) International Library of Group Analysis London, Routledge 1999.

Building on Bion: Roots – Origins and Context of Bion's Contributions to Theory and Practice (edited with R. Lipgar) International Library of Group Analysis London, Jessica Kingsley Publishers 2002.

Building on Bion: Branches – Contemporary Developments and Applications of Bion's Contributions to Theory and Practice (edited with R. Lipgar) International Library of Group Analysis London, Jessica Kingsley Publishers 2002.

Dreams in Group Psychotherapy (edited with C. Neri and R. Friedman) International Library of Group Analysis London, Jessica Kingsley Publishers 2002.

Self Experiences in Group, Revisited: Affective Attachments, Intersubjective Regulations, and Human Understanding (edited with I. Harwood and W. Stone) International Library of Group Analysis London, Jessica Kingsley Publishers 2012.

Previous publications

John Schlapobersky

Author

From the Couch to the Circle: Group-Analytic Psychotherapy In Practice London, Routledge 2016.

When They Came For Me: The Hidden Diary of An Apartheid Prisoner. London and Cape Town, Berghahn Books and Jonathan Ball Publishers 2021.

Editor

Selected Papers of Robin Skynner. Vol. 1. Explorations with Families: Group Analysis and Family Therapy. London, Methuen. Reissued 1988, London, Routledge.

Selected Papers of Robin Skynner. Vol. 2. Institutes and How to Survive Them. London, Methuen. Reissued 1990, London, Routledge.

Author's introduction: Malcolm Pines. Something of myself

At the time of writing, I am in my ninety-fourth year and sixty of these years were devoted to working as a psychiatrist, psychoanalyst and group analyst. When I was an undergraduate at Cambridge aged nineteen, a new world was opened up to me when I started to read about psychoanalysis, and this led me to envisage working as a psychiatrist and psychoanalyst. While still a medical student I applied for training at the Institute of Psychoanalysis and John Bowlby, then the Training Secretary, referred me to Dr Adrian Stephen, who I later discovered was the younger brother of Virginia Woolf; hence my interest in Cambridge, Bloomsbury and psychoanalysis. After Adrian Stephen's death only some eighteen months after I began with him, I was re-interviewed by Donald Winnicott, who referred me to S. H. Foulkes as a training analyst with the Anna Freud group. Whilst a psychiatric registrar at the Maudsley Hospital where Foulkes was head of the Psychotherapy Department, I began a long analysis with him that would eventually lead me to follow him into the world of group analysis and create the institutional framework and foundations for the literature on which this new discipline is based.

I came from a medical family as both my Russian Jewish parents had qualified in Russia, my father in Kyiv (now in Ukraine) and my mother in Dorpat (now Tartu, Latvia). They met while serving in the Russian Army Medical Service in the 1914–1918 war. As a consequence of the revolution and civil war, they left Russia in 1919, and travelled first to Belgium, where my father had family, and then settled in England. My father, who had been an ophthalmic surgeon in Russia, established a medical practice as a GP in the East End of London and my mother devoted herself to the upbringing of the family and the support of my father's practice.

My parents' eldest child, my sister Dinora, was already three when they arrived here. I was the third of three children and, like our parents, all three of us became doctors. Dinora's first degree was in Modern Languages, which she studied at University College, London. On graduating in wartime she went on to study medicine at University College London, at that time evacuated to Exeter. She qualified as a GP and became a distinguished psychoanalyst in the British Psychoanalytical Society. In the course of her long working life, she published a book, *A Woman's Unconscious Use of Her Body* (1994) a pioneering work in psychoanalytic women's studies that is still of value in the field and beyond. My brother Arnold and I read for our first degrees at Cambridge. Arnold became a distinguished chest physician and committed mountain climber. In the prime of his life, he perished in a climbing accident in Snowdonia – a shock for all of us and most of all for his children and wife. Together with Dinora's and Arnold's children, we have been and continue to be a close extended family meeting on regular family occasions.

The inevitable rivalry in being the youngest of three children meant that, like Goldilocks, I was always looking for the right chair. This rivalry played a part in my choosing a medical career in psychiatry, next in psychoanalysis and then in pioneering the development of group analysis. These papers give an account of this journey and of the pioneering spirit that has guided me.

Acknowledgements

My first acknowledgement is to S. H. Foulkes, whom we knew as Michael – my mentor and analyst, the originator of group analysis; and to his co-author James Anthony. The group-analytic network launched and inspired by the radical theorising of Foulkes and Anthony was carried on by those of us who joined the group-analytic practice in the 1960s. I was fortunate to take part in the burgeoning spirit of group analysis.

The next acknowledgement is to my adventurous fellows who founded the Group Analytic Practice in 1964, including Foulkes, Robin Skynner, Dennis Brown, Colin James, Pat de Maré, James Home and Lionel Kreeger, who all contributed to the expansion of group-analytic theory and practice. The next acknowledgement is to those who – with me – founded the Institute of Group Analysis in 1973, including those named at the Practice above; and Vivienne Cohen and Heinz Wolf. It was founded on the premises of our Practice and in 1985 was moved to premises of its own at Daleham Gardens. Robin went on to found the Institute of Family Therapy at our Practice with a different, related network of colleagues, which was also later relocated to premises of its own. Through these many and widening developments, we spread our wings beyond London, to the UK, Europe and beyond.

The next acknowledgement is to my good friend John Schlapobersky. Together we have thought through the theory and practice of group analysis and written about it, resulting in our successive chapters in the *Oxford Textbook of Psychiatry* and a further chapter adapted from this work issued in the German textbook, *Gruppenpsychotherapie und Gruppendynamik*. John has been a great help in getting my ideas into better order and I have benefitted from his remarkable prowess in writing his handbook of group analysis, *From the Couch to the Circle: Group-Analytic Psychotherapy in Practice*.

This book

These papers are my own selection from a larger collection that spans some sixty years of immersion in my primary training and work as a British psychiatrist and psychoanalyst and one of the originators of group analysis – a new discipline in the field. Some of the papers included were published previously; others were drafted as conference or keynote submissions that were not published at the time of presentation. None of them appeared in my previous book, *Circular Reflections*.

I have selected twenty papers that represent the bulk of my written work that did not find its way into *Circular Reflections*. I have benefitted from the active support of my daughter Rosamond, both of my sons, Simeon and Jonathon, the engagement of two archivists, Wendy Russell and Georgia Clemson, literary assistant Louise Crane, a close reading by my friend John Rees, the editorial oversight of my friend and colleague John Schlapobersky, and the active engagement of my publisher, Routledge. There have been two further people who have acted as editorial assistants and reviewed the writing – Kristopher Springer who made a beginning and Christopher Canter who has helped to bring the project to completion; and by an Advisory Panel comprising Robi Friedman, Thomas Mies and Dieter Nitzgen.

Milestones in development

What follows is a more detailed account of the significant events during the course of my working life out of which the papers emerge. I will name the landmark events here. The first was the establishment of the Group Analytic Practice in 1964 and the second the establishment of the Institute of Group Analysis in 1973, in both of which Foulkes joined us. When he passed away in 1975, I led a panel that inaugurated the Foulkes Lectures, the third landmark event. This is an annual memorial lecture that we chose Daniel Abse to inaugurate in 1976. The series celebrates its fortieth anniversary this year. The fourth landmark event was the development of the journal *Group Analysis*. It had its origins in a correspondence journal, GAIPAC – Group Analysis International Panel and Correspondence – that Foulkes established when he retired from the Maudsley in 1963. He called on his networking knowledge to create and edit an international exchange and he invited colleagues from the Group Analytic Practice to edit sections. This was gradually transformed into a published journal, first under the editorial guidance of Harold Behr. I then edited the journal for sixteen years and, as the field widened with the creation of new training institutes in many countries, the international status of the journal grew. It helped to create and consolidate a new scholarship.

The fifth landmark was the International Library of Group Analysis that I established, first with the publisher Routledge and then with Jessica Kingsley Press. I was responsible for 41 titles altogether. The first of the sixteen titles that Routledge issued was Yvonne M. Agazarian and Richard Peters's *The*

Visible and Invisible Group in 1981. The first title in the series once it moved to JKP was my own previous collection of papers, *Circular Reflections: Selected Papers on Group Analysis and Psychoanalysis*, issued in 1997. The series came to an end with Richard M. Billow's *Relational Group Psychotherapy* in 2003.

The sixth landmark event was the establishment of regular meetings for our developing professional bodies, in which I have played an active part. I attended the first Symposium of the Group Analytic Society in Lisbon with Foulkes and others in 1973, when we were hosted by Eduardo Luís Cortesão and his colleagues. The last of the Society's Symposia that I was able to attend – at the age of eighty-nine – was held in 2014, once again in Lisbon, and I was present at every one of the meetings between these dates. They have taken place under the auspices of the Group Analytic Society International, which has been a 'parent' to so many others, including the International Association of Forensic Psychotherapy, the International Association of Therapeutic Communities and other associations. The Society has also spawned the development of Institutes of Group Analysis in many other countries and was one of the foundation stones for the Association of Family Therapists and the Institute of Family Therapy, which held their first meetings at the Group Analytic Practice. There are other vital professional associations, including the International Association of Group Psychotherapy, described below, and the American Group Psychotherapy Association, where the contribution from group analysis continues.

My training background

I belonged in a peripheral way to the Anna Freud evolving tradition in the British Psychoanalytic Society as described by King and Steiner. I describe this as 'peripheral' because my training analyst S. H. Foulkes, although affiliated to the Anna Freud group, ploughed his own path as the founder of the new discipline of group-analytic psychotherapy. This discipline evolved out of the task of treating soldiers in the Second World War suffering from shell shock, known today as post-traumatic stress disorder.

Psychoanalytic training

My own psychoanalytic training followed a narrower path. It began at the British Psychoanalytic Society with an immersion in Freud's writings and was taught by ex-Viennese analysts such as Willi Hoffer, who were amongst those who accompanied Sigmund and Anna Freud in their 1938 flight from Vienna. On their arrival in London, they became members of the British Psychoanalytic Society which, until then, had been 'distinctively British', but they were unwelcome to Melanie Klein. After her earlier arrival from Budapest via Berlin, she had a strongly entrenched group of followers in London whose radical formulations of early childhood development were abhorrent to Anna Freud, her father and her group. There were inevitable struggles for power between the newly arrived Viennese Freudians and the group who preceded them.

In my time the student body of the British Psychoanalytic Society was predominantly Kleinian; the Anna Freudians were a smaller group, but some of us chose to be 'independents': neither Kleinian nor Anna Freudian, and more attracted to such independent figures as Donald Winnicott, Michael Balint and Charles Rycroft. Wilfred Bion was of increasing importance through his pioneering psychoanalytic therapy of schizophrenic patients. I found the training restrictive, inward-looking and excessively focused on the Freud/Klein controversy that split the student body and monopolised the so-called 'scientific meetings' (the fortnightly paper presentations to the whole Psychoanalytic Society). Discussions of the meeting's paper, though often highly interesting, tended to follow predictable party lines.

It was this constricted inward-looking format that encouraged Pearl King and me to initiate the 'Applied Section'. King was a distinguished historian of the Psychoanalytic Society whose background was in sociology. The Applied Section was a forum for psychoanalysts applying psychoanalytic viewpoints to areas of work outside the practice of 'classic' psychoanalysis, in work with institutions, families, brief therapies, social sciences. They were involved in research projects, developmental studies and humanities. In this Section we had a forum for voices other than our own, such as Robert Hinde and George Steiner. I chaired the Section for several years. Some years after qualification, I was in a supervision group meeting with Anna Freud; here I learnt how to use the structural theory that she had developed clinically, which was a valuable lesson. We all greatly enjoyed the Kaffee mit Schlag wheeled in precisely at 9:45 p.m. by Paula, the domestic helper who had come with the Freud family from their Viennese home, 19 Berggasse.

My psychiatric training was at the Maudsley Hospital, then the preeminent postgraduate psychiatric centre in London. Under Sir Aubrey Lewis it had grown into a comprehensive entity with research departments in both basic and applied sciences. I enjoyed the vigorous competitive intellectual life, where we psychoanalytic devotees had to hold our own in case presentations.

The influence of S. H. Foulkes

I began running groups at the Maudsley under the supervision of S. H. Foulkes, who was Head of the Psychotherapy Department whilst he was also my training analyst. After completing his psychiatric training in Frankfurt, Foulkes did his psychoanalytic training in Vienna where his analyst, Helene Deutsch, followed Freud's classical theory in her own orientation. Foulkes then returned to Frankfurt where, in 1930, he took up the position of Director of Outpatient Services in the recently established Frankfurt Psychoanalytic Clinic. This centre shared premises with both the Frankfurt Centre for Social Research and Frankfurt University's Department of Sociology.

Foulkes benefitted from the interdisciplinary nature of institutional life there until forced to leave by the Nazi accession in 1933. Psychoanalysis and Marxist economic theory were dominant influences, and it is remarkable that though both Erich Fromm and Foulkes were members of the same organisations, neither of them has once referred to the other in his papers and memoirs. This is possibly because, as Fromm became such a widely published social theorist, Foulkes chose not to acknowledge their shared history. This dissociation possibly repeats Foulkes's attitude towards the work of Trigant Burrow, who died in the 1920s and had anticipated some of Foulkes's group-analytic theories.

As a Jew, Foulkes had to flee Germany in 1933. He settled in London, where he re-qualified in medicine and then psychiatry, and became a member of the British Psychoanalytic Society. His introductory paper was on introjection, which was his response to the Kleinian school's overemphasis on projection (Foulkes 1990a).

The Cassel Hospital

I left the Maudsley for my first qualifying appointment at the Cassel Hospital which, under Tom Main, had become a psychoanalytic training centre close enough to central London for us to continue our training analyses and attend the Institute of Psychoanalysis. Main was an analysand of Michael Balint and an inspiring teacher and organiser. He was a world leader in psychoanalytic hospital management, research and training, which began with his work at Northfield where he devised the term 'therapeutic community'. He had a distinguished war record as a psychiatrist and had worked with Foulkes at Northfield Hospital in the Second Northfield Experiment. At Cassel, I was a member of the research team set up by Balint to investigate brief psychotherapy; its members were all psychoanalysts, working at either the Tavistock Clinic or the Cassel Hospital. Eventually our work was systematised by David Malan and published as *A Study of Brief Psychotherapy* (1963). I presented our work to the Psychoanalytical Society – with mixed responses, for some saw it as a betrayal: they could not appreciate the value of the economy of endeavour that brief methods could bring to widespread social need.

Russian literature and scholarship has provided another vital thread in these developments. I appreciated and learnt much from the psychologist Vygotsky and the language theorist Bakhtin, whose understanding of speech 'utterances' as the search for responses of the Other enriches the group-analytic theory of speech as dialogue and discourse. They afford lines of enquiry through all my mature writings.

Training in group psychotherapy – the beginning

By now, my interest centered on group psychotherapy, which offered a new way of providing psychotherapy on a far wider scale than individual psychoanalysis. I was leading the formation of the Institute of Group Analysis in

London, setting up an in-depth group-analytic training involving personal therapy in an experiential therapy group not always confined to health professionals, plus theory seminars, supervision and written work. Much was based on my experience of how psychoanalytic training was organised at the Psychoanalytic Society. My papers on training date from this period.

When we established the Institute of Group Analysis in London in 1973, it was the only centre in Europe to offer a dedicated group-analytic training and attracted many therapists from continental Europe. We provided workshop facilities for short-term group-analytic experiences, which led to our first invitation to set up group-analytic training on the continent in Denmark. Following their training in London, some of the trainees who came from other European countries formed their own centres for training in western Europe, the Nordic countries and former Yugoslavia, and then extended further invitations for us to send training teams to their centres.[1]

The spread of group-analytic training

Denmark

I was particularly challenged and stimulated by the invitation to set up group-analytic training in Denmark. Twice I had been invited to participate in their seminars on group analysis; I then insisted that to develop group analysis further they had to undergo a full training. I assembled an enthusiastic team and, for three years, we went regularly every three months to lecture, conduct experiential groups and supervise. We greatly enjoyed this immersion in Danish culture. The Danes then formed their own successful Institute of Group Analysis in Copenhagen, followed years later by another in Aarhus, their second city. Our Danish colleagues followed this with an invitation for us to set up a course of supervision for their individual and group psychotherapy and our team consisted of Murray Cox, Jonathan Pedder, Colin James and myself.

Norway

The Norwegian Association of Psychiatry then wanted to set up their own training. I was invited to an event where the group-analytic model and an American model were compared and was happy that the group-analytic model was preferred. Our first training team there was initiated by Liesel Hearst, who was joined by Meg Sharpe, Harold Behr, Don Montgomery and Gill Nathan. Bryan Boswood joined them later. The Norwegians took over full responsibility for their own training after some five years, and the Norwegian Institute of Group Analysis, Oslo, has been outstanding in both training and research. It has had a considerable influence on the high standard of Norwegian psychiatry. Liesel Hearst went on to play a decisive part in training developments in German-speaking countries, where her contribution is especially valued, in particular at the Seminar für Gruppenanalyse in Zürich (SGAZ) and at the Gruppenanalyseseminar in Bonn (GRAS).

Yugoslavia

Before the breakup of Yugoslavia in 1991–1992 following Tito's death, I had set up and taken part in several group-analytic seminars and for three years was invited to a summer school of psychotherapy in beautiful Dubrovnik, before the savage wars that ensued. At the meeting of the International Association for Group Psychotherapy (IAGP) in Zagreb, Croatia in 1986, there was a strong interest among training institutes in different parts of Europe in establishing direct institute links between their trainers. Those responsible for the initiative found themselves opposed by some out of concern this might represent disloyalty to our existing international associations. I spoke up firmly for establishing direct links, declaring that our loyalty was to a way of thinking, a body of ideas and a mode of practice – and the trainers needed their own international association. The European Group Analytic Training Institutions Network (EGATIN) was established just before the Balkans broke into war. EGATIN is now the umbrella body for training institutes in Europe and beyond. With a membership of some forty training institutes from more than twenty countries in and beyond Europe, it enriches all its member institutes and sets a benchmark for international cooperation.

Russia

Having been raised in an Anglo-Russian home, I have a strong sense of connection with Russian culture. When an invitation to teach group analysis came first from Moscow and then from St. Petersburg, I was eager to go and made several visits. Directly and indirectly, I helped to set up training there, which has since flourished under the auspices of the International Courses Committee of the Institute of Group Analysis in London. I also worked in both Lithuania and Estonia. My colleague John Schlapobersky organised our first workshop in Moscow, which I attended with him and with our colleague Liza Glenn. John continued with these developments for some time and then David Kennard and Sue Einhorn took them forward in St. Petersburg.

North America, AGPA and IAGP

I began visiting North America, participating in meetings of the American Group Psychotherapy Association (AGPA), bringing group-analytic theory and methods which were scarcely known there. Reciprocally, I was made aware of and was impressed by the serious research pursued in university centres. This practice was in contrast to the United Kingdom, where both psychoanalysis and group analysis were taught and practised outside university centres, which had rejected psychoanalytic theory and practice. In the early postwar years, the International Association of Group Psychotherapy was founded principally by Jacob Moreno, who was the main founder and exponent of psychodrama, and by Foulkes. Psychodrama and group analysis are very different in style and theory. However, Moreno and Foulkes had combined to form and lead this international organisation, though Foulkes played a much smaller part. Psychodrama has generated enthusiasm amongst its practitioners and in the international meetings through demonstrations of its practice by gifted therapists such as Moreno and his wife Zerka. These attracted many followers, so that the shared enterprise of the IAGP veered towards the psychodramatic pole. However, towards the end of his life, Moreno wanted to re-establish the more balanced organisation that had originally been set up. As Foulkes's delegate I met Moreno and helped this new chapter to begin. I decided to experience psychodrama for myself and undertook some training to understand these different approaches, which helped me to maintain some balance between group analysis and psychodrama. As president of the IAGP I travelled to Central and Latin America and Taiwan, thereby gaining a much wider understanding of the different cultures and enterprises of our members.

The wider participation in the IAGP led to the formation of the European Association for Transcultural Group Analysis (EATGA), an association of group analysts from several countries who wanted to explore how different cultures, histories, languages and methods of child-rearing could contribute to the fundamentals of developmental processes of our personalities and basic assumptions. At our meetings we formed small groups based on language and geographical areas, such as Scandinavia or the Balkans. People were encouraged to use whatever language they preferred; translation was not offered, but might be provided by other group members. Other experiential groups were formed on the basis of such fundamental, developmental issues as religious upbringing to provide for groups in which persons revisited their immersion in religious communities that many had abandoned.

A wider perspective

When I qualified as a psychoanalyst, I was invited to receive two books of my own choosing, the cost of which had been provided by a psychoanalytic trust fund. My choices were significant: Marjorie Brierley, *Trends in Psycho-analysis* (1951) is a masterly survey of the development of psychoanalysis principally in the United Kingdom; and Erik H. Erikson's *Childhood and Society* (1950) introduced psychosocial development, the study of child development in sociocultural settings. I greatly enjoyed this wider perspective, but soon became aware that Anna Freud did not approve of this widening beyond the limits laid down by her father and by herself.

My interest in the psychosocial, the influence of culture on personality, led beyond psychoanalytic ego-psychology to studies of the self, in particular to the American school of social psychology. This school was led by Charles

Cooley, George Mead and William James, forerunners of Heinz Kohut's Chicago school of self psychology. Aspects of his work resonated with the Independent Group of psychoanalysts in London, and rewarding exchanges took place between ourselves and some Chicago psychoanalysts. When I was asked to outline self psychology to Anna Freud's group, she listened without enthusiasm, finally saying: 'This is very different'. I wrote and presented several papers on Kohut and self psychology, which led on to my discovery of some beautiful writings on intersubjectivity and dialogue. In particular it led to an enthusiasm for Bakhtin, the Russian scholar of language and literature referenced earlier. I particularly liked his dictum that 'speech is an interlocution': the speech act seeks someone to respond and is not complete by itself. Naturally, this is of particular interest and importance for group analysis, where we are all part of the group's speech and response pattern. Mirroring and resonance are basic factors as laid out by Foulkes, and I have enjoyed exploring both the scientific evidence, such as the discovery of mirror neurons, and the literature covering myths such as Narcissus and Echo with their myriad reflections and resonances.

Bloomsbury

While a medical student aged a mere 20 or so, I applied for psychoanalytic training. I was interviewed by Dr John Bowlby, then a Major still in army uniform, who referred me to Adrian Stephen. He was an exceptionally tall man, quiet and gentle, who I later found out was the younger brother of Virginia Woolf. Naturally I became interested in the history of the Bloomsbury group and wrote on Cambridge, Bloomsbury and psychoanalysis. This led to my writing on the history of psychoanalysis in Britain, and how Freudian thinking had impacted British psychiatry. It was at this time that controversies arose around the impact of James Strachey's translation of Freud in the *Standard Edition*. When I became the Chair of the Publications Committee of the British Psychoanalytic Society, I had some influence in encouraging revisions and in 1975 I organised a panel discussion on the Strachey translation at the International Congress of Psychoanalysis in London.

Boundaries and borderlines

Looking back, I recognise how my life situation placed me on a borderline and that I had to contend with problems over boundaries. I was a child of Russian immigrants and had an upbringing in Whitechapel among Jewish immigrants, yet I travelled daily by underground to the City of London School, a public school not then in the class of St Paul's and Westminster. My university training was a pre-medical education at wartime Cambridge, where I studied with self-doubt as to my exemption from the military. Whilst marginality spurred me to excel, it also undermined my achievements. Within psychiatry I belonged to a minority group, somewhat illegitimate to mainstream and academic psychiatry. The Maudsley gave me a good pedigree despite my having chosen psychoanalysis, which Aubrey Lewis told me blocked my academic career. So, when elected to the prestigious presidency of the psychiatric section of the Royal Society of Medicine, I attempted with a Presidential lecture to show how psychoanalysis can contribute to the broadening and deepening of perspectives. Looking back, I see that I was myself seeking legitimation in view of my marginality. I used my speech to survey how the boundary concept had been introduced and used from Freud onwards; how it was used in differentiating neurotic from psychotic disorders and how this was disputed territory, now commanding much attention. The speakers invited to address the Society during my period in office showed how boundary concepts were being applied. The then relatively little-known research scientist Colin Blakemore, the late Sir Colin Blakemore, spoke of his cell biology research; the psychoanalysts Joe and Anne-Marie Sandler spoke on ego boundaries. The boundary concept was stretched wide to fill the year programme and provided an entertaining and informative series.

Pop-up community

Pop-up events are frequent and popular nowadays but were not so in 1972, when I took part in a special psychosocial event in Hoxton, then still a very run-down part of East London. The organiser was a well-known Danish social psychologist who had advertised a weekend community which we would form and live through. We brought bedding, toiletries and a limited amount of money. There were some sixty participants, including young children with their parents. We formed three groups based on income levels: 'wealthy', 'middle-class' and 'poor'. I was assigned to the 'wealthy', a group of seven. Asked to give our group a name, we chose the Magnificent Seven, after an American film based on the Japanese masterpiece *Seven Samurai*. We pooled money to budget for food, which had to be bought and prepared. Being wealthy, we were given the task of acting as capitalists and exploiting our economic power. Among the poor were some who had recently left prisons or psychiatric facilities and who belonged to the less stable members of society. Over the weekend, tensions between the three groups grew strongly. Capitalists were resented and in the final debriefing session, reviewing the life of the community that we had built over the weekend, explosions of anger, frustration and resentment led to fisticuffs. The organiser seemed unable to resolve the situation, so I and another psychotherapist brought us back to the dialogical level.

Psychoanalytic conference in South Africa

A somewhat similar event disrupted the first psychoanalytic congress in Cape Town in 1998, leading to the formation of the South African Psychoanalytical Confederation. The programme of this eagerly anticipated and well-attended event had been put together by those psychoanalysts who had left South

Africa to train in London and now wanted to give back to their native country the skills and knowledge they had acquired. The unbalanced programme was made up of papers given by the returning South Africans. The role assigned to the home team was secondary: to provide responses and to engage in discussions with the visitors. No group events were considered necessary. I was invited to attend and contribute by convening a large group. I invited my colleague John Schlapobersky to join me: it was his country of origin and we had worked together in large groups before on training programmes at the Institute of Group Analysis. The enthusiastic welcoming reception on the opening day soon faded and dissatisfactions were palpable. The organisers alerted me to the fact that tensions and dissatisfactions were riding high and, when some 200 of us gathered in a circle for the large group, I opened the session by explaining that this was an opportunity to speak whatever was on their minds. A long silence ensued. When I enquired what the silence might be about, a response was that if they spoke their minds, there would be blood on the floor. My response was: 'Then let there be blood on the floor'. Speaking began, dissatisfactions were expressed, blockages were opened. The `bloodletting' had happened; the healthy circulation of words and feelings led to better understanding between the organisers and the participants. John introduced a perspective brought from his own knowledge that he read into the dynamics. We seemed to be witnessing a hostile re-enactment of the meeting between the original colonised people of the country and the colonisers from the Netherlands and Britain who came to control and direct them, and there was relief and recognition in the understanding. Subsequent meetings had different structures for their list of contributors, and they had large group meetings built into the programmes.

In conclusion

I entered into group analysis through my relationship with Foulkes as both my department head and my training analyst. His group-analytic theory became the basis of my own theory and practice. His emphasis on mirroring as a key factor in both child development and group-analytic therapy stimulated me to research mirroring. My Foulkes Lecture in 1982 was on this subject, as are several of the other papers in this collection. My aim in these selected papers is to show how group-analytic theory is a nodal point in the network of psychodynamic development. It encompasses psychoanalysis, developmental psychology, neuroscience, ethology, primatology, social sciences and linguistics. I hope my readers will appreciate these explorations. They are enriched through studies of mythology, fairy tales and children's stories that have always provided me with valuable sources of meaning. Chapter 11, 'Listening and the sonorous self', concludes with a study of a beautiful tale by Hans Christian Andersen, and the last two papers in this collection explore the mythologies of Narcissus and Echo and of Perseus and Medusa for the light they shed on vision and hearing in early development and in psychotherapy.

My life's work has summation in lines I quote in Chapter 6 on dialogue and selfhood. José Ortega y Gasset's dictum 'Who am I? I am myself, plus my circumstances' (Ortega y Gasset 1963: 45), I follow with a dictum of my own: how resonant for us indeed is that word *circumstances*, we who are advocates of and toilers in the circle!

Malcolm Pines, Putney, 2021

Note

1 Malcolm Pines was also deeply involved in establishing group-analytic training in Sweden during its formative years. He travelled there with Colin James, Murray Cox, Liesel Hearst and others. He was not directly involved in the formation of their training institute, which may explain why there is no reference here to these important developments. My thanks to Göran Ahlin and Christer Sandahl for this historical information. (Ed.)

Editor's introduction: John Schlapobersky

The papers

The collection opens with a landmark publication in 1982, jointly written with colleagues Harold Behr and Liesel Hearst, 'Group analysis and group-analytic psychotherapy'. It closes with another landmark paper published in 2011, 'Narcissus and Echo: Vision and hearing in early development. Applications to individual and group psychotherapy', which concludes Malcolm's written oeuvre. The twenty papers selected for inclusion from this period of thirty years are organised as follows:

Front matter

Table of contents
Malcolm Pines: Author's introduction: Something of myself
John Schlapobersky: Editor's introduction
Juan Tubert-Oklander: Foreword:
The iceberg and the tip, or who is afraid of the big bad Malcolm?

Section I: Introduction

1: Group analysis and group-analytic psychotherapy

Section II: History and context

2: The historical matrix of group analysis: A perspective from the history of ideas
3: The coherency of group analysis: Its emergence and surrounding, supporting network
4: Forgotten pioneers: An unwritten history of the therapeutic community – Maxwell Jones Lecture 1998

Section III: Development of method and technique in group-analytic psychotherapy

Section IV: Metapsychology, philosophy, mind/body

Section V: Final papers

Section VI: End matter

Group analysis

Group analysis is a clinical and theoretical discipline that is multi-personal in nature and multi-vocal in form and content. We have learnt to read the parts in the whole, to find the whole in its parts, to understand the one and the many, the bearing they have on one another and those many ways in which we call on our own sociability to address and resolve the relational problems that beset us. Today there are departments of psychosocial studies in many universities around the world and the principles of holistic understanding now also embrace many points of correspondence between the social and biological. The many forms in which group and family therapy are being developed and applied, the use of group methods in psychiatry and the helping professions, further points of correspondence between group methods and understanding and the practice of individual psychotherapy – including psychodrama, Gestalt therapy and the arts psychotherapies – are just some of the developmental landmarks in the second half of the twentieth century and now in our present.

Since the time of S. H. Foulkes, who died in 1976, terms like 'matrix', 'resonance', 'mirror', 'figuration', 'translation', 'amplification' and 'location' have come to be in common use amongst clinicians, educators and organisational consultants. They are under continuing development in the group-analytic literature. We adhere to the principle – in understanding change – that one voice speaks for many in the innovations of any time and place. The title of a valuable, earlier compilation of papers in group analysis, *The Psyche and the Social World* (Brown and Zinkin 1994/2000), gives focus to the immanent connection between the psyche and the social world that shapes the double helix of psychological life. It gives the DNA for what it means to be human, rooted and governed both by our individuality and sociability. Each requires the other and together they shape the human condition. We owe the conception of this 'double helix' to Malcolm Pines and I am honoured now to be introducing this compilation of his papers.

Malcolm Pines

Despite our new and developing regard for the complexity of cultural life in social innovation, we must give due regard to the individuals we regard as our pioneers. Foulkes was the father of group analysis and he and James Anthony were its first authors. Malcolm Pines stands first amongst the first generation of group analysts. He laid the foundations for our institutional life, training, literature and international context through teaching, writing, conference work, and editorial work on the journal *Group Analysis* and in the International Library of Group Analysis.

This book represents a late collation of Malcolm's written work, only some of which previously found its way to publication. Despite his generous commitment to the publication of others' work, he came to the compilation of his own oeuvre only late in his life and with the active support of his family and publisher. It is my honour to introduce this compilation to our field which many readers are likely to take up with surprise and delight, as I did when I first read some of the papers of which I had no previous knowledge. Readers will find this surprise and delight in the recorded spirit of Juan Tubert-Oklander's Foreword below. These twenty papers offer the mature writing of a working life that has been pioneering in spirit, innovative in nature, adventurous in scope and generous towards the life of patients, colleagues, students and protégés.

The author of these papers died in July 2021 at the age of ninety-six. I write with responsibility towards his legacy and the memory of his wife who passed away three years earlier; and towards his surviving family. His daughter Rosamond, his sons Jonathon and Simeon and his nephew Jeremy have played an active part in the planning and editorial work behind this compilation. I also carry responsibility towards the fields of group analysis and psychoanalysis in which Malcolm had such influence; towards his colleagues near and far; and towards his critics.

Malcolm was my first teacher in psychotherapy when I began in the field with a placement at the Maudsley Hospital in 1977. The generosity of his friendship has been with me since I completed the Qualifying Course at the Institute of Group Analysis in London in 1981. I edited and introduced the selected papers of Robin Skynner in two volumes published in 1987 and 1989 (Skynner 1987; 1989a) and am now honoured to make a corresponding contribution to the work of Malcolm Pines. This has been more challenging and for a range of different reasons. Malcolm was blessed with wonderful longevity and wrote so much, and over such a span of time, that it took time to identify and select those papers that would make a representative selection fully describing his growth and development. New material would come to light at just that stage when an earlier compilation was put together, only for us to find that these new papers too had to be reviewed and, in some cases, incorporated. The collection includes key papers previously published that are now hardly available for readers in the field. There are many more papers that were prepared as lectures or teaching presentations which have required detailed editorial attention. They have been selected for their current relevance to the field and for the landmarks they reveal in the genesis and evolution of the new field of group analysis that Malcolm helped to cultivate out of the groundwork of his own original discipline – psychoanalysis. A number of these papers provided a basis for the training of group analysts like me, and we grew up on the diet they provided. Many of the others have been waiting for their place in the sun.

This collection

I began working with Malcolm on these papers some five years before he died. The editorial process has been a lengthy one and he showed patience and trust that the work would come together on creditable terms and in time for him to enjoy its reception in the field. Most regrettably he did not live to see this volume. His death marked the passing of the last of the Founder Members of London's Institute of Group Analysis. The membership list of EGATIN, the European Group Analytic Training Institutions Network, records membership of some 34 other such institutes in Europe (at least eighteen in Germany alone) and elsewhere; and these developments now include trainings in China, India, Iran, Israel, Russia, South Africa and other countries too. Many of the training centres carry the name Malcolm devised – Institute of Group Analysis – and they honour the training he helped initiate. He was my first teacher in psychotherapy at the Maudsley Hospital in 1977 and, after I qualified, he became my mentor and friend.

During the editorial process he accepted that I had a primary obligation to see to my own books first and he waited patiently for their issue. He wrote a tribute and validation for the work contained in my own first publication that helped to set me on the path to complete this compilation of his own work. These papers came out of journals, textbooks and Malcolm's own archives. After reviewing a vast collection of material, I put the work for consideration to Malcolm himself and to his archivists, Wendy Russell and Georgia Clemson. They had found many of the papers in one location or another and helped me assemble the first compilation, which then went to Kristopher Springer in the USA, the first of the professional editors recommended by his publisher, Routledge. Kristopher did a lot of the basic work tracking citations, building up reference lists and working on the text itself. When it came back to us, the second of the professional editors, Christopher Canter, undertook a second editorial review making a special contribution by identifying lost citations and dealing with quotations and outstanding queries in the text. He returned to the text in the concluding stages of its compilation and has made a profound contribution to the work. Louise Crane's work as a literary assistant helped consolidate the research and drafting at an earlier stage and she has our sincere appreciation. I have worked through the different contributions to bring all the papers here to the same standard as those Malcolm published previously in books and journals. We have appreciated the expertise and personal support of two other professionals who have made important contributions to this collection. Elizabeth Nokes, the Librarian responsible for the Kings Fund Library serving the Institute of Group Analysis in London and the Group Analytic Society International, has helped to track down publications and citations; and Adeela Sharif who is responsible for the Editorial Office of the journal, *Group Analysis*, has made an equally vital contribution. We extend special thanks to Kate Hawes, Senior Publisher for Mental Health at Routledge, her team and the Production Editor Reanna Young in particular, for their support and expertise throughout this project.

In the last stage of preparation, the compilation has gone to an informal Advisory Panel of readers to review the collection as a whole and each paper specifically. My colleagues in this panel, Robi Friedman, Thomas Mies and Dieter Nitzgen, have been companions in the enterprise and we are deeply indebted to all three of them. They have reviewed each paper as to its merit for inclusion, its location in the series, its originality, the clarity of its writing, the quality of its scholarship, the context it helps to set amongst the other chapters, the light it sheds on Malcolm's own evolution and development, and finally for what it reveals about the dynamics of change in the Weltanschauung of our times. I have made it clear in the endnotes where we have found it necessary to remove illustrative clinical material because we could not see if the necessary consent had been secured for publication. We note that the worth of these papers has been diminished by these excisions and I have tried to write into them – with Malcolm's approval – the necessary applied perspective, taking care with each supplement of my own to make clear who is speaking: author or editor.

The first Appendix provides a catalogue of Malcolm's own publications and unpublished presentations. The second Appendix gives the publication list of the forty-one titles for which he was responsible as the General Editor of the International Library of Group Psychotherapy and Group Process, published first by Routledge. Malcolm then negotiated its transfer to Jessica Kingsley under the new name, the International Library of Group Analysis (ILGA) where the publication series was numbered. Some of the original titles were brought out by the new publisher and the series was finally discontinued in 2003. In 2009 the concept was revived under the new title of the New International Library of Group Analysis (NILGA) edited by Earl Hopper. Malcolm has seen to the publication of the writing of others throughout his life. The series begins with *The Evolution of Group Analysis*, for which he wrote a signal paper, 'The contribution of S. H. Foulkes to Group Analysis', on the life and work of his own mentor and former analyst (Pines 1983b: 265–285).

This collection does not replicate the content of the previous compilation of his papers, *Circular Reflections*, issued by JKP in 1997. It begins with papers that were written before those in the previous collection and goes on to include many others that come after.

Sections and principles for the organisation of the collection

Two principles have been followed in the organization of these papers. The first gives the chronology in which they were written or presented, as best we could determine. The second sets Malcolm's papers in categories.

Section I, Introduction: this is opened with a landmark paper in the field written for a North American textbook, co-authored by Harold Behr and Liesel Hearst and published in 1982. Behr and Hearst relied on this paper for the textbook they went on to write, *Group-analytic psychotherapy: A Meeting of Minds* (2005). This originating paper opens the collection with the consent of its co-authors, and it remains unsurpassed for its clarity of conception and comprehensive scope, despite the passage of time. It serves as the touchstone for the compilation.

Section II, History and context: three chapters trace the history and context of the group-analytic perspective from originating ideas to the development of its coherency and context. The section is concluded with Malcolm's Maxwell Jones Lecture given in 1998. Like many of the papers presented here, it is a much more scholarly and extended study than the original lecture. Written with an elegiac style, it charts the unwritten history of the therapeutic community in a major historical work giving close attention to institutional detail. It laments the discontinuity of these communities and celebrates the sad passage of 'the main line and the good siding' with 'The Slow Train' as 'they all pass out of our life', an elegiac and comic song written and performed by Flanders and Swann who were his friends.

Section III, Development of method and technique in group-analytic psychotherapy: eight chapters trace changing perspective in psychoanalytic and group-analytic theory and technique. This is a core series that will attract the attention of practitioners across this and many other fields. It opens with studies of interpretation, dialogue and response and goes on to advance the idea of the self as a group and the group as a self, assisted by the literature of self psychology and other North American theorists in psychoanalysis. Then he goes on explore, with the help of Bakhtin, the two key concepts for which his oeuvre is best known – mirroring and resonance. From these conceptions he goes on to develop the originality of his picture of a person as a sonorous self and, concluding with 'more about listening', he sets up questions about listening and seeing to which he returns in his final papers.

Section IV, Metapsychology, philosophy, mind/body: In these four papers, Malcolm comes to the metapsychology and philosophy of mind that underpins all his work. Here, once more, the sequence of papers builds a new scaffold of support for novel conceptions that include, in this case, the focus he has given over many years to the close relationship between biology and psychology. The section opens with the 'in-between' – the locus of attention for all group analysts. He builds the understanding of these 'empty' spaces through two endeavours – one in the cross-cultural study of ethnic and spiritual difference and the other through conceptions of the mother-infant dyad in the work of Winnicott and many other students of early development. He goes on to apply the 'in-between' to group-analytic theory and practice on new and original terms, leading to a signature paper in this section, 'From social mind to social brain'. Here he introduces us to the writing of Adam Smith – the political economist of the Scottish Enlightenment – and sets his conceptions of *the mirror of sociability* against those of Foulkes. The consequences are startling and original and, by the end of a long study, he brings us to an understanding of psychogenesis and sociogenesis linked through the sociology of Norbert Elias and the studies made of neuroplasticity by Norman Doidge.

The wealth of scholarship is drawn out to a purpose – to address the question posed earlier in this section by the correspondence between Freud and Einstein. The virtues of group analysis are counterposed against Freud's constitutional aggression with refined arguments and evidence grounded in the developing recognition of the culturally modified brain. He finds reasons for hope in the human condition which he casts in the language of group analysis – we have always been able to amend ourselves. His own mastery of the scholarship of his time has been further advanced since in extended bodies of work by authors like Allan Schore, whose thinking he calls on and anticipates. This section concludes with a comparison of the relationship between the ideas, philosophical positions and clinical stance of Bion and

Foulkes and it summarises Malcolm's own work drawn from the two-volume compilation he edited on the work of Bion.

Section V, Final papers: These are Malcolm's four final papers, written from 2000 onward. The section begins with a major paper on training in group-analytic psychotherapy focused on the training approach of the Institute of Group Analysis in London, where the curriculum, the training structures and outlook were laid down in the 1970s and extended in the 1990s. They have helped to shape the field at large. The other three papers include one masterly clinical study of group analysis and the affective disorders, and two papers on myths, mirroring, Echo and Narcissus, and Perseus, Athena and Medusa, which represent the culmination of his written output. The first of these two is a working draft to prepare the second. They are worth reading together to get the full measure of his constructive vision. The last of these, written when he was 86, is magisterial in scope and immediately relevant to all with an interest in the primary sensory foundations of psychotherapy that belong to the world of sight and sound.

Each paper's context on presentation or past publication is set out in each paper's first endnote, together with acknowledgements and – where necessary – publication permission. Malcolm has first responsibility for the selection of papers in this compilation and I have second responsibility. Our panel of readers have had oversight of the final compilation. His family, his daughter Rosamond and his sons Jonathon and Simeon have played a key part in supporting the archivists and professional editors with the organisation and selection of papers in this collection. Much of this is now in the archive of the Wellcome Trust in London, where it is open for scholars and researchers in the field.

The person: Malcolm Pines

Malcolm has written at length about himself, his person and his family in his dedication and author's introduction. He identified six landmark events in his professional life in which he made decisive contributions that I will summarise here. The first was the establishment of the Group Analytic Practice with colleagues in 1964. The second was the foundation of the Institute of Group Analysis with a related but separate group of colleagues in 1973. The third was the establishment, after the death of Foulkes, of the Foulkes Lectures, a series of annual commemorative lectures that began in 1977, to which he himself contributed in 1982. The fourth was his own contribution to the journal *Group Analysis*, which he edited for some sixteen years. He helped to turn it into a respected, peer-reviewed journal. The fifth was the establishment of the International Library of Group Analysis that was set up first with the publisher Routledge; it was then relocated to Jessica Kingsley Press. The full set of publications in this series – forty-one books in all – is given in Appendix 2. His sixth contribution was the establishment of regular meetings of the Group Analytic Society in the form of symposia convened every three years. He attended the first Symposium in Lisbon in 1973, organised many of those that followed, and attended every subsequent event including the one held in Lisbon in 2014. The Symposium that followed in Berlin in 2017 was the first he could not attend. He was responsible for a seventh contribution: the introduction of large groups to the Annual Meeting of the American Group Psychotherapy Association, which are now a key part of their programme. Large groups are now an integral part of training programmes in group psychotherapy in North America and are widely relied on to address institutional problems and promote fellowship in professional meetings.

Large groups in South Africa and Lithuania

I have worked closely with Malcolm conducting large groups in different settings and will draw on two shared experiences to convey some personal detail about his gifts for the work. He could make incisive observations in a moment to capture and convey human depth, reaching across painful divisions and helping to take group experience across the threshold of liminal change. His leadership role was modest and was expressed with observational eloquence that could bring people to new points of understanding and resolution in a quiet voice. His Maxwell Jones Lecture in 1998, set out here as Chapter 4, will give readers the best account of his own work in large groups.

This compilation of papers charts his own evolution and development as a practitioner. He set a high standard for the role of the group analyst as leader in the large group. As he describes in his own Introduction, he was invited to conduct the large group at the first international conference on psychoanalysis to be held in South Africa after its liberation. He had played a similar role in Argentina some years earlier – a contribution I was not there to witness. He invited me to join him in Cape Town and call on my own knowledge of the locality and history so we could conduct the group together. There was turbulence and conflict of an unpleasant kind during the meeting, arising out of the dominant authority given to psychoanalysts from London in the conference proceedings, many of whom originated in South Africa and had returned for this event. These tensions became the large group's locus of tension and conflict – known as 'the locus of disturbance' in group analysis. Malcolm gave the group 'permission' for the necessary 'bloodletting', but we maintained a close and constant presence, bearing witness to all that followed. Issues were vocalised and, as we worked with the group, it became clear the 'emissaries' from abroad were carrying projections from the locals based on long-standing historical issues arising out of control imposed on the Cape first by the Dutch East India Company and then by the British Empire. But those who stepped into the cauldron from abroad carried their own heedless disregard for the dynamics of colonisation. The history that came to life in matters of the moment allowed all parties to find a sensible accommodation to one another and, as we shed our respective projections, mutual learning became the new order of the day. Malcolm himself summarises the gains and consequences of those events in his author's introduction above.

Years later we shared an equally memorable experience in a large group at the Annual Meeting of the Lithuanian Group Analytic Society, held just outside Vilnius in 2009. We were both visiting speakers, along with Ivan Urlić from Croatia, and the three of us also conducted the large group. The conference centre was located in a beautiful forest setting, but I had a sleepless night brought on by nightmares about my grandfather's siblings and their families, who had all been executed during the Holocaust in 1941 in a nearby forest setting like this one. The killing units of the Waffen SS, the Einsatzgruppen, led the slaughter, marching Jews of all ages out of the towns and villages of the country into forests like this, where they were executed and buried in pits. I have written about these events in earlier publications and have set out to apply the principles of group analysis to the study of war and peace (Schlapobersky 2016). One of my great-uncles died a hero's death taking some of the killers with him, but even the very number of those we lost, was lost with them – young and old, women and children. The personal detail of this horror is now recorded in my own memoir, *When They Came for Me: The Hidden Diary of an Apartheid Prisoner,* (Schlapobersky 2021). After this disturbed night I reported my disquiet to Malcolm over breakfast the next day and found his reaction startling. He told me his own grandparents, his mother's parents whom he knew well and loved and with whom he spent summer holidays in Estonia in the 1930s, had been executed in Riga during the Holocaust in the same wave of killings. I had known nothing of this over the years and I believe few amongst those in his wide range of associations were aware of it.

The atmosphere amongst our Lithuanian colleagues, and between them and ourselves, was warm, convivial and productive. At that stage they did not know – consciously – about our respective histories. Later that morning we led the large group and sat through a despairing, dispiriting silence. Each of the large group conductors offered something, but we could do nothing to help the process open to an exchange of any kind until Malcolm said: 'We seem to be sitting with the silence of the dead and amongst the ghosts of the past'. He was kind, closely attuned, benevolent and enquiring. In the ensuing silence he repeated the observation and later he repeated it again. And then, in a silence that refused to go away, he took the risk of reporting our breakfast conversation to the large group and speculated on whether our own histories might be bound up with theirs. We continued to sit through the kind of silence that can follow a tragedy, after the reported account of a catastrophe. We welcomed the ensuing silence as one in which everyone had joined us. Once we joined them in this way, and from this point of seeming impasse in the wake of these comments, the group came to life, as did the two following large groups. The room filled with historical narrative – with a flood of associations. We could then talk, all three of the visitors: Malcolm about the death of his maternal grandparents in nearby Riga; I about the death of my grandfather's siblings in the same month just kilometres away in a similar forest; and Ivan about his own experience of therapeutic work with survivors of the Balkan wars that had only just been concluded. In our commonality, other people who carried so many stories of loss, injury and betrayal, joined the narrative. The barriers between our histories were set aside and we sat through others' accounts of tragic life histories as if we were amongst our own. When we could find the space to speak again, we talked about how we had broken the silence of dissociation that separates injury from survival. In the large group we all became witnesses and truth-tellers to one another. The stories continued in the large group and beyond; and they continued between ourselves and our hosts – and within their groups and subgroups – for much of the time that followed. Indeed, they continue to this day. Malcolm and I returned to our separate lives in London deeply affected and on easier terms with the homicides that lie in our past, and we were well aware of the benefits that Ivan took home with him too. Our close association with these Lithuanian colleagues continues.

The family and the field

Malcolm's own immediate family includes his three children and the four grandchildren they have between them. He described the close family ties that continued between him and his wife Iris, and his siblings and their families. During his lifetime he was a family and father figure to all the children and grandchildren of these next generations who joined him for the funeral of his wife and then attended his own. They include devoted family members, loving parents and distinguished professionals across a range of fields. His son Jonathon is the Chris Marshall Professor of Cell Biology at the Institute of Cancer Research and a Fellow of the Royal Society.

Many years ago, Malcolm left his wife to take up a relationship with a woman who was in psychoanalysis with him, and he moved out to live with her for some time. I am neither authorised nor informed enough to write about these events and their ramifications in any detail. I write as someone who is now a family friend and who was a witness to the unfolding of very troublesome events. When this relationship broke up, he lived on his own for some considerable period and during this time he made good with his wife and children, who received him back to the family in love and forgiveness. Could he have ever made good with the woman he injured? He resumed a devoted married life with Iris and once again their home became a focal point in the life of their family and relatives. During their later years when infirmity was affecting them both, he suffered from problems of mobility due to both a knee injury and neuropathy. Iris, due to maculopathy, lost much of her eyesight. She provided the mobility for both of them, in which he was compromised; and he provided the eyesight in which she was impaired. Visiting their home was an opening to their enduring care and affection and they grew old together in dignity and shared devotion – to one another, to their children and to their grandchildren.

Repair of the damage that the affair did to Malcolm's professional standing and to the organisations affected has been much more tenuous. When detail of this history and matters associated with it came to light, he resigned his membership of the General Medical Council and British Psychoanalytic Institute, which meant he could no longer practice as a doctor or psychoanalyst. The Institute of Group Analysis which he had helped to found took measured consideration and, in the light of the other organisations' disciplinary action, allowed his membership to continue but denied him the authority to speak, teach or supervise in the Institute's name. It was one of the most painful actions he had to endure but he bore the consequences of his own action with dignity.

He spoke about his misconduct in public on only one occasion of which I am aware. Two of our German colleagues produced a film based on interviews, called *Pioneers of Group Analysis*.[1] Marita Barthel-Rösing and Wilhelm Rösing are reparative historians who use the medium of film. She is both a psychoanalyst and a group analyst and he is a film director. Their film has been shown at professional meetings all over Europe in the last few years. Interviews with Malcolm and with our colleague Liesel Hearst, who between them played the most decisive role in European developments, take up the central part of the film record. It documents the detailed, interpersonal construction of a new field of endeavour and goes on to interview a representative number of others from the generations that follow in the group-analytic field who have made significant contributions. Towards the conclusion of Malcolm's interview, Marita asks him directly about the affair and he speaks openly on camera about the gravity of his misdemeanour. He speaks with sorrow and remorse and those who have watched and learnt of the history from him in this film are deeply moved by the sense of tragedy he conveys, regarding the damage he did to himself, his former patient, his family and the field. What is of most acute relevance to this collection of papers is Malcolm's deeply felt relief on several counts. The first is that his wife and children got over these events, forgave him and went on to do well in their own lives. The children have returned this reparative spirit by taking in hand the challenge of seeing to this record of his written and presented work. Readers will find their love for him in this compilation, and the forgiveness that love can allow. This compilation comes from Malcolm's authorship, from the love and labour of his family and from the close attention of his colleagues. May the creative purpose of a visionary who helped to create a new field come to make good in amends offered for past injury.

In conclusion

Despite the turbulence and uncertainty created in the field by the disclosure of Malcolm's past conduct, he remained the go-to person who was called on to speak at the funerals of his friends and colleagues. The full extent of his fellowship is evident in Appendix 1, which gives a catalogue for the publication of the many obituaries and eulogies he was responsible for down the years.

There is a much more extensive record of these writings in the archive at the Wellcome Trust that can be consulted by scholars.

Malcolm Pines regarded himself principally as a teacher whose quest to humanize the landscape of professional training was realized through group analysis. As a living encyclopaedia, he enjoyed the visits of younger colleagues and continued his communication by email until his last days. Messages of condolence reaching his family from around the world gave thanks for his open soul, love of poetry, inspirational teaching, mastery of writing, gift for friendship and generosity towards the writing of others. I saw him during his last days at home when he told me that he had learnt a lot whilst recently in hospital for pneumonia – to be quiet, not to make demands on his loved ones, and to be grateful for his life. This openness to learning to the very end, and his capacity to describe this, are true marks of his standing. His wife Iris pre-deceased him by three years and he found her absence intolerable. He spent his last few years quietly surrounded by a staggering number of books, music in the Russian classical tradition, and his loving family and friends. He is survived by their children and grandchildren, twelve nieces and nephews, a large extended family and several families of professionals in the field.

John Schlapobersky, Finchley, February 2024

Note

1 Wilhelm Rösing and Marita Barthel-Rösing (2017), *Pioneers of Group Analysis*. Film recording available at https://www.roesingfilm.de/filme/pioneers-of-group-analysis.

Foreword: Juan Tubert-Oklander. The iceberg and the tip, or who is afraid of the big bad Malcolm?

When Malcolm Pines asked me to write a Foreword to his new book of *Further Papers*, I felt honoured and highly stimulated to do it. However, I soon found out that I showed an undue tendency to delay writing it. As procrastination is not one of my regular character traits, I felt that I should take it as a symptom. But a symptom of what?

Symptoms are always multidetermined, and a brief analysis showed that this was no exception. Of the various factors that motivated my postponement, I shall mention two that are directly related to the very nature of Malcolm's book. The first is the enormity of his contributions, concealed by the deceptive simplicity of his discourse. When one first reads any of his writings, everything is so clear and straightforward, but that is just the tip of the iceberg. Then, on a second, third or fourth reading, one finds out that each sentence, each paragraph propels us into an unlimited web of connotations – what Bion (1962) called 'a penumbra of associations' – that paves the path for further queries. In other words, Malcolm's contributions cannot just be read, much less learnt; they can only become a subject for an active dialogue and a shared enquiry. This is the massive body of the iceberg, hidden from direct view by the water surface, and its scale can easily become overwhelming and awe-inspiring for a reader – in this case, myself.

I first became aware of this impact of Malcolm's writing when I read Chapter 6, 'Dialogue and selfhood: Discovering connections'. This is easy reading, like having an amiable chat with an older friend with whom you are not afraid to enter into a light and fluid dialogue – and a creative one at that, always full of surprises. I am sure that this is the sort of dialogue that Malcolm has always fostered with his patients and groups. But just as patients regularly find, after leaving such a session, that this dialogue has dug deep into their very being and continues to haunt them all the way until their next meeting, Malcolm's words in the text went on spiralling inside me for long, so that I soon had to go back to them for a new encounter.

When this happened, I was once again astonished to find out that, as I had noted in a previous article on Malcolm's influence on my thinking and practice (Tubert-Oklander 2010), he had long ago written many things that I had been thinking, teaching and writing during the past few decades. And in this text, written in 1996, he was putting forward some of my more recent thoughts, sometimes in almost the same words. Was this a case of cryptomnesia? This is a common occurrence in writers, whose ideas and writing can contain the words of others heard or read long ago, which they have forgotten about and then reproduced without being aware of it. Or was it just evidence that he and I are soulmates of a kind and follow parallel trains of thought? Perhaps there was a bit of both.

Some of the ideas that presently occupy my mind have been with me since I began to study these matters fifty years ago, long before I ever heard of Malcolm. They were initially, however, vague intuitions that I could not formulate cogently, much less could I convince anyone of their value. Besides, they were clearly at odds with what my elders were trying to teach me. By the time I met Malcolm in 1983, I had advanced quite a lot in their formulation, with the help of my readings of S. H. Foulkes, Enrique Pichon-Rivière, Wilfred Bion and Gregory Bateson, but I still had a long way to go. In Malcolm's lectures I found a man who was thinking through the same questions that obsessed me – indeed, he had been dealing with them for much longer and with many more elements than I. Consequently, he provided me with new words and references that helped me to crystallise and further develop my own thinking. But were these ideas mine or his? Of course, they were both, at one and the same time, since, as Malcolm clearly states in this text, thought is necessarily a relational and social process, as much as a personal one.

This chapter reminds us that for Foulkes (1975) there was an essential identity between the personal matrix and the group matrix, which were just different aspects of a continuum. Thus, Foulkes (1975: 130) wrote:

> Just as the individual's mind is a complex of interacting processes (personal matrix), mental processes interact in the concert of the group (group matrix). These processes relate to each other in manifold ways and on a variety of different levels. The group-analytic group has been termed a psyche group.

Hence, we might say that in every group (and not only in a group-analytic one) the meeting is the concert, the individuals are the players, the group is the orchestra (with or without a conductor), and *mind is the music*. This is the basic teaching I receive from the work of Foulkes, Pichon-Rivière and Pines, and from the reading of all this book's chapters.

Mind is always a collective enterprise as well as a personal one, and human existence is the confluence of the I and the We. Thought is never purely an individual matter, but the outcome of dialogue, both internal and external. Pichon-Rivière (1971, 1995) used to say that thinking is the dialogue within one's internal group and that it both derives from and influences our external dialogues. We all have our inner group of internal interlocutors, which includes both friends and enemies, as well as acquaintances and the wider social group. The members of Malcolm's inner group are most varied and constitute a rather unlikely assembly. In this chapter alone they include James Anthony, Gaston Bachelard, Mikhail Bakhtin, Wilfred Bion, Martin Buber, Norbert Elias, Erik Erikson, Ronald Fairbairn, S. H. Foulkes, Sigmund Freud, Kurt Goldstein, Ernest Hutten, Robert Kegan, Rita Leal, José Ortega y Gasset, Louis Sander, Daniel Stern, Harry Stack Sullivan, Colwyn Trevarthen, Lev Vygotsky, Donald Winnicott and Léon Wurmser.

And when we turn to the other chapters of the book, the list grows immensely. For instance, in Chapter 15, 'From social mind to social brain', his guests include quite a few biologists, from Charles Darwin to Michael Gazzaniga, Jaak Panksepp and Frans de Waal, as well as the major psychoanalytic theoretician Hans Loewald, the founder of social psychology George Herbert Mead, and the great philosopher Maurice Merleau-Ponty. And then, of course, there is also the unobtrusive and unmentioned presence of his parents and siblings, his beloved wife Iris, their children and his friends. Hence, from the group-analytic point of view, which is certainly Malcolm's, a lone thinker is always the representative of a multitude, but there are better and worse such representatives, and Malcolm undoubtedly excels in the task, and does it with a most unusual elegance and flair. (I also have my own internal symposium, which partly overlaps with Malcolm's, and he has been a major figure in it for the past thirty-five years.)

From a slightly different perspective, Malcolm's vast and comprehensive culture, omnivorous reading and open-mindedness make him a master of what his admired Bakhtin calls 'heteroglossia', a dialogue between several languages. Heteroglossia opens the possibility for the growth and change that are regularly blocked by the dogma of 'monoglossia' – the obligatory use of a single language, which is as common in psychoanalytic institutions and communities as it was in Bakhtin's Soviet Union. It is quite obvious that monoglossia is the full opposite of dialogue and, for Malcolm, dialogue is the very stuff of analysis, of thought, and indeed, of human existence. This allows him to conjoin seamlessly psychoanalysis, group analysis, history, political science, literature, mythology, medicine, neuroscience, ethology, sociology, anthropology, poetry and philosophy. The result is a unique polysemic and multidimensional fresco of human existence, which reminds me of the vast depictions of Mexican history and society painted by the Mexican muralists Juan O'Gorman, José Clemente Orozco, Diego Rivera and David Alfaro Siqueiros.

I shall not try to summarise the enormous richness of this inevitably partial selection of Malcolm's writings which I invite the reader to explore (we are still waiting and hoping for the publication of his *Complete Works*). I will only say that this collection provides a privileged opportunity to behold the infinite variety of his enquiries, endeavours and reflections. And, if this expression recalls Mark Antony's passion for Cleopatra, it is quite all right, since one's fascination in reading the works of a master writer like Malcolm Pines has the qualities of a love affair. It is fair to say, like Enobarbus said of

Cleopatra in Shakespeare's *Antony and Cleopatra*, that neither age nor rereading can 'wither . . . , nor custom stale [their] infinite variety' (Act II, scene 2). For I have found that each time I go back to some of Malcolm's writings that I thought I had already mastered, they shine with new meanings, this being the very definition of a classic.

Quite a few years ago, I wrote a brief essay called 'The museum and the workshop: Some reflections on the vitality of texts', which I read in a Colloquium on Analogical Hermeneutics. There, I discussed the difference and contrast between two kinds of texts: some are dead and mummified, forever identical to themselves, worthy only to be preserved in a museum, while a few others, those we call 'classics', are forever vital in their invitation to the reader to engage in an active and passionate interpretative dialogue with them. It brings them back to life and turns their reading into a veritable workshop. I compared the latter to the 'texts' that emerge during psychoanalytic dialogue and I describe this in the following terms:

> I have therefore tackled two different problems, both related to the vitality of texts. On the one hand, I have described the existence of living and fluid texts, whose prototype is dialogue [this being the case of analysis, both psycho-analysis and group-analysis], which are in a perpetual state of renovation, in a reflective situation in which all the participants in a dialogue are a part of the very text, authors and interpreters of it at the same time. We might say that these are texts that write and interpret themselves. On the other, I have approached the paradoxical problem of those texts which are written, and therefore established and immutable, but that nonetheless display their vitality by acquiring multiple shapes and meanings as a function of the reader and the context. Perhaps these are the only texts worth reading, since all others are merely information or entertainment.
>
> (Tubert-Oklander 2009: 55, my translation)

These are the texts we call 'classics', and from this point of view, Malcolm is undoubtedly a classic author. But this poses a major problem. I have been reading and discussing some of his writings with the members of a virtual study group, all of whom are fully trained psychoanalysts and psychoanalytic psychotherapists with ample experience who live in different cities and countries. They were all deeply impressed and delighted on meeting him, but they ask of me a really demanding question: 'Why is it that we had not heard of him before?'

I was hard-pressed to answer it, but I tried, and this is what emerged from the subsequent discussions. Stefano Bolognini (1999/2006), in his delightful collection of narrative portraits, *Like Wind, Like Wave*, suggests that there are two kinds of scientists. There are the public figures who administrate scientific institutions, appear in interviews in the media, have deft political and managerial abilities and a charming and impressive personality that allows them to become idols in the eyes of their audiences. But they are not usually deep thinkers or able researchers themselves and thrive on the work of the teams they lead. Then, there are the true scientists who, more often than not, are rather antisocial, and even weirdos, who pursue single-mindedly the truth about their research aims, subordinating all other concerns and they tend to go unnoticed, and even despised, at least during their lifetimes.

Pretty much the same happens in the arts, a field in which the great ones are often ignored until after their death. Vincent van Gogh hardly sold a painting in his lifetime and Franz Kafka only became the enormous writer that he is after his best friend betrayed his final wish that all his manuscripts be burned after his death. As the great Argentine novelist Ernesto Sabato once wrote, 'In this country of envious people, no one ever gets to be a great man until he ceases to be one'. Surely this is not only an Argentinian trait, but a worldwide scourge.

This is undoubtedly true, but it does not fully apply in Malcolm's case, since he has not only practised, thought, written and taught, but also occupied important positions in psychoanalytic and group-analytic institutions, and acted as a true leader of the group-analytic movement. And he is most certainly not antisocial, but an amiable, gentle and considerate human being. But the truth is that he has fulfilled his elevated positions in an unobtrusive, respectful and modest way, which is a far cry from the narcissistic exhibitionism of most public figures. It would seem that most people are only willing to admire those who despise them or make them feel inferior or inadequate.

So, this is not enough of an explanation. Then, there is the evident fact that Malcolm is far better known in the group-analytic community (albeit unfairly recognised more as a leader than as a theoretician) than in the psychoanalytic community, although he has in the past played major roles in a psychoanalytic institution of which he is no longer a member. The truth is that Malcolm was always somewhat of a foreigner in the psychoanalytic milieu: a true polyglot in a community bent on monoglossia; a committed therapist, rather than a neutral and objective investigator; a group analyst, which is a rather disreputable trait in psychoanalytic environments; an environmentalist; not a staunch believer in the intrapsychic; and an analyst who showed a keen interest in the strangest literature, such as the works of a dissident Soviet philosopher like Bakhtin, or studies on the social behaviour of chimpanzees, instead of sticking to Freud and the anointed texts of our profession. All these sins more than outweighed his administrative and editorial virtues. Finally, he left the institution, and psychoanalytic organisations tend to behave as adolescent bands, in that they declare the inexistence of any member who leaves the group.

But there is still another more important factor, and this is the second cause I mentioned for my own symptom of postponing the writing of this text. It is an emotional one: it is fear, which I have referred to in the title of this foreword. Why should anyone be afraid of Malcolm? He is one of the gentlest persons I have ever met, but the fear is still there, and this demands an explanation.

Most people are *terribles simplificateurs*: they tend to keep things simple in their minds and loathe it when someone faces them with the unfathomable complexity of existence and challenges them to think them through. Of course, when someone uses abstruse and convoluted language, there is always the recourse to say: 'This must be very profound, for I cannot understand it at all, but it is most admirable', and this puts their spirit at rest, since it confirms their belief that thinking is something other people do (an author, a lecturer, a teacher, a sage, or a prophet), so they do not have anything to do with it but follow the leader and mechanically repeat his words, parrot-like.

But when someone like Malcolm comes forward and clearly spells out for us the insurmountable difficulty of the task that lies beyond and waits for us to tackle it, particularly if it calls into question our most hallowed beliefs, the immediate response is fear, and something like vertigo, as if the ground had been removed from under our feet. What he is actually saying is this: 'The world is a maddingly complex place, which we will never be able to fully fathom or encompass with our thought and understanding. I have no definite answers to give you, but only questions. The rest is up to you'. This is a terrifying proposal – to have to think our own thoughts; it is the very same proposal that we should be giving to our analytic patients, and we all fear it. Many just reject it wholesale as nonsense, but quite a few of us are enticed to follow this – the hardest path.

So, who is afraid of the big bad Malcolm? I am, we all are, and I am sure he is also. Fear is the first of the four enemies to be overcome in the path to becoming a man of knowledge, according to Don Juan Matus, the Yaqui Indian sorcerer from Sonora, Mexico, who was the teacher and mentor of Carlos Castaneda (1968/1998). The other three are Clarity, Power and Old Age. Someone who overcomes the first obstacle, Fear, acquires Clarity; then he has to surmount Clarity, which has become the second one, and thus he gains Power, which is the third enemy to be vanquished, and when this happens, comes the final foe, Old Age, which is bound to prevail in the end. Someone like Malcolm, who has managed to keep his youthful spirit well into the tenth decade of his life, clearly qualifies as a Man of Knowledge. From the point of view of my Yaqui namesake, Old Age is bound to come for all of us, that is for sure, but one can accept and manage it for a very brief moment in which the outcome of the whole trip is to bloom and bear fruit, without being defeated before our time comes (although some people are defeated by old age while still in their teens!).

Being a Man of Knowledge is a temporary state. Don Juan describes this in the following terms: 'To be a man of knowledge has no permanence. One is never a man of knowledge, not really. Rather, one becomes a man of knowledge for a very brief instant, after defeating the four natural enemies' (p. 53). This is much the same as what happens with psychoanalysis and group analysis. One is never really an analyst, but a more or less advanced candidate, a would-be analyst in the process of becoming one.

So, Malcolm is, at this very time of writing, a true analyst, a Man of Knowledge and a model for many of us to aspire to. We might well identify him with Faust's final words in the second part of Goethe's grand play:

> Yes! To this thought I hold with firm persistence,
> The last result of wisdom stamps it true:
> He only learns his freedom and existence
> Who daily conquers them anew.
> Thus here, by dangers girt, shall glide away
> Of childhood, manhood, age, the vigorous day:
> And such a throng I fain would see,—
> Stand on free soil among a people free!
> *Faust* – Part II, Act V (Goethe 1890: 495–496)

Malcolm, like Faust, is a tireless seeker after truth. I just hope that the publication of this book places him precisely where he should be, in the company of the Great Ones of our profession, such as Ferenczi, Fairbairn, Winnicott, Foulkes and Pichon-Rivière, all of whom were derided by orthodox analysts.

As to my question about fear, Malcolm is no wolf, but neither is he Little Red Riding Hood, nor a feeble powerless granny in spite of his Kind Grandfather appearance, and most certainly he is not any of the Three Little Pigs! He is the kindest man I know, but he also has sharp teeth and a will of steel, when this is called for. He is what Don Juan would call a 'warrior' and a Man of Knowledge and this book bears witness to this. Read it and enjoy it. Let it unsettle your spirit as it did mine, for it is an invitation for further work, in order to digest its ideas, to make them truly yours and develop them along new paths of your choosing, until you no longer know what belongs to Malcolm and what belongs to you. This is precisely the sort of dialogue in which he loves to engage people.

Good luck and good reading!

Juan Tubert-Oklander, Mexico City, 2021

Section I

Introduction

1 Group analysis and group-analytic psychotherapy[1]

Malcolm Pines, Liesel Hearst and Harold Behr

Introduction

Group-analytic psychotherapy is the term applied by S. H. Foulkes to the form of psychotherapy he developed from 1943 onwards. As a psychoanalyst trained in a classical tradition, Foulkes brought to his work a knowledge of and adherence to many of the basic principles of psychoanalysis, combined with a deep appreciation of the social nature of humans and the profound importance of socialisation processes in the development of the personality. The combination of these two viewpoints led him to the logical application of these principles to small-group psychotherapy in a formal setting. Many of his fundamental ideas were derived from and confirmed by the experience of working as an army psychiatrist at Northfield, a psychiatric military hospital, during World War II, where he laid down many of the fundamental principles of the therapeutic community (Main 1946). This experience of larger groups as well as the small formal psychotherapeutic group laid the foundations for the application of group-analytic principles and settings other than the small group. Group-analytic principles therefore have been influential in the development of large-group psychotherapy and of the therapeutic community and family therapy.

The work of S. H. Foulkes is described in four volumes of his own writings (Foulkes 1948/1984; Foulkes and Anthony 1957/1965, 1984; Foulkes 1964/1986; Foulkes 1975/1986). After his death in 1976, a collection of his papers was edited and published by his wife, Elizabeth (Foulkes 1990a). And there is more about him in the writing of his colleagues (Abse 1974; De Maré 1972; 1977; Kadis et al. 1974; Pines 1978a; 1978b; 1983a; Skynner 1987). The journal *Group Analysis* founded by Foulkes in 1967 acts as an international forum for those sympathetic to group-analytic psychotherapy based on this model.

A knowledge of Foulkes's professional background illuminates the nature of his basic model. Born in Germany, he studied medicine with the intention of becoming a psychiatrist. Kurt Goldstein was a significant influence during his years as a psychiatrist at the Neurological Institute in Frankfurt. Goldstein was a distinguished neuropsychiatrist whose works are best represented in two volumes: *The Organism* (1939) and *Human Nature in the Light of*

DOI: 10.4324/9781003494713-2

Psychopathology (1940). He had made a profound study of the effects of brain injury on the personality and behaviour of patients, which led him to view reactions to injury as always involving the whole organism in its adaptation to disorder of function and its relationship to the total environment. Goldstein evolved his own application of Gestalt psychology, which emphasised figure-ground relation and the study of the total situation of the subject, including the situation of the observer.

> From training and insight acquired in neurobiology as seen by Kurt Goldstein, I held a conviction that the situation in which one works, the situation as a whole, really decided all part processes and their meaning. . . . Naturally in a group the total situation is the group (itself).
>
> (Foulkes 1973: 73)

His emphasis on the study of the group as a whole entity derives from Goldstein's view that the healthy organism functions as a whole and can be described as a system in dynamic equilibrium. The organism has constantly and actively to adjust to its ever-changing circumstances and environmental conditions. Goldstein's emphasis on the nervous system as a network, which represents an apparatus that always functions as a whole, clearly influenced Foulkes in his view that the group also always functions as a whole. This will be discussed further in the section on theoretical foundations.

Foulkes then trained in Vienna as a psychoanalyst and after qualifying returned to Frankfurt, where he was appointed director of the outpatient clinic of the Psychoanalytical Institute. His contemporaries there included Erich Fromm and Frieda Fromm-Reichmann (Jay 1973). The influence of modern sociology on psychoanalysis in Frankfurt was considerable. The Psychoanalytic Institute itself was in the same building as the Institute for Social Research headed by Max Horkheimer, and included Theodor Adorno, Fromm, Herbert Marcuse and others; and Frankfurt University's Department of Sociology, headed by Karl Mannheim, which included Max Wertheimer and Norbert Elias. Joint seminars were held and attended by members of each of these three centres and they enjoyed the presiding influence of Kurt Goldstein. Foulkes left Frankfurt and came to Great Britain as a refugee psychoanalyst. One of his major psychoanalytic papers, 'On Introjection' (Foulkes 1937), was given to the British Psychoanalytical Society.

Foulkes's first analytic group was conducted in the early days of World War II when he was working in a small West Country town, Exeter. The idea of bringing together in a psychotherapeutic group patients he was seeing in individual psychotherapy or psychoanalysis had been developing for many years. His interest in sociology, and in particular the work of the sociologist Elias (1978; 1991/2001; 2000), led him towards a synthesis of the study of society through sociology and the study of the individual through psychoanalysis, and he came to the idea that this could lead to a new form of psychotherapy. In bringing his individual patients together in a group, his intention was to be able to listen to the way in which they communicated with each other, to observe and study this new psychotherapeutic situation. From the first he saw his prime role as facilitating communication and understanding between the members of the group, as well as working with the transference reactions of the individual members of the group towards him as the central figure. In this, his approach differed radically from that of other psychoanalysts and psychotherapists who were experimenting with small-group psychotherapy in those years. He was probably influenced by the work of Trigant Burrow (Burrow 1927; De Maré 1977), which also points in this direction. He was also acquainted with the work of Kurt Lewin (1951), the author of field theory, and related this work to his own:

> Field theory has made a major contribution to the study of group dynamics and social fields which is of interest for a theoretical framework of group analysis. Its concepts of the dynamic whole, of figure and background, of longingness, of tension and conflict, of the various types of leadership and atmosphere, of the time perspective and the here-and-now of cohesive and disruptive forces, of valences and of integrated and leaderless groups, have been incorporated as part of the group-analytic system.
>
> (Foulkes and Anthony 1957: 39)

The viewpoint shared by Foulkes, Lewin, Erikson, Fromm, Sullivan and others is this shift from the study of the isolated individual (Rickman 1957b) to the study of interpersonal relationships and their profound influence on the evolving personality of the child. Early psychoanalytic views had represented individual personality as developing primarily through the impact of primitive instinctual drives on the developing mind, with personality resulting from the outcome of the inevitable conflicts between drive and defence. In classic psychoanalytic theory the influence of society came relatively late in the development of the child, principally through the development of the superego, which represents the internalisation of the parents and the creation of a structure within the mind of the individual, representing the viewpoint of that society of which he or she is a member. In Foulkes's theory the individual and society are artificial abstractions, which are only apparently and semantically separate. The individual is not prior to society. The individual is born into a network of communication processes that inevitably and profoundly affect his or her nature from the moment of birth. 'Psychodynamics are rarely if ever confined within the boundaries of the individual but regularly include a number of inter-connected persons. They are transpersonal manifestations' (Foulkes and Anthony 1957: 39).

In his first book Foulkes (1948) describes both his work in small-group psychotherapy in Exeter and the very significant Northfield experiment. Northfield was a military psychiatric hospital where Wilfred Bion and John Rickman (Bion and Rickman 1943) had worked previously. Closely associated with Foulkes's work, which led to the concept of the therapeutic community, were T. F. Main (1977) and Harold Bridger (1946). This work paralleled but differed significantly from the contemporary work of Maxwell Jones (1968/2013) at Henderson Hospital in that Foulkes's work arose from his position as a psychoanalyst, contrasting with that of Jones whose work was more rooted in community and social psychology. At Northfield Foulkes, together with his colleagues, developed the concept of the hospital as a therapeutic institution. They established two basic concepts of hospital psychotherapy: (a) the hospital should function as a therapeutic community, and its organisation and activities should be firmly in the interest of its task, the restoration of 'sick' persons, and (b) the hospital itself as an organisation can become 'sick' – that is, maladaptive to its task, and in that case needs to be 'treated' (Foulkes 1948). The originality and vitality of Foulkes and his colleagues' wartime experience induced considerable interest in group psychotherapy in some psychoanalysts in North America (1946) and Great Britain – the so-called English school of psychoanalysis. Principal figures here, in addition to Foulkes, are Bion (1962), Henry Ezriel (1973) and John D. Sutherland (1952). It is important, however, to differentiate among these workers. Bion, Ezriel and Sutherland were all considerably influenced by the work of Melanie Klein, Ronald Fairbairn and the object relations school of psychoanalysis. Foulkes adhered more to the ego psychological viewpoint as represented by Anna Freud and her co-workers. Bion, Ezriel and Sutherland developed the 'Tavistock model' of group psychotherapy and group dynamics. Foulkes and his co-workers at the Maudsley Hospital and within the Group-Analytic Society, London, evolved a model that has significant differences in its basic theories and in its techniques (Brown 1979; James 1980).

In 1953 Foulkes founded the Group-Analytic Society – together with James Anthony, Jane Abercrombie, Pat de Maré and others – as a forum for professional persons engaged in group psychotherapy. With a number of his colleagues and trainees he later founded the Institute of Group Analysis, London. This institution now trains a considerable number of persons in group-analytic psychotherapy in a three-year training course. The influence of the society and the institute is now considerable in Europe, though less so in North and South America. There are Institutes of Group Analysis in Lisbon and Rome, and active training courses in group-analytic psychotherapy are being conducted in both Denmark and Germany.

Foulkes founded the journal *Group Analysis*, which began as an international network of correspondents and has since developed into a more comprehensive journal, but it still retains some of the hallmarks of informal communication and the development of a network. Until his death in 1976, Foulkes continued to edit *Group Analysis* and to play an active part in the affairs of the institute. Since his death, the teaching of group-analytic psychotherapy has continued to be influenced by recent work in psychoanalysis, in particular that of Winnicott (1965/1985; 1967/1971), Mahler (1968; Mahler et al. 1975), Loewald (1988; 1989) and Kohut (1966; 1977).

Definitions

Foulkes developed a number of terms to describe both his theory and his practice, many of which have become common parlance.

STRANGER/PROXY GROUPS: Groups consisting of people who have no previous connection with each other.

LIFE GROUP/ROOT GROUP: Persons who are vitally interrelated. The life group has a natural network as a family or extended family.

TRANSFERENCE GROUP: The group-analytic group is usually the group of strangers. Foulkes differentiated between Transference with a capital *T* and transference with a small *t*. All relationships in a therapeutic situation should be called transference (t). In this situation the classic Transference (T) – that is, the specific replication of early patterns of behaviour – will emerge, based on internalised object relations and interpersonal processes.

THERAPY SITUATION (T SITUATION): The therapy situation (*T situation*) is a social situation. All processes and interactions are understood by reference to the situation and to its boundaries, within which old (childhood) experiences and attitudes are reactivated.

FREE GROUP ASSOCIATIONS: The patients' communications in the group become the equivalent of free associations in the dyad. The verbal and nonverbal productions of the group are treated as interconnected communications, as approximations to free association.

GROUP MATRIX: The matrix is a key construct; it denotes a hypothetical web of communication and interrelationships that evolve in a group. It is the common shared ground that ultimately determines the meaning and significance of all events and on which all communications and interpretations are located (Abraham 1973a; 1973b; 1973c; Blake 1980; de Maré 1972).

NODAL POINT: The individual is conceptualised as being a nodal point in a social network, born into and profoundly shaped by its characteristics. The individual is therefore seen as figure against ground, the ground being the social context.

MIRROR REACTION: The patient sees himself or herself, or a part of himself or herself, in particular a repressed part, in the other members. This complex reaction is manifested in many ways and at many different levels of consciousness. The person may quickly recognise and identify (parts of) himself or herself in another person; or the recognition may be resisted in many ways. The ultimate recognition and acceptance of this mirrored part of the self in the other represents a significant therapeutic gain (Foulkes 1964; Pines 1982/1997).

TRANSLATION: This is the group equivalent of 'making the unconscious conscious'. Through the work of communication and sharing, the patients move from less articulate and more primitive forms of expression, such as symptoms, to more articulate forms. Autistic forms of disturbance can be transformed into communications that are based on exchange.

RESONANCE: The considerable degree of unconscious communication between individuals is highly selective and specific. People strike certain tones or chords in each other, and this leads to specific forms of social bonding. The pairings of sadist and masochist, exhibitionist and voyeur, passive-submissive and aggressive-dominant are typical (Anthony 1965; Foulkes 1964). The term is also used in the sense that within the psychotherapeutic group, individuals react to common events in their own specific and idiosyncratic manner; the characteristic reactions of the individual members of the group to such shared events as the arrival or departure of members of the group, breaks in continuity and other group-specific events will evoke resonance.

POLARISATION: This represents the splitting-off of complex reactions into their elements, which leads to group members taking on and representing sharply contradictory attitudes. This typically emerges in divergent attitudes towards issues such as sex, age and dependency. In their combined reaction they bring to light the total complexity of reactions to this particular stimulus. The group, as it were, will speak through one individual who expresses one element of a reaction and the others can thereby dissociate themselves from the other elements. Scapegoating is one example of such polarisation.

Theoretical foundations

The theory of group analysis rests on the premise that the essence of human beings is social (Hopper 1980; Napolitani 1981). The individual is an artificial, though plausible, abstraction; each person is basically and centrally determined by the world in which he or she lives, by the group, by the community of which he or she forms a part. Inside and outside, individual and society, body and mind, fantasy and reality, cannot be opposed: all separation is artificial isolation. The individual is a part of a social network, 'a little nodal point as it were', and can only artificially be considered in isolation, like a fish out of water.

It follows from this that the neurotic position is in its very nature highly individualistic. It is group destructive in essence, for it is a result of an incompatibility between the individual and his or her original group. Because of this incompatibility, instead of being a nodal point in his or her network, he or she becomes a focal point of disturbed interpersonal processes.

The neurotic symptom is a disturbed expression of the patient's conflicts, never experienced in articulate language and therefore inaccessible to memory or to expression. Via a symptom, the patient communicates fundamental and unconscious conflicts.

> Symptoms in themselves autistic and unsuitable for sharing, exert, for this very reason, an increasing pressure upon the individual to express them. As long as he cannot express them in a more communicable way, he finds no real relief. . . . He must set forth to work again and again until he has transformed them into socially acceptable, articulate

> language. Understanding by other members of the group can only occur when the energies (libido) invested in these symptoms can be transformed into exchangeable value (cash, as it were).
>
> (Foulkes 1948: 169)

The proper study of the individual is within his or her natural group, particularly the family. If the psychiatrist were to go out into the patient's life, he or she would find that the patient's problems – as presented in the clinic – represent only one aspect of the patient, compared to those seen in their actual life. The psychiatrist would discover the *location* of the disturbance in some aspect of the patient's life situation and interpersonal relationships. Psychological disturbances are *located* – that is, take place between persons – and can never be wholly confined to a person in isolation.

In the group-analytic situation, disturbances can be located and traced in their effects on the dynamic processes of the group. For instance, if a patient overcomes silence for the first time when the conductor is absent, the speech inhibition is partly located in the therapist. However, if the patient can speak when alone with the therapist, the problem is with others.

The therapeutic process itself is identical with working towards an ever more articulate form of communication. This is achieved by (a) the group process – the patient's active participation in a mutual process, that of making himself or herself understood and of understanding the attempted communication of others, and (b) the conductor seeing 'meaning in action' in the dynamic events of the group and taking them as his or her frame of reference. The medium through which he or she works is communication with words, and the ultimate aim is expression in articulate verbal language that can be understood and shared by all.

The *main aims of therapy* are insight and adjustment. 'There is a relationship between the two: insight promotes adjustment, adjustment facilitates insight, insight without adjustment does not go very far, adjustment without insight is incomplete but it can work. Adjustment seems to be the more fundamental from a therapeutic, insight from a scientific point of view' (Foulkes 1964: 87).

The processes of insight and adjustment are illustrated as follows:

> As the group is a social situation the anti-social, destructive aspect of neurotic behaviour is forced . . . out into the open and does not receive the sanction of the group. . . . The individual in his healthy socially adjusted aspect is supported and allowed to develop and flourish in the group. While by mutual understanding and tolerance a good deal of hitherto neurotic behaviour can be modified and liberated for creative efforts, on the whole the neurotic formations of each individual are felt as a disturbance. . . . The individual in his neurotic aspect is set upon by the others, a process in which he participates actively in his turn, when he attacks the other man's neurotic defences and thus, by the way, his

> own. The group destructive energies can thus be used for the undermining each other's neurotic position whereas the constructive forces combine and support each other. . . . Disruptive forces are consumed in mutual analysis, constructive ones utilized for the synthesis of the individual and the integration of the group as a whole.
>
> (Foulkes 1964: 90)

By adjustment, Foulkes means the process of inner psychological change, the restructuring of the inner world, derived from and reflected in character and interpersonal relationship. He does not mean compliance with the therapist's authority and norms, or merely fitting in with the group's current attitudes. He warned therapists against undervaluing the enormous power of their own authority, that the group unconsciously strives to supply what they want. The therapist, as in other analytic situations, has to recognise and to work through the unconscious compliance of the patients (Foulkes 1971).

A basic law of group dynamics

The deepest reason why these patients, assuming for simplicity's sake, psychoneurotics, can reinforce each other's normal reactions and wear down and correct each other's neurotic reactions is that collectively they constitute the very norm from which, individually, they deviate. This is because each individual is to a large extent a part of the group to which he belongs. This collective aspect permeates him all through to his core. Persons in the group have much more in common than they know at first. They are struck by their differences, which provoke hostility and fear, but later on they find more and more common ground and less and less contradiction between individuality and community. The sound part of individuality, of character, is firmly rooted in the group and wholly approved by it. The group therefore respects and supports the emergence of and the free development of individuality. Neurotic peculiarities and symptoms are relieved as the process of communication develops and brings about shared experiences. Neurotic symptoms disappear 'into the common pool' as soon as they become communicable, and their individual ingredient is now free for group syntonic, socially acceptable employment. Neurotic behaviour tends to diminish in the group and normal behaviour tends to be supported. These processes are not conscious, but a group is forced to act in this direction by the very fact that it can only grow by what it can share and can only share what it communicates and only communicate what it has in common, for example, language in common – that is, on the basis of a community at large (Foulkes 1948: 29).

The conductor's first aim is to facilitate participation on the part of the group's members. He or she recognises and accepts their dependency needs but does not collude with them. The conductor's aim is to 'wean' them – that is, to work through these needs. Interpretations should come from the group itself; the group is the instrument to be used whenever possible.

The conductor's activity must be discriminating, encouraging the liberation of the group from passivity and dependency. If patients are brought into a situation they are continually helping to create and to shape, they become more aware of their own reactions and contradictions. They meet themselves in the situation they have helped to create and for which they now have to accept some responsibility. The less structured the therapeutic situation, the more the patients must extend themselves and become engaged to cope with it.

The group-analytic situation

The group-analytic situation can usefully be considered in the following manner:

1 Structure. Patterns of relationships that are relatively stable and continuously arise out of the interactions of the members of the group. These patterns of relationships take shape as habitual roles taken up by the individuals, as configurations between several members of the group. Alliances, subgroups and divisions are examples of these. (Psychic structuring represents processes with a slow rate of change [Rapaport 1960].)
2 Process. There are processes with a more rapid rate of change representing the dynamic component of the group, which is in constant flux, and this manifests as the interaction of all the elements of the situation, including the reciprocal relationships, the communications, verbal and nonverbal.
3 Content. It is through the analysis of this manifest content, transmitted through structure and process, that latent content emerges, which is necessarily determined by the structure and process already described. The group analyst pays as much attention to structure and process as to content.

The patterns of relationship that are relatively stable and continuous – that is, the structure of a group – can be altered by planned and deliberate interventions, as by Moreno's use of the sociogram, which shows the participants the nature of their relationships. By contrast, the group-analytic method facilitates the gradual evolution of awareness as the ongoing patterning of relationships becomes evident for the members themselves.

Individuals in the group will inevitably participate against the background of the total network of communications that has evolved in the group. This total network of communications is what Foulkes called the group matrix (Abraham 1973a; 1973b; 1973c). The matrix is a slowly developing, specific group phenomenon in which the meaning of individual neurotic responses can be mapped out against the group context. This brings in the dimensional aspect of foreground and background, a phenomenon that Foulkes emphasised from the perspective of Gestalt psychology. The individual's contributions and participations stand out against the background of the group as a whole and represent his or her unique style of participation.

Thus, in group-specific terms, individual and group resistance manifest as attempts to break the mandatory framework of the group-analytic situation – for instance, by late-coming, absenteeism, irregular attendance, socializing outside the group and so on. Transference resistance in the group situation by virtue of its repetitiveness and exclusiveness tends to block group processes and thus becomes an issue for the group as a whole.

Therapeutic factors

Many factors are similar to those of psychoanalysis and psychodynamic psychotherapy: greater consciousness of what were previously unconscious forces, catharsis, working-through, insight and analysis of defence mechanisms. Besides these, there are therapeutic factors that are group specific, arising out of the group situation in itself with all its social factors and forces.

Therapeutic factors in the group-analytic situation can be differentiated from group-specific factors. Therapeutic factors are as follows:

SOCIALISATION: Through the process of sharing, through the experience of group acceptance and belonging, the patient is brought out of his or her isolation into a social situation in which he or she can feel adequate. 'He is a fellow being on equal terms with the others' (Foulkes 1964: 33–34).

MIRROR PHENOMENA: The patient can see aspects of himself or herself reflected in the image, behaviour and problems of the other members of the group. Through this, he or she is enabled to confront various aspects of his or her social, psychological and body image through identification with and projection onto the other members of the group.

CONDENSER PHENOMENA: Even deep unconscious material is expressed more readily and fully in the group through the loosening and stimulating effects that the persons have on one another. Symbolic meanings of dreams or symptoms that manifest themselves through such formations as phobias can be more readily understood and worked with collectively, through the pooling of associations in the group. It is as if what the group members hold in common through their dreams and symptoms can suddenly be understood, the symbol having acted as a 'condenser'.

EXCHANGE: The members of the group often have a lively exchange of information with each other that leads to understanding both of self and of the meaning of emotional interactions and problems; this also can lead to chain phenomena and resonance. Each member of the group will reverberate to a group event according to his or her currently displayed level of development. Thus, for example, if a theme evolves in a group that has to do with violence, one can see how some members withdraw defensively, others display a marked interest in the behaviour of the other persons – that is, sharing the use of projection – while others can be self-revelatory about their own fantasies. Group themes around issues such as parting, loss, grief, mourning and so forth are rich sources of information as to the prevailing fixation and developmental level of group members and of the group as a whole.

GROUP AS SUPPORT: In any therapeutic situation there will always be a balance between the integrative and analytic forces at work. Analysis and interpretation inevitably arouse anxiety and can lead to further defensive activity on the part of the individual. The individual's awareness that he or she is not alone in his or her attempt to resist, as well as to uncover his or her inner world, both gives him or her support and lessens some of the inevitable narcissistic mortification that arises through the acceptance of interpretation. The group members will support each other through painful periods and actively help each other towards the integration of their conflicts. Often one sees patients accepting interpretations and comments from other members of the group that they would resist accepting from a therapist. This is because the person giving the interpretation or confrontation will often offer himself or herself as a person to be identified with, as if saying 'I know from my own experiences, I say this as one who has the same experiences as yourself and this is how and why I understand you so well'.

COMMUNICATION: 'Working towards an ever-more articulate form of communication is identical to the therapeutic process itself' (Foulkes 1948: 169). The therapeutic process 'from symptom to conflict' is synonymous with a growing capacity for communication. The therapist's role is to facilitate the processes of communication in the group; the process of *analysing* takes precedence over that of *interpretation*.

> The conductor strives to broaden and deepen the expressive range of all members, while at the same time increasing their understanding of the deeper, unconscious levels. The zone of communication must include the experience of every member in such a way that it can be shared and understood by the others, on whatever level it is first conveyed.
>
> (Foulkes 1964: 112)

'Neurotic and psychotic disturbances are always linked with blockage of the system of communication, socialisation, of the patient and the aim of analysis is precisely to translate the autistic symptom into a problem which can be verbalized' (Foulkes 1964: 112). Each patient benefits through working towards a freer expression of conflicts within the group situation, both his or her own and those of his or her peers. 'The language of the symptom, although already a form of communication, is autistic. It mumbles to itself secretly, hoping to be overheard; its equivalent meaning conveyed in words is social' (Foulkes and Anthony 1965: 259–260). 'The group has to go downwards and to deepen its understanding of the lower levels of the mind by broadening and deepening its vocabulary until every group member also understands these levels' (Foulkes and Anthony 1957/1965: 263).

Selection of group members

The group-analytic situation can accommodate a wide range of persons and problems, provided that they can meet the minimal requirements of the analytic approach. The prospective group member will be required to reflect on and react to the interpretive interventions made by the conductor and the manifold communications emanating from the group members. The person under consideration must possess a minimal ability to tolerate confrontation, the forced interaction of a relatively closed environment, and the frustration of slow, gradual and oscillating change. There must be a willingness and ability to enter into the treatment contract – that is, to attend regularly: once- or twice-weekly sessions over a two- to three-year period – and to keep the 'rules' of the group (see below).

In the selection interview, the therapist will attach less significance to traditional psychiatric categories, such as psychosis, neurosis or personality disorders, and pay more attention to the ability to communicate in a group and the capacity to develop insight and motivation for change (Foulkes 1964). However, sometimes even the apparently unmotivated patient who nevertheless stays in the group may derive considerable benefit from it.

Contraindications

Patients with severe character disorders whose symptoms are ego-syntonic would not only fail to benefit from group-analytic psychotherapy but might well be destructive to the group itself. Certain socially very isolated individuals, without the necessary supportive network outside the group to sustain them in the intervals between group sessions, do not do well in group analysis. Other patients who are doubtful candidates are those with grossly unrealistic expectations of the group, its conductor and therapeutic processes. They may perceive the group as powerfully destructive or as magically healing. Patients with overwhelming attachment needs, such as drug addicts or alcoholics, would be excluded from typical heterogenous group-analytic therapy group, but they might do well in a homogenous group, often within a hospital or ambulant clinical setting (Arroyave and Pangbourne 1976). Generally speaking, the earlier and deeper the psychogenic trauma, and the more disorganised the personality, the more cautious will the group conductor be when considering such a patient's inclusion. Some group-analytic therapists consider that severe early deprivations such as spatialisation, maternal depression, institutional upbringing and so forth warrant prolonged individual preparation or a combination of individual and group therapy. For such patients, the group is yet another depriving experience (Wolff and Solomon 1973).

The therapist is, of course, a member of the group, albeit one with a special position and a central function. His or her own emotional reaction to a prospective group member is therefore of some importance. A candidate who evokes feelings of strong dislike or disagreement in the therapist that persist after careful self-scrutiny might well do better in another therapist's group. A patient who has reached a severe block to progress in one therapist's group may well benefit by transfer to the group of another therapist.

Selection for group analysis is selection for a particular group. Each group will vary in its characteristics and as to the problems that they are more ready or able to accommodate. A comprehensive group therapy program will therefore include several groups, each of which will over time acquire its own distinct character. For instance, one group will have acquired the capacity to work intensively, in depth and analytically and will therefore be relatively intolerant of the patient who is defensive and unaccustomed to psychotherapy or who is timid and needs much support. By contrast, another group will well understand such vulnerability and the need for slow and gradual exploration.

Composition

The notion of the optimal composition of the group-analytic therapy group is based on the Foulkesian concept that the therapeutic process is identical with an ever-widening and -increasing communication process. This is the benefit each person receives from working towards a free expression of his or her conflict in a group.

The group that best promotes such communication is one with the widest possible span between personality types, 'a mixed bag of diagnoses and disturbances' (Foulkes and Anthony 1957/1965: 66). In this atmosphere of lively diversity, the all-important cross-transferences, mirror reactions and other group-specific phenomena occur and manifest themselves freely and clearly. The limiting factor here is the conductor's and the group's ability to contain the tensions created in such a group, without endangering its cohesion and integrity. It can also be said that the more diverse the group in its composition, the more necessary does it become for one variable to be held in common, such as intelligence or educational background (Foulkes 1975).

In composing a group with optimal diversity, it becomes important to avoid isolation, for whatever reason, of any one of its members. For example, the inclusion of an elderly patient in a group with an age span of between twenty-five to forty-five years of age would not be indicated; similarly, a person who holds extreme religious or political convictions would likely be isolated in a group of people with broader-based views.

If the therapist works with the model of a closed group, the decisions as to composition will be accomplished at the group's formation. If, on the other hand, the model is the slow-open group, the important problem of the group's composition remains throughout its life. The aim is to hold the size fairly steady, to synchronise carefully both departures and arrivals of patients, and thus maintain the richness and diversity of the group's experience and the highest degree of flexibility. In such a group, there is a remarkable capacity to allow the emergence and expression of bizarre thinking and borderline and psychotic manifestations; these are received, held and eventually modified, thereby moving from the idiosyncratic to the 'common sense' of the group as a whole (Foulkes 1964).

The composition of specialised, more homogeneous groups follows similar principles. These include groups for adolescents, adoptive parents, psychotic patients, phobic patients, alcoholics and sexual deviants. These groups, although homogeneous in the diagnostic sense, allow for a wide latitude in such variables as personality attributes, modes of expression of conflict, and defensive organisation. Patients in this range with sufficient ego strength and initiative may well be better placed in a heterogeneous group, which may benefit from their inclusion. There is some evidence that the inclusion of one or two patients with borderline personality organisation in a group of neurotic patients has mutual benefit for both parties. The borderline patients activate strong responses in the neurotic patients and the neurotic patients help the borderline patients modulate the intensity of their affective swings and to strengthen their capacity for secondary processes (Pines 1975; 1978c).

Size

Most group analysts find that they work comfortably with six to eight patients in a group since both patient and therapist are able to encompass eight to nine persons within their visual field so the group can remain a face-to-face resource. While the group as a whole is seen to provide the therapeutic momentum, it is always the individual who is the object of the therapy. Too large a group militates against intimacy and the feeling of containment and reduces the impact of each individual contribution. Face-to-face contact also becomes more difficult in a larger group, and the constraints of time may not allow each member sufficient opportunity for self-presentation.

Too small a group, a group of, say, four or five participants, may lack the vital function of representing the social norm and emotional normalcy from which each individual in the group deviates. There may also be a sense of lack of group identity so that therapy in very small groups of three and four members can take on the quality of individual psychotherapy *in* the group (Gosling 1981).

Since an equal sex distribution is desirable, a group of eight participants with their conductor is the preferred size. Nevertheless, rigidity and uniformity of attitudes on the part of the conductor in his or her capacity as administrator are anti-therapeutic. The exact number of group members should at all times be considered in the light of the group's needs at a given stage of its development.

For the group members, the field of action in which the ever-increasing and -deepening communicative processes take place, the matrix, is well served by the size of a group of eight. Such a group offers a favourable environment in which to experience, partake of, and influence both intrapsychic and interpersonal phenomena. The group of eight facilitates what Foulkes (1964: 82) called 'ego training in action'.

From the conductor's point of view, a group of eight makes it possible for him or her to pay attention to the totality of the group and its communicative processes. At the same time, it allows the conductor to attend to the individual's contributions, both verbal and nonverbal, and to locate them in the context of the group communications.

Medium-sized groups composed of ten to fifteen people are widely used as experiential groups in training courses, workshops and seminars. Such groups are constituted mostly of professional therapists working in a wide range of settings. The manifest aim is a learning experience about group dynamics and self-awareness, and they do not aim to be therapy groups, although the therapeutic benefit is marked. Such groups are usually closed, although in courses running to several years, a slow-open pattern has been preserved.

These groups are marked by a tendency to cohere rapidly and to develop an awareness of group dynamic processes such as subgroup formation, pairing, scapegoating and idealisation of the group and/or the conductor. The here and now of the group life becomes the main preoccupation. Because of their therapeutic potential, there is now a growing interest in the formation of medium-sized groups as therapy groups (De Maré 1980).

Group setting

The group-analytic setting is the physical environment within which the group's therapeutic task takes place. The conductor as the 'dynamic administrator' supplies, creates and maintains the setting throughout the group's life. He or she guards the group boundaries and negotiates between it and the wider social environment. The setting provided will differ with the wider system within which the group functions: a hospital, therapeutic community, clinic or private practice. In every case the conductor should, if possible, provide a reasonably sized, quiet room free from outside interference, with an identical chair for each member arranged in a circle. The chair should be comfortable and allow for a full view of the occupants. A central table small enough not to obscure the view of the group members acts as the group's centre, while the circle of chairs represents the group boundaries. The table, or the group itself, may come to signify a transitional object (Kosseff 1975), supplied as it is by the conductor and invested with meaning by the group. Sometimes the group culture prescribes that the conductor's seat be fixed, and the patients group themselves in a more or less permanent order every time. In other groups the conductor and the group members choose different positions in the circle each session. In either case, the choice of neighbour and the proximity from the conductor are significant communications that are subject to translation from the nonverbal into the verbal, the unconscious into the conscious modality of experience. By keeping the setting as steady as possible, the significance of changes within it becomes available to the group members. In a hospital setting, the maintenance of the group room, its availability for the sessions on the appointed day and hour, are signs of the nature of the dynamic forces surrounding the group that can work towards its integrity or destruction. It is the task of the conductor as the administrator to guard the boundaries and negotiate between the group and its environment.

The room itself should be entirely free of interruption from extraneous sources for the duration of the session. It is surprising how often this is difficult to achieve, yet it is vital for the success of the therapy. Colleagues have to be worked with and their understanding and cooperation won. The wider network in which the therapy takes place is potentially both enriching and depleting of the therapeutic process. A closed group meeting regularly in an institutional setting generates its own institutional dynamics, and the conductor, both as administrator and in his or her role as guardian of the boundary, has to ensure that the wider network accepts the existence of the group. It is the conductor's responsibility to create the venue for the group, prepare it for the sessions and protect it from intrusions.

This meticulous concern for the physical setting is linked to the notion of the psychological boundary of the group. If the boundary is intact in a physical sense, this sets in motion a liberating process within the group that enables the individuals in the group to reach into themselves and through the group matrix towards others within the group, without the additional anxiety of having to look outwards in a vigilant manner. Members can attend fully to what is going on within the group (Chance 1980).

In groups of young adolescents, the group-analytic process is often facilitated by introducing paper and drawing or modelling materials. The way in which these materials are used provides additional opportunities for communication and gives to young people who have difficulty in verbalising the chance to involve themselves more actively in the group process.

Children's groups typically have play materials built into their structure. The circular table is divided into parts, each of which becomes the child's own territory. In this way the autistic play of a child can progress into shared play, providing something of the equivalent of the adult group communicative process.

The medium-sized (median) group setting

The medium-sized experiential group of between ten and fifteen participants is used in training courses, workshops and ongoing seminars for the training of group analysts. The members are drawn from professionals with a working background in and some experience of dynamic psychotherapy. The training takes place in discontinuous meetings over one or more years, and the groups can be closed or run on strictly group-analytic lines as open groups. In such a setting, the experiential group is the central part of the course, with theory and supervision given in medium-sized groups of up to twenty-five members. Although the participants do not primarily come for therapy, the experiential groups prove to be powerful therapeutic agents for psychotherapeutic and restructuring interventions. Such seminars and courses are being more widely used in the training of group analysts. The use of medium-sized experiential groups has proven to be the most important factor in the success of the training (Abercrombie 1963; 1969; Pines 1980; Rafaelsen and Linnemann 1980).

The large-group setting

The ward group as the unit of therapy is part of the practice of therapeutic community work, and meetings of sixty persons or more are increasingly being used as a form of therapy. In training courses at the Institute of Group Analysis, London, large groups of over one hundred persons have been convened and studied. The results of this work have been described in *The Large Group* (Kreeger 1975).

Foulkes (1948) wrote in his first book that group treatment is the resolve to take a *larger* part of the external world, and of a person's associations, into the field of direct observation. The recent development of the unstructured large group as an experimental and therapeutic medium is a natural extension of the increasing expertise in small-group psychotherapy. In this context, large groups comprise anywhere from 35 to 150 participants, seated in concentric circles, meeting together for 1½ hours at fixed intervals. There may be more than one group conductor present. The conductor's interventions in this setting are considerably more influential than in medium- and small-sized groups. At the same time, the conductor in the large group is more truly a participant member who will use interventions and self-disclosure to facilitate self-awareness and individuation processes on the part of the individual group members. In large groups the multiplicity of relationships makes reality-testing especially difficult. Projections and feelings of invasion of the self can abound and psychotic-like mechanisms can be released, sometimes with dramatic heightening of anxiety. The large group in its early phases can be experienced as a persecutory environment by the individual members, who can feel oppressed and endangered in their very existence and unable to voice their half-formed thoughts. This may lead to depressive states or to their counterpart, euphoric evasiveness. Members appear to be faced with opposite choices, such as total withdrawal versus engulfment by the group, security versus depression, submersion versus perilous exposure. It is remarkable, however, that some individuals may often find their voice for the first time in the large group and that social anxiety and phobic reactions may be considerably alleviated in this setting. The strength of this experience reveals some of the significant differences between small- and large-group processes. By contrast, some persons who have found it easy to voice their thoughts and to engage in the interpersonal processes of the small group find themselves lost in the large group.

Gradually the reciprocation between the small- and large-group processes enables the individual to come into contact with and to master anxieties and conflicts that would not be revealed in either of these two contexts in isolation. It is for this reason that these two situations, small and large groups, are juxtaposed in training situations – 'The negotiation of a way across the gap, the working through and the infiltration by the delicate filaments of communication between the interface of these two worlds constitutes, amongst many other factors, psycho-social therapy' (De Maré 1975: 158).

This presents both the hazard and the therapeutic potential of the large group. Such groups now form a regular part of therapeutic communities, psychiatric hospitals and group training programs. The large group represents a new thought system with great potential and wide application both in psychotherapy and in the community at large.

Frequency, length and duration of small-group sessions

Group-analytic sessions of ninety minutes are held once or twice a week, over a period of two to three years and often longer. Group analysis is therefore prolonged, thorough and demanding on the patient, the group and the group analyst since reliability and continuity are of its very essence. The aim is a deep and lasting change in both internal object constellations and the resulting external relationships and perception of the environment. It is by its nature slow and the investment in time and commitment is considerable. At the other end of the scale there is the danger of 'group addiction' – that is, interminable group analysis with resulting loss of independence, self-reliance and ego integrity. Foulkes likened the treatment to a spiral staircase with exits. Where termination takes place will depend on the individual's personal aims and expectations. This is one reason why the preferred pattern of groups is the *slow-open* one: individual members leave in their own time and the group as such continues, often over a very long time. It can develop a long and detailed history that is part of the group's culture, and this enters the matrix and thus the individual's internal group life. The *closed group* is one in which people start and finish together. Intense work can be done in such a group, which can achieve an idiosyncratic group culture and strong interpersonal relations. It is left to the conductor and to external circumstances whether the slow-open or the closed group is the preferred medium of therapy. The open group usually forms in hospitals with a rapid turnover of patients and in universities and other institutions (Bramley and Andry 1977), in which the comings and goings are determined by the nature of the institution rather than the therapeutic needs of the individual. However, it is a group pattern that attracts interest and invites experimentation exactly because of its community-oriented structure. Clinical experience and research are needed to validate the open group's therapeutic potential.

The functions of the therapist in the small group

Two distinct functions pertain: (1) *Dynamic Administration*: see section on 'Group setting' above. (2) *Therapeutic Activity*: we distinguish between leadership, analysis and interpretation. As a *leader* the therapist is not primarily concerned with the formation of a 'good, efficient' group. The therapist is not out to create a team, to encourage good morale, friendship or bonhomie. As a leader, he or she puts the group as a whole into the centre of his or her attention; the leader tries to let the group speak, to bring out agreements and disagreements, repressed tendencies and resistances against them. The leader activates and mobilises that which is latent in the group and helps in the analysis and interpretation of process and content and of interpersonal relationships. The leader encourages the active participation of the group members and uses their contributions in preference to his or her own. Inevitably, the leader has a powerful effect on the evolving culture of the group. He or she emphasises the 'here and now' aspects of the situation and stands for an attitude of tolerance and appreciation of individual differences. The leader helps the members of the group become active participants in the process of group maturation through which individual change takes place.

The group will always look first to the therapist as to an omniscient and omnipotent figure from whom they expect magical help. In that sense, the group may experience the therapist as a father figure or, when in a regressed state, as the primordial mother. Foulkes did not go far in the discussion of the symbolism of differences between the therapist as the father and the group as the mother (the writings of Schindler 1951; 1966 and Slater 1966 explore these subjects). He paid much attention to the process of maturation that occurs as the group is gradually weaned from its dependence on the therapist as leader. As Foulkes put it, one cannot be weaned from something that has not previously been there or was never established. To begin with, therapists should accept the 'exalted' position into which the group puts them, not because it gratifies their own wishes for power but because from this position they can lead the group into a process of analysis, insight and more appropriate adult behaviour. Leaders first accept the positions the group chooses to confer on them, realizing that this gives the group security. It is a position they accept in order eventually to relinquish, to change from being a leader of the group to being a leader in the group. Eventually, the group replaces the leader's authority by that of the group itself. Thus, there is a modification of the individual superegos. The power of the leader is based on projections of the superego components of each person's personality. Gradually, as the group weans itself from dependence on the leader who uses their power in a benevolent and releasing way, leadership becomes an ego-based activity rather than a superego one.

Interpretation is one of several interventions available to the group conductor. The therapist attempts to foster the group's abilities to understand and to interpret their own situations, reactions and behaviour and to develop the self-analytic functions of the group. The conductor waits – in the matter of interpretation – until they have evidence that the group is not able on their own to understand the dynamic processes and unconscious meanings of the events of the session. If the conductor waits sufficiently long, they will more often than not find that the group can themselves evolve or resolve the dynamic issues of the session. Often what the therapist says is to elucidate what has not yet been said by any one member of the group. This rather humble activity that often does not rank as 'interpretation' may be a crucial element of therapy. The therapist's actions may be subsumed under the heading of 'activity', which may include reflection on group events; bringing events from the background into the foreground; linking communications; clarifications; confrontations with individuals; drawing the group's attention to events that are being ignored, such as the silence or withdrawal of a previously active member; pointing out the configurations that are developing within the group, of which subgrouping, pairing or scapegoating are examples. Often the therapist will feel that their most appropriate role is to remain silent, thereby becoming the projective and containing element of the group situation.

The dictum to which Foulkes worked is that *interpretation is used when analysis fails.* Complementing this activity, the therapist may interpret his or her understanding of the unconscious processes to the group as a whole or to individuals within the group. Communication may become more sensitive and deeper as the group matrix develops and the process of therapeutic change is therefore, in a sense, silent and not solely based on interpretations. What may be fundamental for the individuals in the group is the way in which their relationships to each other alter and develop over time. The members of the group are often extremely sensitive to this and develop keen awareness and insight into these often very subtle developments. Frequently in a group, patients will comment that they are now able to say things to each other that they would not have been able to say previously. The alteration in these role relationships and interpersonal relationships provides the 'moveable context' of the group-analytic situation that De Maré (1972) has contrasted to the 'unchanging context' of the psychoanalytic situation. In psychoanalysis the relationship aspects are kept constant so that transference will appear against the unchanging context. In the group-analytic situation transference relationships are explored and analysed to free the individuals from the transference-bound repetition and thus enable them to develop sensitive, less distorted and more mature forms of relationship. Thus, a good deal of the therapeutic processes that have been called 'ego training in action' represents the silent working through in the new situation of previously pathological and unresolved conflicts.

The conductor allows the interpretation to come to him or her from the contributions of the patients. Basically, the therapist's interpretative activities can be differentiated into the following three types: (1) interpretation that enables unconscious processes to become more conscious, (2) interpretation of resistance and defence, and (3) interpretation of transference reactions.

The group members' interpretative contributions as co-therapists to one another are essential components of the therapeutic processes although, if and when this interpretative culture becomes a manifestation of resistance, it has to be dealt with as such. The culture slowly evolves, partly based on identification with the conductor, but as Foulkes emphasised from the start, group members' reactions to one another often represent unconscious interpretations that need to be made conscious.

The group analyst is free to make interpretation to individuals as well as to the group as a whole, as interpretations are always significant for the group as a whole as well as for the individual. Thus, they can be addressed to any particular individual, they can refer to any configuration of relationships within the group or between the group and the conductor, they can be concerned with the 'here and now' or can range over the whole history of the group. They should preferably be based on the available experience of the moment and on the level at which the emotion is most active.

The conductor directs his or her interpretation towards the following:

1. Ongoing group interactive processes, such as group regressions, fantasies, subgroupings, pairing, mirroring, and so forth
2. Repetitive conflict situations
3. An understanding of the past experiences that spring to the mind of the patient in their association to the group situation
4. Current experiences in the life of the patient both within and without the group
5. 'Boundary incidents', events taking place at the interface between the ongoing group and the outside life of the individuals comprising it

There are no essential distinctions between processes inside the group and those going on outside, for inside and outside are false dichotomies. Boundary incidents therefore can involve the relationship of a patient to any member of his or her own social group and even to his or her body, as manifested in illness, psychosomatic or otherwise.

Transference

In group-analytic theory and practice, therapists do not confine their activities to interpretations, nor are their interpretations always direct to transference or particularly towards themselves as the central figures of the group. To do this would be to maintain the therapist in the role of the central figure, as a projection of superego fantasies on the part of the individuals. The therapist in the group is in a face-to-face situation. He or she is part of the group as well as 'outside' the group and is far more visible to the group members than the unseen analyst in the psychoanalytic situation. By virtue of this situation, *who* he or she is, his or her personality and his or her responses to the group situation will affect the group processes (Foulkes 1964). *What* he or she is is intrinsically part of what he or she does. The mutative changes are therefore not confined to the effects of transference interpretations; the mutative experiences may arise out of confrontations between members of the group or between the group as a whole and the therapist, and not solely from interpretative activities. Foulkes therefore opposed the argument that only transference interpretations are mutative, and because he did not draw a rigid distinction between events occurring within the group situation itself and those occurring outside, he felt free to pay attention to these 'external' events. For him the equation for therapy was T = (t + X), where T stands for the total therapeutic situation, t for the transference and X for the current interpersonal and life situation of the patient outside the group. In Foulkes's (1975) view, a situation had developed within psychoanalysis where the transference can swallow up the neurosis. By this he meant that the transference process, which should be the main vehicle of liberation for the individual from his or her neurotic conflicts, can become so powerful and so resistant to change that it largely replaces the illness and does not give way to a healthy resolution (Cortesão 1974; Leal 1968). This could arise from a faulty technique, that of exclusive attention to the transference, that could have the effect of infantilizing the patient and maintaining him or her in a dependent, neurotically gratifying position and one which also gratifies the therapist's unconscious countertransference. It was in response to this faulty development that Foulkes developed his therapeutic equation.

Ground rules

There are a few basic rules to which the prospective group analysand is expected to adhere. Members are expected to attend every session, to arrive on time and to stay for the entire session unless unavoidable circumstances arise that prevent this. Individuals are expected to inform the group of their intended absence in advance, or in the case of unexpected absence, they should let the conductor know. The conductor prepares the individual at the outset for the possibility of departure from the group, by imposing the expectation that he or she should give advance notice of his or her intention to leave the group at least a month before he or she plans to do so. This allows for a period of working through the termination of therapy and pre-empts a disruptive departure that may have repercussions on both the group and the departing member.

Group analysis carries with it an implicit expectation that significant events and experiences in the individual's life situation should be honestly disclosed to the group. No subject, topic or theme is proscribed and all expressions of feeling are invited. Events that the individual feels to be important should be shared with the group in a time and manner determined by the individual's own level of comfort and spontaneity. The rule of honest disclosure fosters a respect both for the individual and the group. By virtue of regular, full and sustained participation in the group, members gradually introduce into the group all facets of their personalities and, in this way, they develop a pool of material that contributes to the formation of the group matrix.

The translation of early primitive modes of expression into interpersonal terms by talk that makes change possible, allows the corrective emotional experience of the group. For this reason, group members remain seated throughout the session. They are expected to communicate through talk and minimal activity. They do not touch one another as a rule, except for an occasional neighbourly gesture of comfort or consolation in moments of distress. Abstinence from physical contact provides the momentum to overcome emotional blocks verbally, or to remain with the feelings that have been mobilised in this way until an understanding of their meaning can be reached.

For similar reasons, anxiety-reducing activities like smoking, drinking or eating during sessions are not accepted as a constructive part of the group culture. While there may be no blanket prohibition on these activities at the outset, when they do occur, the conductor intervenes to create a group climate that will lead the group towards an explanation of the defensive significance of these activities, both for the individuals engaging in them and for the group as a whole.

Members are asked not to socialise with one another outside the group. When this does happen, people are generally encouraged, through the open atmosphere of the group, to examine the significance of such extra-group contact by telling of it in the group and reflecting on its meaning. Strict confidentiality and respect for the privacy of disclosed material is asked of all the members, as it is only in an atmosphere of mutual trust that therapy can take place.

Generally, it is the conductor who decides on matters pertaining to the composition of the group, such as the introduction of a new member. However, the conductor is careful to prepare the ground by mentioning in the group any proposed changes in the structure of the group. He or she does this in advance and listens carefully to the response from the group at both the manifest and latent levels; he or she regards the feelings generated by these changes as important material for therapeutic work in the group.

A decision to leave the group is taken by the individual member, but again the conductor and the group play an active part in helping the individual towards this decision, by examining the significance for the individual and the group of his or her departure. The breaking of ground rules is in itself an important communication, albeit on a primitive level, that will be offered for the process of translation in the group.

Limitations of group therapy

Group-analytic psychotherapy takes place in an artificially-created, highly specific environment. It is an uncovering, intense and prolonged process that requires some ability, both practical and intrapsychic, to sustain the stresses and demands created. It requires stability of abode and a minimal degree of economic and social continuity and support to enable the patient to maintain the therapeutic contract. If the problems that bring the patient into therapy are too pressing or too acute, the thoroughness and inevitable slowness of group analysis may be unacceptable or inappropriate; a symptomatically oriented treatment regimen accompanied by support and environmental interventions may be preferable.

The group-analytic therapy group is essentially a verbal communication network. Gestures and body language have an important place, but the aim is to translate these and other primitive communications, such as acting-in and acting-out, into verbal communication – that is, language. The limitations of the process are clear: it requires the mental ability to use words and language – that is, to conceptualise. This ability might be insufficient, as with mentally defective patients, those with a low intelligence, those with organic brain impairment or those with certain psychoses that result in speechless withdrawal. An extreme example would be autistic children who, though they may be physically in one room together, cannot form a group. However, the conductor must at all times be in touch with the meaning of an apparently noncommunicating patient. In an adolescent group one youngster, who was known to the conductor to be of high intelligence, sat mute in the group for one whole year, resisting all efforts by others to draw him into conversation. At the end of the year, he declared his intention to leave the group. The group reacted with shock and set about dissuading him from leaving, pointing out the importance he had for the group and the love they felt for him. The group heralded new vigour and self-confidence in the group and elicited verbal participation in the young man.

Group analysis requires highly trained group analysts. The careful selection, the duration of the postgraduate training of three to four years and the training requirements (a personal group analysis, theory seminars and supervision) will inevitably produce a limited number of group analysts. There is thus at all times a limited number of trained group analysts – a scarcity in relation to the effective as well as the potential demand for such therapists. The economic relationship of scarcity and supply does, and will for some time to come, make group analysis a relatively expensive mode of psychotherapy, either for the individual patient or for the community who, in a public health service, pay for such treatment. This is a limiting factor of some significance that could be overcome only by a radical change of view in individual and community mental health (Behr and Hearst 1977; Renier 1976; Sharpe 1977).

Research

Group analysis presents a consistent and coherent conceptual framework for personality development and for a congruent method of psychotherapy for disturbances of personality.

CONCEPTUAL FRAMEWORK. The outline has been presented already. The validity of this model is strengthened by current investigations into personality development, principally in early childhood, which increasingly emphasises the interactional nature of in infant-parent relationships and their profound effects on the emergent personality of the child. This applies both to normal and to abnormal development. This area has been reviewed by Robert Emde (1980; 1981) from the psychoanalytic field, and it is clear that with the current emphasis upon interaction, communication and context, there is growing support for the basic group-analytic model.

THE THEORY OF THERAPY. Current psychoanalytic theory recognises that the psychotherapeutic situation itself silently replicates the earliest transactions of the parent-child relationship, the primary matrix and psychological force field from which personality formation grows and differentiates. It is increasingly recognised that the process through which structural changes in personality can be brought about is this repetition of the early situation in a new context, that of psychotherapy. The group-analytic situation shares with psychoanalysis many of the fundamental characteristics of the primary matrix, although there are many distinct aspects of the group as opposed to the dyadic situation. The common features are (a) a relatively unstructured situation that exists within clearly defined boundaries of time, space and authority, (b) a relatively neutral therapist whose viewpoint includes the total therapeutic situation including his or her own role, (c) encouragement of free group discussion/association, (d) translation of unconscious processes and contents, (e) acceptance, recognition and working through of transference and countertransference, and (f) an appreciation of the developmental function of psychotherapy and the need for time in which developmental processes can evolve.

Research on specific mechanisms of the group-analytic situation

Group-analytic theory has emphasised the significance and importance of such concepts as the 'matrix', which relates to the developmental aspects of group-analytic psychotherapy, and of 'mirroring', which applies to a specific therapeutic mechanism.

MATRIX: Abraham and her co-workers (1973a, 1973b, 1973c) developed a special technique that brings out the unconscious meaning of subjects' self-reports. They demonstrated that the existence of aggressive phenomena related to the group matrix could be experimentally demonstrated. They attempted to investigate Foulkes's definition of the matrix as the unconscious operational basis, the common shared ground that includes verbal and nonverbal communication, and attempted to demonstrate how it can be seen more objectively.

MIRRORING: These processes are being given much attention today, both theoretically and empirically in dyadic and group-analytic psychotherapy. They have become particularly prominent since Kohut drew attention to the 'mirror transferences' that regularly appear in the psychoanalysis of a narcissistic personality disorder. He also emphasised the great significance of empathic mirroring responses by the mother in laying down the healthy narcissistic substrate of the normal personality. Other writers who have demonstrated the importance of mirroring processes in personality have included Lacan (1977), Winnicott (1967/1971), Lichtenstein (1977) and Mahler (1968; Mahler et al. 1975). Empirical research has been described by Lewis and Brooks-Gunn (1979) and by Abelin (1980).

EVALUATION: The evaluation of group-analytic psychotherapy through rigorous research is an important yet still elusive task. The theory of group analysis embodies concepts derived from such diverse disciplines as Gestalt psychology, psychoanalysis and sociology. Yet, because these concepts are distinctive and new in themselves, they require further definition and refinement and must be tested against clinical practice of group analysis. All research procedures alter the field of practice, particularly when single aspects are isolated and examined apart from the whole. The part cannot be viewed out of context of the whole, nor can it be described or treated in such a way without imposing some injury on the validity of the investigative process. This general problem for research in psychodynamic psychotherapy has yet to be overcome.

Notwithstanding, research into group analysis is advancing along two fronts. The first of these, designated as informal research, is taking place through the writing and presentation of group-analytic approaches; the material accumulated in this fashion contributes to a pool of information out of which the original group-analytic concepts are further refined and new concepts begin to emerge. This work is regularly reported in the journal *Group Analysis*. A more formal and systematic approach is needed where the established procedures of empirical research are employed. A notable pioneering work is that of Dick (1975/1983), whose ten-year study of outpatient analytic group therapy showed a high rate of positive change. This is in marked contrast to Malan's (Malan et al. 1976) rigorous follow-up of groups conducted on the 'Tavistock model', where the results proved to be much less satisfactory. The lesson from this seems to be that the group-as-a-whole techniques, where they are applied formalistically and without much regard to the individuality of the patients, do not prove therapeutically effective. Group-analytic psychotherapy, although a therapy conducted in and by the group, consistently puts the individual into the foreground.

As yet, there is little to report other than the Dick and Malan studies. The research facilities in the United Kingdom have not yet applied themselves to a systematic study of group-analytic psychotherapy which takes account of the training and experience of the therapist and the detail of dynamics both of the experience of the therapy groups, and of the settings in which the work is carried out.

Ethical considerations

The viewpoint that is the basis of Foulkesian group analysis is that human nature is essentially social, not individual. Foulkes put it that our social nature is an irreducible basic fact. The group itself becomes a token representation of the surrounding community and its culture which is called into the consulting room, where it comes into active cooperation within the treatment situation (Foulkes 1964). This face-to-face stranger group actively participates in its own treatment. Personal revelations, intimate feelings, fantasies and thoughts, irrational behaviour patterns and relationships outside the group with spouses, lovers, parents and children all become the common property of the analytic group. This requires a trust in the group members' discretion and ethical behaviour of a high degree, and in practice this trust is hardly ever misplaced: the group culture is such that this common group property remains within the group. Yet, the only group member whose training and professional attitude ensures absolute secrecy and discretion is the group conductor. Thus, by taking a larger part of the external world and of the person's associations into a field of direct observation, as Foulkes stated, and combining this field of vision with that of the personal, intrapsychic one, the individual is exposed to the community. 'Common sense', the sense of the community, is applied to the individual's internal psychic life. On the face of it, this raises the existential question of being required to share information with others, which is essentially individual and personal and at times hidden from one's own awareness, and having it scrutinised by them in the light of shared communal experience. This demand can be justified only if humans, social beings, are conceived of as situated in a network of relationships so that intrapsychic change is synonymous with change in relationships: so expression takes the place of repression. The individual in the group sets forth to transform symptoms that are unsuitable for sharing into socially acceptable, articulate language. In this way a common area is created within which each member of the group develops his or her unique personality and becomes an individual in his or her group. This common area in which everyone has a stake is the only, and at the same time the safest, assurance that the most basic group law, that of absolute trust and confidentiality, is kept.

Since the group represents the wider community from which it was formed, one could conceive of a community that is immoral, depraved, unethical or psychotic in structure. We are nowadays only too familiar with this possibility and cannot discount a situation in which one would be practicing group analysis within such a community. The basic assumptions and the philosophy of such a society would run counter to those of group-analytic psychotherapy, indeed to all psychoanalytic therapies. The tension between the individual's self-centred needs and impulses and the needs and impulses of those surrounding him or her requires resolution if the personality is to survive intact. The group member has to engage in the processes of identification and empathy with his or her peer members in order to find a solution for his or her own needs, which their needs curtail. In a society where such empathy is reserved for one section only, group-analytic therapy as described here is inconceivable (Garland 1980). The taking back of the projections and projective identifications that create the society's divisiveness in the first place would be made impossible; the deepening and widening of communications and relationships, the essence of group treatment, would be distorted and undermined. It can be said, therefore, that group analysis in the true sense can exist only in a democratic society, based on the recognition of the intrinsic value of every one of its members, irrespective of colour, sex, social status or intelligence levels. Sanity and wholeness, empathy and understanding, psychic responsibility – the achievement of these depend on such values being upheld, however imperfectly and gropingly, by the society within which the therapy group functions.

Summary[2]

Group-analytic treatment takes place in a face-to-face stranger group of eight or so members who meet regularly with their conductor for the purpose of psychotherapeutic treatment, usually once or twice a week. Placed in such a group, the individual re-establishes his or her typical conflicts and behaviour patterns, endowing the conductor, the group members and the group as such with properties of seminal persons in his or her past and present life. He or she 'uses them' as personifications of his or her inner object constellations – that is, as transference objects. In the analytic group, the individual is conceived of as a nodal point in an interrelated network, influencing and influenced by the transpersonal processes that form the dynamic field, the matrix.

Individual disturbances are seen as disturbances in communication, originally in the network of the primary group, the family. The analytic group creates a framework and a unit of observation within which the individual's disturbed communications can emerge and be taken into the field of observation. The therapeutic process within this framework is identical with the ever-widening and -deepening process of communication.

The analytic group has its group-specific dynamics, which are distinct from the sum of the individuals that form the group. Thus, we speak of a 'group as a whole'. Within this group, all mechanisms known from psychoanalysis are present and are translated into group-dynamic terms. For example, displacement can be expressed in the attack on a group member instead of the conductor, splitting in subgrouping, polarisation and so on. The group itself symbolises the 'internal objects' of its members including part-objects, transference objects and other whole persons and can be perceived at various levels of the conscious, the preconscious and the unconscious. The group-specific dimension is expressed in concepts such as mirror reactions, resonance, location and polarisation.

Group analysis takes place in the group-analytic setting that includes the selection of group members, the time, place and frequency of meetings, the 'rules' and attitudes of the members and the analytic attitude of the conductor which make up this situation. Implicit in this is the manner in which the conductor deals with members' contributions, the relationship between the conductor and the group as a whole. The members' free and unguided contributions become the group associations, the dynamic equivalent of free association in the psychoanalytic dyad. The patients' relations one with the other are treated as transference relations, and here we distinguish between true transference – that is, repetition – and transference expressed as responses, impressions and experiences in the group. Both are accepted as communications and subjected to translation from the purely individual, autistic level, to a communicable level of exchange. This proceeds by clarification, explanation, confrontation and interpretation – processes which are by no means undertaken by the conductor only but in which every member of the group participates.

The group therapist is called the conductor to indicate his or her special position and function in the group which is ill-expressed in the word 'leader': the conductor leads the group only in specific states and situations. He or she sees his or her task as helping the group to realise its own therapeutic potential and to participate actively and responsibly in the resolution of its problems. We can consider the therapist-conductor in his or her three aspects: (1) what he or she is – his or her personality, professional training, receptivity of the group's communications and respect for the unique individuality of its members; (2) what he or she represents – the primary transference figure for the group members in its unconscious aspects, such as the superego, the ego ideal or the punitive primordial parent figure; (3) what he or she does – his or her reactions to the group's needs at various stages of development, at times actively, at others passively, always within the group context. He or she directs his or her attention to the individual member or the group as a whole in the knowledge that that which is relevant to one member concerns others albeit at times on other psychic levels; the individuals and the group's process are inextricably related.

The group-analytic group has been used in clinics, hospitals, therapeutic communities and in training courses in group psychotherapy. The small, slow-open group is adapted to meet specific needs and settings into closed and open groups. The special needs of patients such as psychotics, the severely deprived, addictive patients or special groups such as children and adolescents are treated in variants of the analytic group, and these are usually homogeneous and are sometimes offered as combined group and individual treatment.

The analytic group is an excellent training and observation forum in which the social aspects of the individual can be taken into the field of vision. The individual can thus be observed and treated in his or her true nature as a social being rather than in the abstraction of his or her individual isolation.

Notes

1 This is an edited version of a paper published as a chapter in *Group Psychotherapy: Changing Approaches*, edited by G. M. Gazda (1982), pp. 132–178. The two other authors of the chapter, Harold Behr and Liesel Hearst, have given their consent for its issue here. Harold Behr has provided written authorisation. The verbal authorisation from Liesel Hearst was extended with written authority by her daughter, Daniela Pountney, her literary executor, after her mother's death. Behr and Hearst's own book, *Group-Analytic Psychotherapy: A Meeting of Minds* (2005), owes much to the work they did with Pines in this originating publication. Grateful thanks are extended to the editor of the book in which this paper was published, Dr G. M. Gazda, for his permission to allow its publication here. (Ed.)

2 In its original form, this chapter contained clinical illustrations of a group at work at this point which illustrated many of the dynamics described, all of which has been removed. The book as a whole contains many passages that serve this purpose, and permissions could not be confidently secured for this chapter. (Ed.)

Section II

History and context

2 The historical matrix of group analysis

A perspective from the history of ideas[1]

In 1939, a German Jewish psychoanalyst who had left Germany in 1933 began to practice group analysis in the small English city of Exeter shortly after moving there. S. H. Foulkes was soon caught up in military psychiatry, where he had ample opportunity to put his ideas and experience into practice. He elaborated his theoretical ideas in his first book in 1948.

Thus, the practice of group analysis began in England, geographically far from Frankfurt and from Vienna, where Foulkes had trained and worked, and in relative professional isolation. This is often a necessary condition for original work; compare the example of Ronald Fairbairn (1949, 1994) who was contemporaneous in Edinburgh. But no man is an island, and Foulkes's work has to be set in the context of the European ideas of his intellectual and social inheritance. We must situate him in history, figure against ground which, as he himself insisted, was a basic component of group-analytic theory.

This is a review of some strands of the European nexus of ideas about 'mind, self and society', to borrow the felicitous title of a great American work by Mead (1934, 1964), who contributed significantly to philosophy, as did his contemporary John Dewey (1954) who also emphasised the inseparable connectedness of self and society. But this paper was prepared for a European occasion, and here I wish to give the European context of thought that I believe contributed to Foulkes's concept of the matrix.

In *Consciousness and Society*, Hughes (1979: 12) defines the aim of his classic text as 'detailed studies of the inter-relationship of thought in relatively brief periods of time'. I attempt to cover roughly the same time scale, focusing on Germany, France and Britain. I differ from Hughes in not being able to pay attention to Italy on this occasion and I do not focus on psychoanalysis itself. My focus here is on the intertwining of psychoanalysis and group analysis, one representing the dimension of individuality and the other that of plurality.

Nineteenth-century Germany psychology and philosophy have such a rich history that it is possible to touch on only a few significant figures and trends. German philosophers insisted that the study of the mind must be that of an understanding of the whole person, situated in a nexus of 'objective reality' – that is, in culture: culture as language, art, myth, religion, custom, law.

DOI: 10.4324/9781003494713-4

Wilhelm Wundt (1915), best known as the founder of experimental psychology, devoted his greater efforts and dedicated his mature years to the study of what he called 'folk psychology', a social psychology of cultural values showing how the mind is connected and reciprocally interrelated with others.

For the great historian and philosopher Wilhelm Dilthey (1914/1988), the individual is interpenetrated by sociohistorical reality – recall here Foulkes's words describing how the individual is penetrated through and through by the colossal forces of society, and his ideas of transpersonal processes (Foulkes 1964: 176; Foulkes and Anthony 1965: 142). Dilthey is best known for his delineation of the distinction between the human sciences and the natural sciences, the *Geisteswissenschaften* and the *Naturwissenschaften*; note the powerful word *Geist*, the soul, the spirit, that does not refer only to the mind. This German word conveys a world of ideas that does not translate easily into Anglo-Saxon or French vocabulary, dedicated as they are to empiricism and to logic. Debate about this word has intensified with a renewal of attention to James Strachey's use – or misuse – of it in the *Standard Edition* of Sigmund Freud's works.

Dilthey laid down the principles for historical understanding which appear to me also to be basic to the principles of group analysis. First, all human manifestations are part of an historical process and should be explained in these terms; second, different ages and differing individuals can only be understood by entering imaginatively into their specific point of view; and third, the historian is bound by the horizon of his or her own age. How the past presents itself and the perspective of present concerns become a legitimate aspect of the meaning of that past. This gives context to our own countertransference responses and frames our notion of empathy. The first point is represented in group analysis by Foulkes's insistence on understanding the historical development of our personalities, for which he drew on the work of Norbert Elias.

I cannot elaborate further here on Dilthey, whose work is beginning again to receive historians' attention after some decades of obscurity, except to say his work considerably influenced Max Weber, the seminal figure of modern sociology. Among historians I would select the Spaniard José Ortega y Gasset (1963), who perhaps has encapsulated Dilthey's and his own philosophy of history through the dictum, 'Who am I? I am myself, plus my circumstances.' How resonant for us indeed is that word 'circumstances', we who are advocates of and toilers in the circle!

Though we do not find the word 'matrix' itself in these writings, there is a sense of it and we do find such concepts as nexus, interpenetration of the individual by culture, the reciprocal interrelationship of people, the whole notion of networks, and of the individuals as nodal points interpenetrated by culture.

In a study of what he calls 'Supra-Individual Super-Consciousness', Müller-Freienfels (1935) refers to writings that begin with the psyche as an organic whole, connected with society and not with the concept of the single individual. Foulkes (Foulkes and Anthony 1957/1965/1983) referred to the social unconscious, that of which we are completely ignorant because we are born into it, which reminds me of how Balint (1959) would say that until removed from it, the fish is completely unconscious of the water it swims in, as is the human being of the air that they breathe, until the airways are threatened. These ideas played a prominent part in German thought, which has been overshadowed by the attention paid to the development of psychoanalysis. I have left aside the contributions of Jacob Moreno which antedate Foulkes, but Moreno (1932; 1934) was immersed in the same German intellectual culture.

Now to France, a country which we do not nowadays readily think of in connection with group therapy before the Second World War; yet we are wrong in this. Firstly, the psychology of the unconscious was born in France through the study of hypnosis, first by Franz Anton Mesmer, and then by Jean-Martin Charcot, Hippolyte Bernheim and Pierre Janet. Hysteria was the model illness that revealed the power of the unconscious. France is also the country of the French Revolution. Paris was the first modern city. It lived through the turmoil of the storming of the Bastille in 1789, then the uprising of 1848, then the Franco-Prussian War of 1870 followed by the bloody suppression of the Commune of 1871. French philosophers and psychologists beginning with Gustave Le Bon and Gabriel Tarde were the first to recognise and codify the immense forces of the masses, 'crowds and power', to borrow Elias Canetti's title (Canetti 1984; Burrows 1981).

Le Bon wrote: 'The substitution of the unconscious of crowds for the conscious activity of individuals is one of the principal characteristics of the present age' (quoted in Nye 1975; Widener 1979). Le Bon (1895/2019), who died in 1931 at ninety years of age, achieved great fame and influence from his book *The Crowd*. Freud (1921) took this as the basis for his book on group psychology, *Group Psychology and the Analysis of the Ego*, and Theodore Roosevelt kept it by his bedside. Both Hitler and Mussolini recognised the force of Le Bon's ideas, and that tower of French culture, General Charles de Gaulle, was brought up on these ideas as was his generation of French soldiers – Le Bon was in their military curriculum. A yet unwritten piece of group history is that Le Bon was consulted by the French military command in the First World War over issues of morale, thus predating the British and American experience of psychiatrists in the Second World War.

Le Bon likened the psychology of the crowd to that of the unconscious that liberates great passions. It can be used either destructively or creatively, producing heroism or bloodthirsty cruelty. The crowd seeks domination; it obeys the single-minded leader as the hypnotic subject does the hypnotist. Le Bon warned of the great forces that modern industrial society was accumulating as the age of the crowd replaced that of the individual. His distinction between the intellectual and affective selves was well ahead of its time, though not elaborated as a developmental psychology, other than to emphasise that the seeming unity of the self is an illusion, and that personality consists of the agglomeration of many part-selves. Tarde (1903), who was more academic than Le Bon, developed further ideas on imitation that are in many ways the equivalent of Freud's concept of identification, and he saw this as the basis of personal psychology.

French society had many powerful historical reasons for acknowledging and studying social psychology (Moscovici 1985). First was the French Revolution, which continued turbulence and instability of the French political system under pressure from the sense of a growing menace from rapid industrialisation and the growth of cities. In the Paris of Baron Georges-Eugène Haussmann, the boundaries between rich and poor were eroded as the city was rebuilt. This led eventually to a significant political movement called solidarism that dominated French politics in the 1890s and the first decade of the twentieth century (Zeldin 1979). Its major exponent was Léon Bourgeois, statesman, Nobel Peace Prize winner of 1920, and a founder of the League of Nations after the First World War. Under the influences of solidarism, France began to develop a sophisticated modern system of welfare and taxation (Hayward 1959). What was the background and what were the tenets of solidarism? The French Revolution had legislated for the maximum freedom of the *abstract* individual. This had led to the dominance of privileged groups: liberty, equality and fraternity had simply become slogans and, in reality, illusions. The dogmatic ruthlessness and pious optimism of nineteenth-century laissez-faire economics, influenced by a social Darwinism of the survival of the fittest, had led to social atheism. The prized notion of liberty could only be maintained by one in good health where the illusion of self-sufficiency could be maintained. But that liberty, which then seemed to be the supreme and unqualified good, disappeared in illness. Then the security that comes from solidarity with neighbours is infinitely more desirable than is impotent liberty in the hands of the isolated and ineffective individual. The political science of solidarity attempted to recognise and fill the psychological and social space between the individual and the state, for if both individual and state claim sovereignty, there is a neglect of the supreme fact of the social life.

This introduces the 'in-between' analogous to Donald Winnicott's (1951) transitional space between subject and object. Here in the space between the individual and their society is the space for culture and interconnectedness. As Samuel Butler (1903: 317) said, 'Extremes are alone logical, and they are always absurd, the mean is alone practicable and it is always illogical'. The logic of cognition, combined with the logic of affect, can produce a new form of logic. Bourgeois's solidarism opposed social Darwinism by maintaining that association, not competition, is the predominant characteristic of life, along similar lines to Pyotr Alexeyevich Kropotkin's (2008) *Mutual Aid*. Rights and duties were emphasised. The just man freely accepts both limitation on liberty and increased social duties, as they are the consequences of essential interdependence. We are born into society as 'debtors', dependent on others as we are again in old age. We are debtors through our essential dependency: 'From the very date of his birth man is a debtor, born a debtor of human association. He takes his share of the inheritance built up by his ancestors. At birth he begins to benefit from the immense accumulated human capital' (Hayward 1961: 29). Of course, in between we repay our debts by nurturing our own families and entering constructively into society, paying our way and accepting that social relationships consist of a plurality of reciprocal ties of solidarity (Hayward 1961).

I suggest that here, in French social thought, we can see the concept of a family matrix, a social network, a matrix of interrelationships, a recognition of the vital part that small groups play in human life, all set in the context of a civil society where this term was coined. For those who are inclined to such speculations, there is an opportunity to connect such ideas as Heinz Kohut's self-object theory that describes the babe who is born strong because the responses of others are a part of his or her own self; and Winnicott's (1957: 134–140) notion that there is no such thing as an infant alone. Perhaps these ideas find a reflection in Bourgeois's statements?

Finally, from France, in the early years of the twentieth century, there is a school of writers who call themselves 'unanimists' (McLaurin 1981). They were reaching out for a way of expressing the connectedness of the human psyche and held the view that a group is not only a collection of individuals but assumes its own psychological presence. Its principal figure was Jules Romains, a novelist who described how one day in Paris, surrounded by pedestrians, traffic, the life of the street, the life of the city, he could suddenly grasp all this through a sudden flash of super-consciousness. He tried to express the way in which the life of a village, the experiences of a group of companions, reflects the dynamic of connectedness – each person only has his or her full existence within the group setting. Romains had knowledge of Émile Durkheim's sociology, of current anthropology and of developments in social psychology, and tried to integrate this knowledge with his artistic intuitions. We remember here the 'oceanic feeling' that Romain Rolland communicated to Freud, and which Freud responded to reductively by seeing it as an aspect of narcissism (Abraham 1991).

In nineteenth-century Britain, individualism had swept all aside. In France, the Catholic Church had resisted the distortion of Darwinism that had led to unbridled individualism, but the Church of England was a weak barrier in comparison. However, British psychology, much influenced by the great and good William James, began to evolve a more sensitive appreciation of the dynamic nature of mind and of society. This led to such works as Graham Wallas's (1908/1921) *Human Nature in Politics*, in which he examined the irrational self-interest in voting behaviour. Nineteenth-century British reformers believed that once the people had the vote, they would use their political power to better their conditions, but in practice, the voters did not behave as enlightened, middle-class rationalists. Wallas saw that people responded to symbols rather than to social reality. He was a founder of the London School of Economics and had great influence. He wrote that the primary processes of thought are unconscious but that understanding will help us to 'see through' to reality. The capacity to 'see through' is a form of mistrust that leads to reality-testing. Compare this with Freud's (1927) statement in *Future of an Illusion* that the voice of the intellect is a soft one, but it does not rest until it has gained a hearing. Wallas's words are more penetrating and would no doubt have impressed Bion: 'We are born with a tendency under appropriate conditions to think, which is as original and independent as our tendency, under appropriate conditions, to run away' (Wallas 1908/1961: 39).

Sofer (1978) has differentiated between what she calls revolutionary and revisionist social scientists over this period in England. She uses 'revolutionary' in Thomas Kuhn's sense, that of radical, category change, whilst 'revisionists' are those who see no need or possibility for radical change. Sofer describes a movement of economists, philosophers, psychologists and social scientists who saw the need for major changes in British society but were opposed by those who basically felt that no change was possible and wanted to maintain the status quo. Among those seeking major change, the preeminent figure was Wilfred Trotter. He is an intriguing figure, a great neurosurgeon in his maturity and before that a fiery revolutionary and a boon companion and later brother-in-law of Ernest Jones. In his 1916 book, Trotter presented his pessimistic view that 'herd instincts' are basic to humanity and that the masses have to be governed by an elite that can channel these instincts to higher ends.

Trotter, like Le Bon, achieved much esteem, though we do not know if prime ministers kept his book at their bedsides. But his ideas of group mentality, the pervading social force of group psychology, did influence opinion formers for a decade or more. These included the Bloomsbury Group, that interconnected network of upper-middle-class, mainly ex-Cambridge intellectuals, such as Desmond McCarthy, who translated Romains's novel, and Leonard and Virginia Woolf. The Bloomsbury Group broke the Edwardian mould of social and psychological conformity and complacency. Leonard Woolf was a social reformer and politician and intellectually concerned with group forces. Virginia seems to show in her novels, for instance *The Waves*, the sense that individuals are so intermeshed that they are like the waves of the sea, inseparable from their watery matrix. She mentions Trotter in her diaries and, in November 1917, recorded a conversation with Roger Fry: 'Old Roger takes a gloomy view, not of our life, but of the world's future; but I think I detected the influence of Trotter and the herd and so I distrusted him. Still, stepping out into Charlotte Street . . . I found all this sordidity made me think him rather likely to be right' (McLaurin 1984: 37).

Virginia Woolf was present at Melanie Klein's first lectures, given in 1926 at the house of Adrian and Karen Stephen, Virginia's brother and sister-in-law who were psychoanalysts in training. During the 1920s and 1930s, a British 'new psychology' was developing (Rose 1985). This had bypassed the isolated group of British psychoanalysts who were dictated to by Ernest Jones and not allowed to mix with outsiders, and these new psychologists had begun to uncover family and group dynamics. The Tavistock Clinic, the Child Guidance Centre and the medical section of the British Psychological Society were centres of the exploration of group forces. Ian Suttie, who integrated sociology, psychology and anthropology and who influenced John Bowlby and Winnicott, published his influential book *The Origins of Love and Hate* in 1935. Rigid though the psychoanalysts were, they had begun to appreciate the complexity of the individual in a social setting through Klein's emphasis on early object relationships. It was in this context, far from Vienna and Berlin (that still adhered to instinct theory) and their individualistic focus, that Foulkes arrived. He gave a paper on introjection to the British Psychoanalytical Society, published in 1937, and tried tentatively to show his knowledge of classic psychoanalysis and the appreciation of the importance of early object relations. But not until he moved to Exeter, and there faced his own history and his own developing ideas, did he give utterance to these ideas and act on them. There, the matrix of group analysis was born:

> Each individual member is actively brought up against the first basic problem of social life; his relationship to other people and to the group as a whole. He has to solve this actively. The clash between his own egotistic needs and impulses and the restriction imposed by the group, as expressed in the formula 'the individual and the group' is replaced by the co-operative formula, 'the individual in the group'. . . . He is a participant in a double process dwelling in both camps of this conflict; he must tolerate the wishes and desires of others, if his own claims are to be tolerated, and he must restrict in himself, what he feels he cannot tolerate in others.
>
> (Foulkes 1964: 58–99)

Note

1 This paper was given as the keynote address at the Eighth European Symposium on Group Analysis, 'Mistrust in the Matrix: Conflict, Cooperation, Creativity in Groups and Institutions', Oxford, September 1990. Mistrust is the evolutionary basis of survival, for seeing through, for not being cannibalised or taken in. For me (MP), the title of the symposium acknowledged that beyond our local differences – the narcissism of petty differences, as Freud (1930) called them – it was a sign of the strength of our European network that we could meet and debate this most central issue and, despite our mistrust, establish our matrix with greater strength through our interconnectedness and reciprocity. (MP)

This is an edited form of the paper first published as *The Matrix of Group Analysis: An Historical Perspective* in *Group Analysis* 24 (2): 99–109, 1991. Acknowledgements are made to the editor of the journal for consent to its publication here. (Ed.)

3 The coherency of group analysis

Its emergence and surrounding, supporting network[1]

My aim in speaking with you on this privileged occasion is to present group analysis, originating from the work of S. H. Foulkes, as a comprehensive and coherent account of becoming, remaining and failing in that lifelong difficult task of being a relatively healthy human being. This is to live in reasonably good, tolerant relations to oneself, our inner society, and towards others, our external society. In group analysis, the social aspect is essential, for humans are social beings deeply permeated throughout their lives by society, which shapes and forms us. Group analysis originated from Foulkes's experiences as a neurologist, psychologist, psychoanalyst and social historian. Naturally, he was influenced by the networks of which he was part during his formative years. Let me describe some of these influences.

Michael Foulkes (as he later liked to be called but originally Siegmund Heinrich Fuchs) was born in Mannheim into a prosperous middle-class Jewish Rhineland family, one that had not experienced strong anti-Semitism and that had seemed well-accepted in their local community. He was the youngest son and presumably somewhat indulged, and he was athletic as well as studious. His was a sports-loving family; his elder brother captained the city football team and was a celebrated goal scorer in Germany's national football team for which he played in the Olympics. Foulkes served in World War One as a wireless operator on the western front and then underwent medical studies first at Heidelberg and next at Frankfurt University.

He was drawn to neurology and psychiatry and was profoundly influenced by two years of work in Frankfurt under the direction of Kurt Goldstein. This neurologist and psychiatrist had organised and directed the hospital for the treatment of brain-injured soldiers in the German army. Goldstein was an inspiring leader and was both a researcher and clinician. His major work is *The Organism* (Goldstein 1939/2000), which he wrote in the Netherlands where he took refuge from the Nazis after his arrest and deportation before emigrating to the United States. In this work he showed that the response of the brain-damaged patient to his injury is a consequence of the psychology of the patient together with the disturbance of the whole central nervous system in response to localised cerebral damage. Goldstein was influenced by Wertheimer and, like him, became a pioneer in Gestalt

DOI: 10.4324/9781003494713-5

psychology. He collaborated with Adhémar Gelb (Goldstein and Gelb 1918) in the development of subtle psychological tests that revealed the functional impairment of his patients, such as the loss of capacity for abstract thought. Foulkes absorbed from Goldstein the holistic Gestalt approach, which teaches that an entity is not to be understood as an assemblage of parts but has to be seen in its wholeness, in context, as an organism in constant adaptation to its environment. The evolutionary thrust of this approach, of functional adaptation, I shall return to later in considering human evolution in groups.

Foulkes met dynamic psychology again in his contact with Paul Schilder, who was a pioneer in psychoanalytic neurology and psychiatry. Schilder (1999) is best known for his monograph *The Image and Appearance of the Human Body*, in which he showed how our body images are profoundly social as well as libidinal. It is noteworthy that Schilder was so convinced of the importance of social factors in psychological development and in psychological illness that he anticipated Foulkes by working with small groups, though his approach was more individual than group-centred.

To train as a psychoanalyst, Foulkes moved to Vienna, where his analyst was Helene Deutsch, a close protégé of Freud's. Vienna was at the centre of psychoanalytic development. Freud had produced his structural theory, Wilhelm Reich was teaching character analysis, and there was a dawning recognition of and research into early child development and the importance of the mother-infant relationship and of the influences of society in human development.

After his psychoanalytic qualification, Foulkes returned to Frankfurt where the founder of the Psychoanalytic Institute was Karl Landauer, a leading psychoanalyst. He was another influential figure in Foulkes's intellectual development (Landauer 1914; 1924; 1931; 1936). He was one of this circle of Jewish clinicians who did not leave when they could – apparently he could have left early in the Nazi accession but he chose to remain and then had only the Netherlands as his option for flight. There he and his family were apprehended in 1943, and though he perished in Bergen Belsen, his wife and some of their children survived. There is yet insufficient knowledge about his important contribution in the 1920s and '30s. What we do know of is the new confluence of sociological, principally Marxist theory, with psychoanalytic theory through shared discussions between psychoanalysts and sociologists of this time.

The pre-group-analytic circle included psychoanalysts Landauer, Heinrich Meng, Erich Fromm, Frieda Fromm-Reichmann and Foulkes. The sociologists and social psychologists had association in two different circles. One circle was based at the Goethe University's Department of Sociology under the influence of Wertheimer and Gelb and included Norbert Elias, Kurt Lewin and Karl Mannheim. The other was based at the Frankfurt Institute for Social Research which, like the university Department of Sociology, shared premises with the Frankfurt Psychoanalytic Clinic. This circle included Theodor Adorno, Max Horkheimer and Herbert Marcuse. It is to Elias that we now turn, for with him we meet the historical approach to psychology and the profound influence of society on individual psychology.

Elias, whose centenary was celebrated in 1997 with many international meetings, is an influential figure in contemporary sociology. His influence is mostly in continental Europe, especially in the Netherlands, where he spent the last years of his life, and in Germany. His best-known work is *The Civilizing Process* (Elias 2000) which Foulkes enthusiastically reviewed in the *International Journal of Psychoanalysis* (Foulkes 1938: 263–266; reissued Foulkes 1990b: 79–82). Elias and Foulkes developed a relatively close friendship in the UK in the early years after the Second World War when Elias was in London. As an early member of Foulkes's circle, he even thought of becoming a group analyst himself, and with Foulkes, Abercrombie, Anthony, de Mare and others, they founded the Group Analytic Society.

The essence of Elias's (2000) approach is as follows:

1 The evolution of society profoundly affects individual psychodynamics.
2 The civilising process can be followed in European society from the thirteenth century onwards.
3 It is revealed through the 'descent of manners', the changing instructions given to young people as how to behave in courtly society. This establishes protocols for the correct way to deal with bodily and libidinal economy through matters such as eating, disposal of waste matter from the body, sexuality, cleanliness, hygiene, and how to behave so as to obtain recognition and favours from one's seniors.
4 As individuals are instructed to civilise their behaviour, restraints are imposed on impulses; the strength of the social within the individual increases, and where id was ego begins to appear.
5 Society gradually monopolises the sanctioned use of violence through instituting laws and punishments, and a state emerges which – in contrast to the person of the monarch – gradually becomes the sole determinant for capital punishment. As the central power increases, individuals are no longer allowed to attack or defend themselves impulsively against their fellows. In return for giving up their impulses, for their self-restraint, they receive the protection of the law. The authority of the state, in whatever form it took, is to be both revered and feared. The superego of the individuals becomes increasingly powerful as an internal force, as individuals undergo education and learn social compliance with the law.
6 Figuration: This is Elias's term for conceptualising 'persons' as profoundly social, always existing in chains of relationships, interdependent within those increasingly longer chains that modern society evolves, where our daily needs can only be met through actions of myriads of unknown others.

Through Elias's influence on group analysis, we have learnt to constantly examine and question the meaning of ideas that give primacy to individual process. He describes how it has come to pass that in the developing discipline of psychology, we need to examine and question the primacy of projection over introjection and all those postulates of psychology, including psychoanalysis, that have not yet accepted the depth of the social within each one of us. Individuality is indeed a slippery concept, and we can trace how different societies construe this term, may even have little use for it, for there are societies where the essence of the person is in their connectedness with their family, kin, clan, with their human and non-human environment.

The group-analytic concept of the individual being constituted to a profound degree by social factors has received much encouragement from current research in child development, in a deeper study of the nature of communication and in current psychology and neurobiology. Here, I shall sketch out something of what personally I have found to be important. The focus of attention in research is on the exquisite sensitivity of caregiver-infant relationships. Only close observations with open eyes and the appropriate technical equipment has revealed the processes that are present both pre- and postnatally.

1. Infants' attention can be attracted by adults very soon after birth. They will imitate adult facial gestures such as tongue protrusion even one day after birth.
2. Imitation involves active scanning of the visual environment for what the infant finds interesting.
3. The most interesting things are the facial expressions and the sounds coming from fascinating adult caregivers.
4. Infants are constantly and actively seeking the response of others to their own actions as well as responding to the activities of others.
5. Successful completion of units of activity between infants and caregivers gives pleasure, while unsuccessful ones give displeasure.
6. Human activity can be conceived of as essentially 'dialogical', involving partners in mutual synchronised and interesting activities. In the absence of such activities, development falters, is arrested or regresses.

These processes affect infant development in the most profound manner. They affect bonding, attachment and mentalisation (i.e., the development of mind and the awareness of being in a society of persons who are like-minded but also different). They also affect the acquisition of social and emotional intelligence as well as cognitive development. On the neurological level, there is increasing evidence that neuronal networks forming the basis of mind are deeply affected by the early processes of infant/caregiver relations and actions.

Through these advances, we see how profoundly infant mental and emotional development is indebted to 'good enough' environmental responses. Understanding these early influences is important, but it also makes us aware of how difficult it may be to influence such early factors by psychotherapy. We must accept the limits of our powers, but we can also see that this information can reinforce our belief that as human development is so profoundly social, we may be able to reach to very basic and early levels of human nature through our group-analytic work. For instance, the realms of psychosis and delinquency are opening to group-analytic techniques adapted to the special conditions of these disorders.

I cite here the pioneering work in forensic group psychotherapy of the late Murray Cox and his colleague in the field, Estela Welldon. Cox established the psychotherapy service at Broadmoor Hospital, a high-security special hospital in Berkshire for those with severe mental illness who are also dangerous (Cox 1978/1995; Cordess and Cox 1996; Cox and Theilgaard 1987/1994; Schlapobersky 1996). Welldon established the group therapy programme at the Portman Clinic in London, a centre associated with the Tavistock Clinic specialising in outpatient therapeutic help for forensic patients (Welldon 1992; 1997; 2012; Hakeem 2009). In 1990 Cox gave the fourteenth Foulkes lecture, 'The group as poetic playground: From metaphor to metamorphosis', and in 1997 Welldon gave the twentieth Foulkes lecture, 'Let the treatment fit the crime' (Welldon 1997) in which they shared decades of pioneering work at their respective centres. In 1997 we held an international symposium in London on the psychotherapy of schizophrenia and other psychoses. Encouraging news is coming through about group psychotherapy for these conditions, and there is important work under development elsewhere (Kanas 1996; Stone 1996).

I turn now to other aspects of human development that are to do with language and that also encourage the group-analytic enterprise. I shall be drawing on Russian psychology, on Lev Vygotsky and Mikhail Bakhtin. Vygotsky, a Jewish researcher of genius, gave a great developmental thrust to a social psychology of infancy and childhood that has significant differences to the Piagetian model. Vygotsky (1981: 164) was influenced in his thinking and research by Marxist theory, as were the Frankfurt sociologists. He claimed that higher mental functioning in the individual is rooted in social life, that 'human psychological nature represents the aggregate of internalised social relationships that have become functions for the individual and form the individual structure'. Note that he writes not of object relations but of social relations, and when he writes of how social relations have become functions for the individual, we can see similarities to the Kohutian and self-psychological ideas of the internalisation of self-object functions and self-object relationships that were recognised decades earlier by Vygotsky. There are two axioms from Vygotsky's work that I present because I consider them both relevant and revelatory for group analysis. The first derives from his insistence on a genetic psychology – that is, in tracing psychological phenomena to their origins. On the basis of his research, he asserted that

> any function in the child's cultural development appears twice on two planes. First it appears on the social plane, and then on the psychological plane. First it appears between people as an interpsychological category, and then within the child as an intrapsychological category.
>
> (Vygotsky 1981: 163)

The second of Vygotsky's axioms – set out below – is most apposite to group-analytic theory and practice. We call on the group to aid in the psychological development of its individual members through the capacities of the group as a whole, which are greater than those of any one of its members. Groups have a potentially greater store of human experience and mentalities to draw from, though the negative of this must not be neglected: the anti-developmental components of group life named 'anti-group' by Morris Nitsun (1996). Vygotsky's second axiom is what he called the zone of proximal development, which he defined as 'the distance between a child's actual developmental level, as determined by independent problem solving, and the higher level of potential development as determined through problem solving under adult guidance or in collaboration with more capable peers' (Vygotsky 1962/2012: 86). The individual, isolated child as the object of study is a laboratory and educational artifact, for the natural situation of a child, as we have all experienced, is to be with helpful others, our 'more capable peers'. Anxiety in the test situation of the school of life will always hamper our capabilities, and in psychotherapy we have to make judicious decisions about the appropriate balance between exposing patients to the anxiety of the group-analytic unstructured situation, finding the challenges that they are capable of solving for themselves and recognising when conductor interventions are appropriate. We are in the area so sensitively described by Winnicott (1968) with his concept of 'being alone in the presence of another', which becomes the basis of internal security. This is, as Vygotsky (1962/2012) wrote, an inter-psychological event that has been internalised and appears as intra-psychic.

I have been greatly stimulated by another Russian thinker, Mikhail Bakhtin. Vygotsky and Bakhtin wrote under Leninism and Stalinism and were influenced both positively and negatively. Bakhtin, a philosopher of language, was indeed sent into internal exile under Stalin, and knowledge of his work was suppressed for many years. His approach has been named 'dialogical' – it is congruent with the view of human development now coming from psychoanalysis and other sources which I find most natural and convincing. Bakhtin's view of language is intrinsically social. In this, his theories are in opposition to those of Saussure and Chomsky, which have gained wide acceptance in the West, and he opposes them on much the same grounds that led Vygotsky to oppose Piaget's tenets. He gives primacy to the social over the individual. For Bakhtin, the fundamental unit of language is not the word or even the sentence but the 'utterance' (Bakhtin 1981; Holquist 1981; 1990). He argues that 'speech is always cast in the form of an utterance belonging to a particular and speaking subject and outside this spoken form it cannot, it does not exist' (Bakhtin 1981: 71). Bakhtin, as cited in Wertsch (1991: 50), puts forward the view that the voice that is speaking, the voice that is responsible for the utterance, always exists in a social milieu and addresses the other, seeking a response. The speech act has its reality – it turns to someone else who becomes a link in a chain of communication. 'Utterances are not indifferent to one another and are not self-sufficient; they are aware of and they mutually reflect one another' (Bakhtin 1986: 81). You can see the parallel with Foulkes's belief that the conversation of a group is a series of linked communications, of unconscious responses and interpretations that we try to hear and to understand (Foulkes and Anthony 1957/1965/1983). As far as I know, Foulkes had no direct knowledge of Vygotsky or Bakhtin, though he was keenly interested in the nature of communication and in the constraints and facilities of language. We must assume that this kind of thinking had found its way into his Weltanschauung through those of his associates – like Goldstein – who had closer association than he with the thinking and ideas of their colleagues in the Soviet Union at the time.

According to Bakhtin (1981), we are constituted through dialogue, through what he has called 'the architectonics' of self. There is a form of auditory mirroring, which is a crucial way in which we gain information about ourselves through the verbal responses of the other, their intonations, spoken and unspoken messages. From earliest infancy, we are in search of understanding, which is mediated through the other. Any true understanding, according to Bakhtin, is dialogic in nature, for as we listen and try to understand, we are laying down a set of our own answering words, and 'the greater their number and weight the deeper and more substantial our understanding will be' (Voloshinov 1986: 102). This statement encapsulates beautifully those moments in group analysis when the utterances of a speaker are met with deep resonances from others in ways that constantly amaze me with their deep and often compassionate understanding; with the telling of experiences from another life at another time; that, speaking from 'the zone of proximal experience', come to illuminate dark areas of the speaker's mind, areas that they do not have access to on their own but that are given back to them through the responses of others.

Though Bakhtin confines himself to spoken and written language – he wrote masterfully on the novel in *Epic and Novel* – we can apply his principle of dialogism to the dialogical relations of infants and caregivers that characterise early life. Before speech, we have what have been named 'proto-conversations'. These are the amodal sensory communications revealed in the applications of psychoanalysis to infancy, which have shown that good mothering involves vocal motor gestures and games between infants and adults (Stern 1998). We join in and show interest and give attention to the infant's vocalisations and gazes. When we show the infant that we are doing something interesting and amusing with them (e.g., looking at the same toy together), we are joining it imaginatively, we enter turn-taking with the infant and cross the solipsistic space between two separate biological organisms. By these actions we begin to form the intersubjective realm and the intersubjective experience that is crucial for the development of mind. This is what gives the child the beginnings of a realisation that it possesses a mind, is a minded person, who can find like-minded persons in the other(s) who are at times alike but at other times different. This is the crucial stage that seems not to be reached in autism and is significantly lost or impaired in psychosis.

The sources I have drawn on from developmental psychology, from language and from neurobiology are, in my viewpoint, powerful arguments for the assertion that group analysis is a theory and praxis in its own right, which draws on developments in its own clinical field and in adjacent ones to create a distinct and coherent discipline. Each discipline, as does each one of us, has a unique viewpoint. No two of us have had the same life experiences, so each one of us can enrich the life experience of the other. This is what Bakhtin (1981) called a 'surplus of vision'. Thus, we celebrate 'heteroglossia', as he called it, the meeting in language of minds who express themselves in their own ways, as opposed to 'monoglossia', the single language that tries to impose itself as *the* authority, *the* truth. Bakhtin also wrote about what he called the 'authoritative voice', a voice based on the assumption that utterances and their meanings are fixed, not modifiable as they come into contact with new voices. He described the authoritative voice as one that demands that we acknowledge it, that we make it our own; it binds us quite independently of any power it might have to persuade us internally. We encounter it with its unconditional allegiance, and instead of functioning as a generator of meaning or a thinking device, it allows no play with its borders, no gradual and flexible transition, no spontaneously creative styling variants (Bakhtin 1981).

We meet this in the authoritarian father, dogmatic teachers, the authoritarian state, fundamentalism and the ideological voice. It is a voice that can only be totally affirmed or totally rejected; one cannot divide it up, agree with one part, partially accept another part, utterly reject a third portion. We have met this voice in dogmatic systems of psychology, in some aspects of psychoanalysis and, it can be argued, even in some schools of group analysis.

In contrast to the authoritative voice is the 'internally persuasive' voice which is half ours and half someone else's. It allows for dialogical inter-animation, for interplay; it is a voice that accepts that we live in a world that is always ambiguous, from which our words can reveal a certain but temporary clarity:

> Such a word awakens new and independent words, it organizes masses of our words from within, and does not remain in an isolated and static condition. It is *not finite*, it is *open*; in each of the new contexts that dialogize it, this discourse is able to reveal ever newer *ways to mean*.
>
> (Bakhtin 1981: 346, emphases original)

Those of you who were privileged to know and to learn with Foulkes will recognise that his was that internally persuasive voice that allowed new thoughts to arise and arrive. I hope that I am facilitating such new thoughts and meanings for you by sharing in those ideas that have given rise to new thoughts in me.

An instance of these new thoughts is in my approach to that verbal intervention that we name 'interpretation'. Nowadays, I see this as the insertion of the therapist through words into the mental life of an other or others, as an internally persuasive voice, a voice in the circle, one that is less authoritative than previously. Readers will find an account of these perspectives in Chapter 5, 'Aims of a wandering psychotherapist – Interpretation, dialogue, response', where I look at an aspect of the complex interactive field. This encompasses myself, within the group as a whole. My intentions are to awaken new and independent words, new forms of meaning. The verbal intervention is one particular way of being with the group, for the presence of the group conductor is of itself a powerful intervention in the group process, presenting himself/herself as a focus for the mobilisation of unconscious forces that permeate the social life of the group.

To end with, I will introduce you to some of the very stimulating ideas found in Merlin Donald's (1991) *Origins of the Modern Mind*. He brings together findings from neurobiology, anthropology and cognitive psychology to describe the evolution of the mind of *Homo sapiens* from that of our ape ancestors and argues that encephalisation, the increase in brain size and structural complexity in humans, is an adaptation to the demands of social living where complex relations have to be established, monitored and maintained. The members of the social group acquire the ability mentally to represent themselves, others and the complex social structure of the whole group. Each evolutionary stage in society has its own neurobiology. The ape and early hominid lived episodically, dominated and entrapped by the present; the appearance of mimesis, the ability to imitate and thereby to re-present the past in the present, is the next stage and involves groups in ritual. The next stage is the mythic, where questions are asked and answered about the fundamentals of human existence through religion and legend. With each of these stages, there is an adaptive biological alteration affecting not only brain structure but many other bodily structures. However, when we reach the present stage of modern man, reaching back now to our Middle Eastern and African ancestry, to the people who invented writing in its various pre-phonetic forms (e.g., cuneiform, hieroglyphics), what is added to the biology is the technology of graphic representation. Through the use of these visual symbols, the next adaptation is the creation of external memory. Now information is preserved and transmitted and potentially widely available. The availability of external graphic memory is an essential step to analytic thought, leading on to theory, the forms of thought which we have inherited from ancient Greece. Theory is anti-mythic – things and events have to be stripped of their previous mythic significance before they can be subjected to 'objective' theoretic analysis.

I say this knowing well that the subjective element is always present in so-called objective analysis. Similarly, the mythic is always with us and connects us deeply to shared beliefs and to human experiences that cannot be reached through higher mental functions. Foulkes acknowledged the deep presence of the Jungian archetypal level in human mentality, which our Jungian colleagues are exploring with us: our work is in the circle, the symbolic container, the archetype of the great mother who is both active and passive, creative and destructive, which we can journey both backwards and forwards in company (Foulkes 1964: 15).

I end with this because we need to balance constantly both the mythic and the analytic modes of understanding. What we should beware of is re-mythologising what has been demythologised. We create our mythic ancestors – Freud, Jung, Moreno, Foulkes, Bion – and we form cults, followings, antagonisms, to assert the truth and superiority of our own particular myth. But though we must respect our ancestors, it is unwise to regard them as graven images, nor should we worship them.

Note

1 This paper was given as a keynote lecture to an early meeting of the Israeli Association for Group Psychotherapy in Jerusalem in 1996, with the title 'Group analysis and its surrounding and supporting network'. The meeting took place under the auspices of Ada Abraham and Benny Rippa, who helped to lay the foundations for group analysis in Israel. This is an edited form of the paper published in 2002 under a revised title, 'The Coherence of Group Analysis', in *Group Analysis* 35 (1): 13–26. It was then reissued in German in a special edition of *Gruppenpsychotherapie und Gruppendynamik*: Pines, M. (2013). 'Die Kohärenz der Gruppenanalyse, psychosozial 131: Symbolbegriff und Symboltheorie in Psychoanalyse und Gruppenanalyse', 26, H. 1, 9–18. Acknowledgements are made to the editor of *Group Analysis* for consent to its publication here. (Ed.)

4 Forgotten pioneers

An unwritten history of the therapeutic community – Maxwell Jones Lecture 1998[1]

If the idea of running a psychiatric hospital as a therapeutic community can be given a date of birth, it was May 1946, when the *Bulletin of the Menninger Clinic* published the famous collection of papers from Northfield (Main 1946). Still earlier, Maxwell Jones (2013) had published his own first article on group psychotherapy in 1942, in the *British Medical Journal*. Tom Main's article in the 1946 *Bulletin* went on to announce the birth of the therapeutic community concept. In this lecture I shall speak of the processes that preceded the birth he announced in May 1946 and I will look at its lineage and parenthood. The therapeutic community method is rightly regarded as an important contribution to modern hospital psychiatry, but its antecedents are to be found in pedagogy, therapeutic education, social medicine and the changing human relations that took place between the two great European wars.

Both the Cassel Hospital and the Tavistock Clinic came into being at the end of World War I. The Cassel was established to meet the increasing needs for psychotherapy for traumatised war veterans and the Tavistock to meet the needs for the civilian population (Griffiths and Pringle 1997; Main 2001; Schlapobersky and Pines 2009). The traumatised nation that had lost millions of young men in battle and illness was left with broken families who found little comfort from outmoded religious rituals. Grief and mourning filled people's thoughts and writings; attachment, identification and the work of grieving took on a new importance in psychodynamic thought that was developed by Ian Suttie in 1935 at the Tavistock Clinic, followed by John Bowlby's work on delinquents and their family backgrounds (Suttie 1935/1988). Social psychology studied organisations and developed theories, amongst them Kurt Lewin's (1951; 1977) social field theory, that could encompass group phenomena. Social support systems – pensions, panel doctors and municipal hospitals – represented the emergence of 'therapeutic society', one in which life stages, birth, childhood, marriage, parenthood and ageing would become legitimate areas for the exercise of therapeutic attention and authority. I shall focus on group psychotherapy, therapeutic education and changes in hospital psychiatry and do honour to the forgotten pioneers who developed these new ideas and practices. I shall then reach out to Mill Hill and Northfield, the birthplaces of the therapeutic community movement.

DOI: 10.4324/9781003494713-6

Context and the therapeutic community movement

First, I will look into the context of psychoanalysis in Freud's work at the end of the nineteenth century and the social and cultural history out of which his thinking developed. The concept of unconscious processes was emerging in philosophy, psychiatry and the arts; the darkness of the mind was being explored as the limitations of positivistic science were increasingly recognised. This was the epoch of Darwin and Spencer showing the physical and social evolution of mankind, and of Hughlings Jackson, the Queen Square neurologist so much admired by Freud, who enunciated his 'doctrine of levels': the lower centres and primitive activity of the central nervous system were suppressed by its higher levels so long as the system was intact. He described how damage to higher centres released the activity of the lower and Freud adapted this model in his dynamic neuropsychology. The drives of the id, of our primitive uncivilised impulses, are held in check – he said – by our educated civilised egos (see Critchley and Critchley 1998).

European culture feared the forces released by the French Revolution that had overthrown monarchies and religions. The revolution revealed the power of the id crowd, of the people's armies led by a charismatic demagogue. In Austria, Freud grew up in a patriarchal authoritarian society. His psychological models were inevitably moulded by his social context, by his unconscious acceptance of and rebelliousness against current social forces. His focus was on the neurotic patient, for whom he fashioned the new intimacy of the psychoanalytic situation. This, he believed, was free of the influence of society. Later we shall consider how society was hiding under the couch (Redl 1966; Redl and Wineman 1965).

For twenty years Freud's co-workers came from similar social and ethnic backgrounds, so he seized the opportunity to work with the Zurich group headed by Bleuler and Jung, through whom he intended to conquer the world of academic psychiatry and psychology. About then, his work was becoming known in England and America, and the Americans began to study in Vienna and Zurich. In 1909, Freud, Jung and Ferenczi famously visited Clark University in Worcester, Massachusetts. Trigant Burrow met them in a theatre interval in New York and was so inspired by their work that, with the encouragement of Adolf Meyer at Johns Hopkins Hospital, he took his family to Zurich for his own personal analysis for a year (Burrow 1984; Pertegato and Pertegato 2019).

Vienna, a frontier between West and East, saw the emergence of related but different psychologies to Freud. This was the home of Jacob Moreno, the originator of group psychotherapy and later psychodrama, and of Alfred Adler, the socialist general practitioner who moved the psychotherapeutic situation into society. Social psychotherapy began here – the social space for the therapeutic community concept. Elsewhere I have written of the Apollonian-Dionysian dimension of psychotherapy (Pines 1997). Freud, for all his revolutionary ardour, was the classicist rooted in the Western intellectual tradition, who guarded psyche and society from being overthrown by the barbarians who are always at the gate. Apollonian, he created a tightly controlled group, closed to outsiders. The Dionysians, Moreno and Adler, moved into the forum and mixed with the crowd and the proletariat. They were social reformers. Adler pioneered parental guidance for disturbed children, and Moreno, through group discussions, organised the disenfranchised prostitutes of Vienna into a movement through which they gained civil rights. In the 1930s Wilhelm Reich opened his sexology clinics to bring his version of psychoanalysis and Marxism to the workers. Here, psychodynamic thought and practice moved from the individual to the group and out into the wider field. Reich took this synoptic vision with him on emigrating but struggled in different Scandinavian countries, failed to gain access to the UK and eventually joined several of his colleagues at the New School for Social Research in New York. But his radical spirit and his unboundaried approach towards his patients, especially in sexual matters, earned notoriety and cost him the regard and trust of many. As his later work focussed largely on sexuality, he became increasingly controversial, especially with his construction of orgone box accumulators, devices that his patients sat inside to harness the reputed health benefits, leading to newspaper stories about sex boxes that cured cancer. He is parodied in Woody Allen's film *Sleepers*. The tragic undoing of a professional life in which he began as the deputy director of Freud's outpatient clinic in Vienna and ended up dying in prison on a conviction brought by the FBI for the fraudulent sale of sexual devices should not blind us to his extraordinary influence. He coined the term 'sexual revolution', and during the student uprisings in Germany, rioters threw copies of his *Mass Psychology of Fascism* at the police.

Returning now to the German- and English-speaking worlds in the inter-war period, field theory, replacing the closed systems of nineteenth-century science, was becoming the new scientific paradigm (Lewin 1977). Organism and environment were seen to develop in equilibrium; Cannon's (1932) homeostasis and Gestalt psychology (Wertheimer 1959) were precursors of systems theory. The neurologist Kurt Goldstein outlined the functional unity of the central nervous system, moving neurology beyond Freud's. Goldstein showed how the response to injury in the central nervous system is not solely the release of low-level activities; it is an adaptation of the whole person, central nervous system and personality, to injury. He organised his post–World War I centre for the treatment of the brain-injured in Frankfurt as a helping community where patients and their families were encouraged to aid each other in rehabilitation. Goldstein presided on benign terms over the community while carrying out his great neurodynamic research. His young assistant S. H. Foulkes imbibed his teaching and later adapted it to group psychotherapy and the therapeutic community. Goldstein's integrated approach, his holistic thinking and philosophical interest in orders of adaptation and resilience were jointly developed with his cousin Ernst Cassirer, then professor of philosophy at Hamburg, who visited the Frankfurt clinic for regular seminars. Foulkes and Cassirer influenced a whole generation of innovators that included Fritz Perls, who was another of Goldstein's medical assistants and who went on to develop Gestalt therapy. Goldstein's clinic grew through the 1930s and he moved on to establish an even larger and more influential clinic in Berlin until the Nazi accession in 1933, when he was amongst the first to be arrested. At that stage Nazi policy against communists was even more stringent than against Jews, and though Goldstein was both, it was still possible to secure his release on negotiated terms. He took immediate deportation as the only option and his move influenced those circles of which he was part to disband and move towards immediate departure. This included Adorno, Cassirer, Fromm, Foulkes, Horkheimer, Perls and others. Those who could not make the move then were trapped and later perished. Goldstein moved to Amsterdam where, on a Ford Foundation scholarship, he completed the book that has shaped the thinking of generations of neurologists, group analysts and others interested in holistic thinking – *The Organism* (1939/1995). He went on to settle in the United States and, like others in his family and his other colleagues in exile, seeded a visionary approach taken up by generations of followers including Foulkes in the UK, Maslow in the United States (Maslow 1943; 1954; 1962) and Oliver Sachs and others (see foreword to Goldstein 1939/2000).

A significant Austrian innovation recognised and appreciated by Maxwell Jones came from August Aichhorn, a Viennese schoolteacher who was put in charge of reformatory schools and had to deal with a group of violent young men between the ages of seventeen and twenty. They proved incorrigible, and their teachers despaired of altering their behaviour except through imposed discipline. Aichhorn, deciding to take charge of the situation, allowed aggression full rein, believing that if it is not opposed it will reach a climax and resolve harmlessly, which is what happened. The boys' behaviour became ever more violent and destructive as they sought punishment to justify the hatred of their teachers. The local community was so alarmed by the destructive behaviour that it sent for the police, but Aichhorn stuck to his guns. He stood by calmly as a boy threatened to cut another's throat, recognising this as more a performance than a dangerous intention. The boy threw the knife to the ground, howled and wept with frustrated rage, then fell into a deep slumber. Eventually all twelve boys followed suit; the violence had reached its climax. For three months alternating episodes of peace and rage followed as the boys began to develop emotional bonds between themselves and their workers. The identification of each boy with the all-loving leader created emotional bonds between members of the group as a result of their common attachment to the leader; the groundwork was laid for the positive response to the attitudes and expectation of the therapist. The capacity for empathy with the delinquent can lead to a successful use of transference which encourages essential ego strengthening, advancing towards an increasingly independent ability to learn and to develop more mature relationships. Anna Freud, recognising the importance of Aichhorn's work, encouraged him into analysis with Paul Federn. His pioneering book

Wayward Youth, with a foreword by Sigmund Freud, was translated in 1935, after which Jones must have noticed it and followed this model (Aichhorn 1925/1955; Eissler 1948).[2]

The therapeutic community movement in the British context

Now I shall explore the question of why and how therapeutic community work emerged in the British context in the early 1940s. What was the facilitating environment for the maturation of this concept? My thesis is that the situation of psychotherapy in psychiatry in Britain from the 1920s onwards forms the matrix for therapeutic community work, based on factors which I will set out below. Further historical detail is furnished in the endnotes.

Britain saw the development of an eclectic form of psychotherapy strongly influenced by psychoanalysis; this, combined with a recognition of societal forces, characterised the English school of psychotherapy. Notable figures included Hugh Crichton-Miller at the Tavistock Clinic, T. A. Ross at the Cassel Hospital, which was originally a hospital for the treatment of battle trauma amongst officers, and W. H. Rivers, a psychiatrist, experimental psychologist and anthropologist. He was the medical director of Craig Lockhart, a World War I therapeutic community for officers just outside Glasgow and is the hero of Pat Barker's war fiction trilogy, *Regeneration, The Eye in the Door* and *The Ghost Road*. His contribution corresponded to the work of Freud in Vienna and Goldstein in Frankfurt, who were working with corresponding populations on the other side of the conflict. Rivers's most decisive contribution was to open British psychology and psychiatry to the influence of Freud.

British psychiatry was emerging from its earlier lethargy when all mental illness was thought to result from organic degeneration. Hospitals began to open their closed wards, admitting voluntary patients. The Maudsley Hospital was founded to admit only voluntary patients. The social democratic influence was changing the status of the psychoanalytic patient: he was regaining personhood.

Psychoanalysis and psychodynamic psychotherapy lived in a state of creative tension with each other. Ernest Jones, the Napoleon of psychoanalysis, with his field marshal Edward Glover, isolated psychoanalysis from any other form of psychotherapy. Psychoanalysts were banned from working at the Tavistock Clinic, that seat of eclecticism where Ian Suttie (1935/1988) wrote *The Origins of Love and Hate*, interweaving psychoanalysis and the social. John Bowlby's (1965; 1969; 1973; 1980) research on delinquency, childcare, the growth of love and attachment theory stems from the same sources. The barriers between psychotherapy and psychoanalysis finally ruptured in wartime when the psychoanalysts John Rickman, Dennis Carroll and Foulkes, under the wise leadership of J. H. Rees from the Tavistock Clinic, came into creative contact with wartime psychiatry at Northfield. Bion, Sutherland and Bridger, who trained as psychoanalysts after the war, worked at Northfield during the war before qualifying under the good governorship of Tom Maine, Alfred Torrie and Emanuel Miller. These were distinguished psychiatrists and psychotherapists and were not psychoanalysts (Harrison 2000).

London was much unlike Vienna in social structure and climate. It had a sturdy democracy that resisted both Mosley's fascism and Harry Pollitt's communism and had moved towards social democracy and social medicine. Industrial psychology explored social dynamics at work. The first professor of occupational psychology at London University was the psychoanalyst Millais Culpin. The innovative Peckham Health Centre harnessed social forces in social medicine. British psychoanalysts, in contrast with Vienna, were mainly British-born Christian persons of middle-class origins; the Tavistock Clinic was dubbed the 'Parson's Clinic' by the Irish Catholic Maudsley professor of psychiatry Edward Mapother, an anti-psychoanalyst. The Bloomsbury group supported psychoanalytic ideas. Virginia Woolf's younger brother Adrian, who wanted to reach the Lighthouse, was the psychoanalyst Adrian Stephen, my own first analyst. James and Alex Strachey came from that same group of Cambridge intellectuals and psychoanalytic ideas were permeating society. The eminent, influential psychoanalyst John Rickman, who served in a Quaker relief unit in Russia during World War I, collaborated with Bion in the first Northfield experiment and was well versed in sociology and anthropology. Object relations theory explored connections and disconnections in the psychic life of infants. Society shaped and was in its turn shaped by the psyche.

The influence of progressive education described in Bridgeland's (1971) *Pioneer Work with Maladjusted Children* features 'twentieth-century originals', of whom Homer Lane is the archetype. Lane, of vigorous New England Puritan stock, had been influenced by the great educational philosopher John Dewey. Several schools in America had introduced self-government, and in 1913, Lane came to England to advise on the foundation of a 'republic' to be run on similar lines. Little Commonwealth, as it was called, was a home for post-school-age adolescents referred by the courts or their own parents. In 1918, following allegations of sexual impropriety made against Lane, the withdrawal of Home Office support meant closure. Under the influence of psychoanalysis, he had been experimenting in an amateurish way with the psychotherapy for some of the girls, and there were further allegations without evidence. He was brought to trial on the charge of failing to register as an alien and agreed to go into voluntary exile, dying in the United States in 1925. Auden (1936), one of his admirers, wrote as an epitaph that 'Lawrence was brought down by smut-hounds, Blake went dotty as he sang, / Homer Lane was killed in action by the Twickenham Baptist gang'.

The combination of self-government and an inspiring personality has been the model for other pioneers of schools for the maladjusted. Lane used what we now call group therapy with shared responsibility fifty years ago; any commonwealth meeting was 'an occasion for searching group analysis' and their meetings were converted into therapeutic groups.

David Wills was the first British social worker to train in the United States. He was also influenced by Lane and took part in the Q Camp experiment, where psychoanalysis was introduced into residential treatment for maladjusted youths. Two forgotten pioneers, the psychoanalysts Marjorie Franklin and Dennis Carroll, pioneered this work. Carroll's book gives a brilliant account of his experiences in Hawkspur Camp, founded in 1936 and closed in 1940 because of wartime conditions. It was sponsored by the Q Camp committee whose convenor, Dr Marjorie Franklin, was a pioneer of psychoanalytic insights into delinquency. She was a member of the British Psychoanalytical Society who had trained with Ferenczi in Hungary. She was consultant psychiatrist at the service that later became the Portman Clinic and at the British Hospital for Functional Nervous Disorders, the first outpatient hospital for the neuroses. She came from a wealthy banking family and maintained the Planned Environmental Therapeutic Trust, which today houses important archives of the therapeutic community movement. Craig Fees, the enthusiastic archivist of the trust, has given much help to me in assembling material for this lecture. I am particularly grateful for his information on Marjorie Franklin and Dr Dennis Carroll, also a consultant at the Portman Clinic. These historical sources are most accessible in Whiteley's (2004) 'Evolution of the Therapeutic Community'.

Dennis Carroll was Edward Glover's right-hand man – a brilliant scientist, he trained as a psychoanalyst in the 1930s. He pioneered psychoanalytic work with delinquents and criminals together with Glover and was a co-founder of the Psychopathic Clinic, now known as the Portman. Carroll has not left many writings, but the records of the Portman Clinic show how central a figure he was in teaching and research. He was an active, enthusiastic supporter of the Hawkspur experiment, and there is an as-yet unexplained connection between Hawkspur, Carroll, Bion and Northfield. Bion was a staff member of the Psychopathic Clinic before the war and had contact with Carroll, who went on to become commanding officer at Northfield, though not at the time when Bion and Rickman were there. We can at this stage only speculate whether Bion knew about Hawkspur and the methods of therapeutic community in progressive education.

After the war, Carroll worked for the Home Office and the United Nations. He presided over the Third International Congress of Criminology in the year of his sudden death, aged fifty-five. Glover, who gave his funeral eulogy, described him as a physician, a psychoanalyst of distinction, one of the most brilliant psychiatrists of his generation, and finally a pioneer in and ultimately a master of a new science – the psychology of crime. Glover described this as a field of study running from the frayed edges of social life down to the deepest layers of the individual mind where conscience is born or, as sometimes happens in delinquents, where it lies stillborn (Glover 1931).

David Wills had a deep understanding of the light that psychoanalysis could throw on disturbed behaviour. He understood the enormous power of positive and negative transference. The boys sought in him the loving parent they had not had, and with great skill and understanding he lived through the 'corrective emotional experience' they sought. They attached themselves to him and his wife; time and time again they would test his capacity to go on loving in the face of delinquency and bad behaviour. But he knew they sought punishment out of a great sense of guilt, and he fashioned a system of discipline that would meet these needs. The authority for discipline was vested in the camp committee to which he was consultant. The campers were paid wages for their work, and punishment was largely fines for breaches of behaviour.

Wills provided the essential nutrients for psychic development advocated by the school of self-psychology that Kohut and his followers established. They delineate ways in which caregivers, guardians of emotional development in infancy and childhood, act to provide emotional nutrients vital for the secure growth of a child's sense of self, as 'self objects'. The self object is defined as the intrapsychic experience provided by objects – persons who are needed to sustain the sense of continuity, cohesion and eventual coherence of the self.

These self object functions provide opportunities for mirroring, idealisation, twinship, adversarial experiences and effectiveness. Mirroring gives the child the opportunity to glow in the loving and appreciative gaze of the loved one: a child's idealisation gives glory to the perfection of the parental person; two people who pair find common humanity in this twinship; and the adversary can be an opponent who, though combative, pits strength, creates and holds limits and can say no. Effectiveness can arise out of discovering how cooperation enhances one's own strength and that two together can make one.

The 'protective shell' in which these boys lived was made up of their hatred of the world about them, which they could only shed on discovering that when they were given freedom, not discipline or control. They discovered in progressive increments that they had to begin to discipline themselves. The camp committee, which they themselves had created, offered the opportunity for self-government and eventual self-discipline. Garland's (1982) fine paper, 'Taking the Non-Problem Seriously', describes how in group analysis it is not the presenting of a problem that gains sustained attention but rather, a range of problems that the patient creates for himself or herself and for others in the setting of the group itself. At the camp, delinquency was the symptom that brought them there, but what emerged was the underlying dis-ease, the disorder of not being whole. The need for punishment arises out of tremendous feelings of guilt. So stealing is an appeal for affection and running away is an attempt to escape from intolerable inner conflicts. Wills anticipated Bion's work at Northfield, where he required that soldiers face the consequences of their behaviour as a group. The soldiers found that by projecting authority onto superiors, they deprived themselves of their own powers. Carroll, the psychoanalytic adviser to Hawkspur, was a commanding officer at Northfield; his own commanding officer had shown him a publication about Hawkspur and advised Bion to try these new methods. So Hawkspur came to Northfield! The progress of the Hawkspur boys, after initial careful assessments, were monitored by Wills, Franklin, Carroll and the interesting Dr Norman Glaister, who merits separate mention as another forgotten pioneer.

Glaister first appears in Franklin's account of how the Planned Environmental Therapy Trust came into being. He was one of only two who in 1928 came to meet Marjorie Franklin in response to her advertisement in the *Journal of the Royal Medical Psychological Society*; the other, to my surprise, was the analyst Adrian Stephen. Glaister, then medical superintendent of Northumberland House, a private mental hospital, was especially interested in the study and implementation of experiments in community living. He was already involved with the Grith Fyrd Pioneers (meaning Peace Army in Old English), an organisation which offered camp life to young men at a time of massive unemployment and demoralisation. He was interested in social innovations early in his professional life. There were three great influences in his life: first the evolutionary philosopher Herbert Spencer (2000), then, from 1919, Wilfred Trotter (1916) through *Instincts of the Herd in Peace and War* and finally the physicist and philosopher L. L. Whyte. Through Trotter's influence, Glaister believed, at the same time as Trigant Burrow, that the problems of the day had outgrown the capacity of the single mind of any one person, that only a coordinated group of unlike minds – a 'multimental' group – would be adequate to the social situation of the current time. He tried to create a 'living social organism', reorganising a pacifist camping organisation for adults and children. This Order of Woodcraft Chivalry was organised into guilds which were led by Keepers of the Fire. Glaister became grand keeper for several years, until the usual disagreements of utopian organisations led to splits and he left. Then he joined Sir Richard Acland's Common Wealth, a left-of-centre political party.

The last stage in Glaister's evolution was through meeting L. L. Whyte, through whom he recognised the next stage in evolution to be social and not biological. This was something Spencer had proposed earlier. Multimentality could be the first achievement of a new stage of symbiotic psychosocial relationships. Glaister founded the Braziers Park School of Integrative Social Research in Oxfordshire, which continues to study the art and science of living in practical ways and explore the advantages and problems of living in a group.

There were many experiments in social living in the 1920s and '30s, including the kibbutz movement in Palestine, Burrow's camp in America and Glaister's Order of Woodcraft Chivalry – all were feeling their way towards new forms of social organisation. The Peckham experiment was an important study of the nature of physical and mental health which took the family as the basic unit of human life and the small community as the next stage beyond the family. The Peckham experiment influenced Harold Bridger's organisation of social living at Northfield. Joshua Bierer's Social Club at

Runwell Hospital, later his development at the Marlborough Day Hospital and Pat de Maré's Social Club at St George's Hospital and his contemporary leadership of the median group movement are – in their different ways – facets of the same movement towards multimental social organisations.

The *Wharncliffe Memorandum*: A missing document

Early in World War II, the psychoanalyst John Rickman, then stationed at Wharncliffe Emergency Hospital, drew up the *Wharncliffe Memorandum*, a blueprint for the hospital treatment of neurotic and battle-scarred soldiers. This document, which has since gone missing, was probably the basis for the first Northfield experiment. I have found notes of a visit to Wharncliffe in January 1941 by the eminent psychiatric geneticist Eliot Slater in the archives of the British Psychoanalytical Society. He was no friend of psychoanalysis but reports of a scheme of physical rehabilitation for neurotic soldiers initiated by Rickman. He describes it as a new system for the occupational therapy of soldiers suffering from neuroses, consisting in the widest possible application of the principle that, as the occupation of a soldier is soldiering, the best occupational therapy should be soldierly activities. Extensive use is made of greater classes in physical training, grenade practice, route-marching, classes in map-reading, strategy, signalling and so forth. The scheme was initiated by Sergeant-Major Bryant. The method was extended with new techniques added through Rickman's imagination and enthusiasm (Whiteley 2004). Slater later wrote to Rickman of how impressed he was by this visit and describes a new convalescent hospital established nearby. Half its beds were for convalescent general military cases and half for psychiatric cases, filled from both Mill Hill and Sutton, who should return to the army. He proposed introducing this scheme of paramilitary training as a form of psychiatric rehabilitation, based on Rickman's work (Rickman 1957a; 2003; Whiteley 2004).

In the rest of his letter Slater states that the great majority of neurotics do not make good soldiers and are a source of weakness rather than strength to the army and that the greatest obstacle to the success of the neurotic as a soldier is an absence of goodwill. It would indeed be a brilliant discovery if the missing *Wharncliffe Memorandum* should ever turn up.

Early developments in the United States

I shall begin in America with Dr Trigant Burrow in the 1920s and the 1930s, when he explored the dynamics of small and large groups under what he called 'laboratory conditions'. Neglected and opposed for much of his life by his former fellow psychoanalysts, he significantly influenced Foulkes, who had read his papers in German in the 1920s.[3] He was a remarkable man. He qualified in medicine after a PhD in psychology and worked closely with Adolf Meyer at the Phipps Clinic of Johns Hopkins University, Baltimore, where later Harry Stack Sullivan began his pioneer inpatient group therapy with young male schizophrenics.[4] Meyer encouraged Burrow to meet Freud and Jung on their visit to America in 1909.[5] Burrow was to later write approvingly of Jung to his mother (Burrow 1924–1927; 1984). Inspired by his experience in Zurich, Burrow returned to New York in 1910 and set up as a psychoanalyst in Baltimore. In 1911 he joined Brill, Ernest Jones, Adolf Meyer and others to form the American Psychoanalytic Association. He became its president in 1925, but after that his career as a psychoanalyst went into decline because of his involvement in what he called the 'laboratory method of group analysis'. Meyer asked him to resign from the university, though their relationship remained cordial.

For twelve years Burrow practiced psychoanalysis and published many important papers in which he pioneered the exploration of early infant-mother fusion and separation experience.[6] Sadly, he was removed from membership of the American Psychoanalytic Association in 1933, ostensibly because of the divergence between his views and those of American psychoanalysis. The cause of the divergence, of the opposition and exclusion, was not only Burrow's research into group analysis – he was the first to use this term – but because he spoke out trenchantly to psychoanalysts about their own group behaviour. He argued that we need to rid ourselves of the idea that the neurotic individual is sick and that we psychopathologists are well. We need to accept a more liberal societal viewpoint that permits us to recognise without protest that the individual neurotic is in many respects not any sicker than we ourselves. We lose count of the circumstance that the neurotic in his private substitutions and distortions has merely failed to ingratiate himself in the collective confederacy of substitutions and distortions which you and I, with no less an eye to our self-protection, have had the cunning to subscribe to, under the cover of our arbitrary pseudo-group symptomatology. Burrow challenged what he called the esoteric practice of closeting a patient in our private consultation room to hear a story of ineptitudes and maladjustments that are due to social interpositions and substitutions common to the race and therefore identical with one's own. And he concluded that by inviting patients to meet us in secret conferences, we place ourselves outside all relation to their medical and scientific significance (Burrow 1924–1927).

Burrow insisted that consensual observation is synonymous with scientific method. It is only in the group laboratory situation that sexual fantasies, family conflicts, the social mask become the materials for observation in groups of up to twenty people. He insisted that through unconscious social resistances psychoanalysts have not exposed themselves to public examination of their own psyches. At the fifteenth annual meeting of the American Psychoanalytic Association, also in 1925, he described how the social mind is characterised by what he called substitutions and improvisations that remain unchallenged amongst members of our own profession. He went on to describe how we disguise the fact that neurosis is social and that it can only be understood through social analysis. He challenged his colleagues to face their complicity in complexes that are as neurotic – in our organisations – as those found in the work of personal analysis. He published this challenge in a paper for the *British Journal of Medical Psychology* (Burrow 1927a).

> He bore the ensuing opposition of his fellow psychoanalysts with dignity. In several letters to Freud, he asked him to accept and to understand that the extension of psychoanalysis to a group situation was a natural extension and comparable to the step that Freud himself had made in his pioneer work. He even asked Freud to seek within himself the origins of his resistances to understanding Burrow's work, an invitation which Freud declined to take up (Burrow 1924–1927; 1984).

How had Burrow come to this method of group analysis and in what way did it anticipate the therapeutic community method? He had become dissatisfied with the emphasis psychoanalysis places on an individualistic assessment of human behaviour. Disorders in behaviour were for him essentially social or interrelational and demanded observation and study in the dynamic group setting. He entered into mutual analysis with his associate Clarence Shields, an analysand who had challenged Burrows by asserting that the resistances that the analysand experienced in the analytic situation were intrinsically related to the social situation of psychoanalyst and patient. According to Shields, Burrow himself, though presumably an analysed and unneurotic person, would discover in himself those same resistances if he submitted himself to analysis by his patient. Burrow accepted this challenge, and discovering the correctness of this assertion, he began his exploration of the individual in the group situation (Burrow 1926; 1927; 1992; Pertegato and Pertegato 2019).

The social image is the result of upbringing and education through which the individual conforms to the expectations of family and society and becomes distorted and divorced from his spontaneous and more authentic self. This fictitious social image is reinforced and supported by the need to present an image that would be supported by significant others. This exploration was remarkable and anticipated developments that took place twenty or thirty years later by Schilder (1938; 1999) in America, by Foulkes in England, by Lacan in France and after World War II by the encounter movement. Burrow also realised early on that these social deceptions are not the property of any one individual but of the group as a whole – a microcosm of the wider society. He wrote:

> Under no circumstance does the procedure consist in the analysis of the individual by another individual or individuals. Whatever manifestations a student may present, in no circumstance is he made answerable for it as though it were a reaction particularly to him. Whatever it may be, the manifestation is viewed as the expression of a latent content that is

> common to the group as a whole. Under no circumstance is the reaction of anyone regarded as isolated or separate.
>
> (Pertegato and Pertegato 2019: 183)

Comparing his experiences in group analysis with his previous experiences as a psychoanalyst, Burrow wrote further:

> For many years it was my daily experience in personal analyses to pursue diligently the secret fantasies and symbolic irrelevancies of the individual unconscious, hunting them out from their remotest crevices with meticulous painstaking. . . . In group analysis, however, the patient is made witness to the situation wherein these irrelevancies and secret excursions constitute a latent tendency that characterises fully the social group about him. It becomes gradually plain to him that his adoption of a code of symbols possessing only a private latent meaning is a general social condition.
>
> (Pertegato and Pertegato 2019: 185)

In the same paper he wrote, 'With the gradual maturing of the group method, the cherished reminiscences and private ruminations of the individual have come finally to be wholly disregarded. The only concern which occupies the group-analysis is the immediate interrelationships socially of the members composing it as expressed in the symbol of their momentary interchange' (Pertegato and Pertegato 2019: 186).

Emphasis is on the total exploration of the here and now of the whole group, including the conductor. Burrow's words resonate with the ringing declaration of Tom Main's 1946 article on the therapeutic community, where he writes of the social arrangement of the hospital where the patients are robbed of their status as responsible human beings. Here Main challenges what he calls the anarchical rights of the doctor in the traditional hospital society that have to be exchanged for the more sincere role of member in a real community, responsible not only to himself and his superiors but to the community as a whole, privileged and restricted only insofar as the community allows or demands. The doctor no longer owns his patients; they are no longer captive children, obedient in nursery-like activities but have 'sincere' adult roles to play (Main 1946).

Burrow and his students anticipated and worked on this some twenty years earlier. The emphasis on the group as a whole and on the here and now became watchwords in the writings of Foulkes, Bion and their schools. Foulkes was, I thought, the only one in the United Kingdom to acknowledge the influence of Burrow on his thinking, stating that he had been impressed by Burrow's writings when he had first read them in German in the 1920s. In conversation with Richard Crocket of the Ingrebourne Centre, he recounted how Burrow had influenced his work.

Burrow's earlier psychoanalytic papers written from 1914 onwards are novel and anticipate the work of Kohut and the school of self psychology when he writes of the 'preconscious' experience of the infant which remains part of our psyche throughout life. By preconscious he does not mean Freud's preconscious, that which is accessible to consciousness, but that which is prior to consciousness, when the infant is at one with the mother. The preconscious mode is one of experiencing the feeling growing out of the infant's primary identification with the mother. For the infant's mother is the infant's love 'subject' rather than love 'object' – there is not only a primary physiological unity between infant and mother in the womb but a psychological union, a pre-objectless state, manifested in later life in states of quietude and self-possession. The break in physiological and psychological union with the mother through birth is restored when the infant nourishes at the mother's breast and experiences a semblance of organic unity, completion and satisfaction.[7]

Burrow's later work led him into physiological research, where he sought to uncover the mechanisms through which individuals isolated from each other experience tensions which can be recognised and measured by muscular patterns of the forehead and eyes. He attempted to show how these patterns could be relieved through relaxation following the emergence of conscious awareness of them. Here again, he anticipates the practice of transcendental meditation and yoga and other methods of stress recognition and release.

Returning to the UK – Foulkes, Jung and Withymead

Foulkes published his first paper on group analysis co-authored with Eve Lewis in 1944. It was reissued as the first chapter of his book *Therapeutic Group Analysis* (Foulkes 1964: 20–37). The paper describes clinical work in Exeter over two years with fifty patients, some of whom had previously had individual therapy while others at a local child guidance clinic had not. In this prescient paper the authors outline the following therapeutic factors:

1. Fostering social integration and relief of isolation
2. Mirror reactions
3. Activation of the collective unconscious
4. Exchange

There is a Jungian note in the reference to the collective unconscious. Lewis was a Jungian analyst who worked at Withymead, the pioneer therapeutic community in Exeter, where Foulkes himself was working. Withymead was founded in 1941 by Irene and Gilbert Champernowne[8] and was described by the Jungian analyst Anthony Stevens as 'The Jungian Community for the Healing Arts'. It treated 240 adults between 1942 and 1954, when it closed as a result of financial and group-dynamic difficulties. I find this coincidence intriguing – that Foulkes did his original group-analytic work in Exeter with Lewis who later, if not at the time, was working at this psychotherapeutic community. Did some influence diffuse from Withymead to Foulkes before he joined the Royal Army Medical Corps and went to Northfield? Another coincidence and possible connection is that Gilbert Champernowne worked at Mill Hill at the same time as Maxwell Jones. Did that experience contribute to the building up of Withymead?

The presiding genius at Withymead was Irene Champernowne, a Jungian analyst who had trained with H. G. Baynes, the pioneer Jungian analyst in London, and later with Jung in Switzerland. Before that, she had been considerably influenced through contact with Alfred Adler in Vienna and had worked with a group of Adlerians in Munich between 1930 and 1936. She had a PhD in psychology and was a woman of commanding personality and strong will. These characteristics contributed to both the creation and destruction of Withymead as a healing community.

Neurotic and psychotic patients were admitted, as were some who came seeking healing without identifiable illnesses. All the staff had been in personal analysis – presumably Jungian – and art therapy was prominent. This included painting, modelling, pottery, music, movement and dance. Psychotherapists and art therapists worked closely together; of central importance was a weekly staff meeting in which the progress of each patient was reviewed, where staff dissensions were worked through, if necessary late into the night. Irene Champernowne referred to the group meeting as 'the ego of the community' where the 'shadow of the community' – negative feelings and disruptive influences – could be confronted and analysed. Stevens describes Withymead as an organisation that was anti-bureaucratic in spirit, in contrast to the traditional mental hospital. The latter exemplified what the sociologist Max Weber termed 'rational bureaucracy', an organisation instituted so that its functions could be performed routinely, providing standardised, mechanistic solutions to problems that were economical in time and effort. This form of rational bureaucracy when applied to large mental hospitals resulted in Goffman's 'total institutions' which turned patients into objects and fed into administrative machinery, worked on by routine operations. Withymead, by contrast, set out to be and to remain small, with a maximum of forty-five patients, so that personal contact could be preserved.[9] It set out to be a sanctuary where self-healing could take hold and regression could be understood, held and contained. The critique of the Withymead approach advanced by Bernard Zeitlyn and Robert Hobson challenged its spontaneity, and its spirit of cultivating 'self-actualisation'. Hobson (1979: 232) went so far as to call this 'the therapeutic community disease'.[10]

Irene Champernowne was aware of potential dangers in a therapeutic community and believed that she had created and maintained a healthy community, though in the end there was bitter division in the staff. Stevens asserts that for as long as the Champernownes remained firmly in control, Withymead remained comparatively healthy. The authority of Irene and her husband, Gilbert, as charismatic leaders of the community was accepted; therapeutic group and community meetings, other than the crucially important staff meetings, were not instituted. The community did not have a political intent, and Stevens (1993) asserts that Withymead was a genuine community, not a synthetic one. The centre was not run as a democracy: administrative decisions were taken by the management committee and clinical decisions were taken by the staff meeting. The staff believed that they were qualified to carry full responsibility for the welfare of their patients and that it would be counterproductive to politicise these functions by giving patients voices in the organisation of the community in the pursuit of democracy.

The Champernownes believed strongly in Jung's view that individuation was a personal pursuit and could not be achieved in a group. For this reason, Irene opposed more recent developments in the therapeutic community movement because she considered that it gave value to the terms not of the individual but of the group. Group treatments focus attention on processes going on outside the individual patient rather than inside the psyche. They focus on the behavioural manifestations of neuroses rather than their intra-psychic roots. The therapeutic potential of the group and its healing influence worked indirectly by individuals participating intimately in the life of the community whose therapeutic responsibility was vested in the staff meeting. But there was much that her vision of Withymead held in common with therapeutic communities.

> In the intimacy of its social organisation, Withymead resembled not only the extended family but a small tribal clan of the type that human beings have lived in since our species began. Withymead thus satisfied the archetypal nostalgia that all of us share for life in such small intimate associations of people, and this goes far to explain its compelling attractiveness.
>
> (Stevens 1993: 105)

Stevens concludes that for a community to possess therapeutic influence, it needs to go some way towards fulfilling the archetypal demand for intimate relationships within the context of a small and enduring group. Within the limits of the adaptive design of the human psyche we are equipped genetically for life in small communities, and as Burrow emphasised, we are in danger of becoming ill through membership of our large Western-style societies that have no closer bonds of affiliation than society at large.

I move on now to the decline and fall of Withymead. As it ran into increasing financial difficulties, though subsidised by the Elmhursts of Dartington, the community was driven to incorporate administrators and medical directors and to seek patients from the National Health Service. Gilbert had by now died and the matriarchal influence of Irene was increasingly challenged by the patriarchal input of medical and administrative males. Divisions took place along gender lines, the innovators being men, the women guardians of tradition. Women began to accuse men of ganging up together in a cowardly fashion, organising a 'masculine conspiracy' to destroy the essentially feminine nature of the community, while men blamed women for allowing irrational prejudices to blind them to economic reality and the need for change (Stevens 1993: 229). 'As the men increasingly took us over, imposing full medical cover, nurses, administrators, hospital routines and so on, the worse everything became, and the spiritual core of the community, which carried the despair and the sickness of the patients, was destroyed' (Champernowne in Stevens 1993: 229).

Stevens describes a movement to replace the matriarchal unity of the community with a differentiated order of paternity, but Irene, the mother, and through her the community, resisted men with increasing ferocity until they ejected her, thereby destroying the fabric of the culture. Male attitudes, essentially pragmatic, were concerned with the realistic demands that society made on Withymead – to set its financial, administrative and clinical house in order. Women, unconsciously prompted by the male archetype, were primarily concerned to protect the ethos of the community. Their actions were determined by intuition and 'inner knowledge' and they responded at times with 'Amazonian belligerence'. Schism rent Withymead because the protagonists worshipped different gods; the more fervently they asserted their faith, the more widely were the gods forced apart. In 1966 the management committee asked Irene Champernowne to resign, and its calamitous financial position led to its closure in 1967. A poignant note is that the search for a medical director, a psychiatrist who could understand and work within the ethos of the community, had discovered a young GP just taking his diploma in psychiatric medicine who would have been ideally suited had they been able to afford his salary. He was the late Murray Cox. Based at Broadmoor Hospital in the years that followed, he established its first Department of Forensic Psychotherapy and went on to become one of the leading pioneers in forensic psychotherapy with a worldwide influence until his untimely death in 1997 (Cox 1978/1995; 1990; Cox and Theilgaard 1987/1994; 1994; Cordess and Cox 1996).[11, 12]

I shall end on a sentimental note, a roll call of therapeutic communities and their initiators. Many have passed out of our lives; happily some live on. Do you recall some of the words of *The Slow Train* of Michael Flanders and Donald Swann, immortalised in song in 1957 and repeated whenever we have need to deal with loss through laughter?

> No more will I go to Blandford Forum and Mortehoe
> On the slow train from Midsomer Norton and Mumby Road
> No churns, no porter, no cat on a seat
> At Chorlton-cum-Hardy or Chester-le-Street
> We won't be meeting again
> On the Slow Train

. . .
The Sleepers sleep at Audlem and Ambergate
No passenger waits on Chittening platform or Cheslyn Hay
No one departs, no one arrives
From Selby to Goole, from St Erth to St Ives
They've all passed out of our lives
On the Slow Train, On the Slow Train
https://www.youtube.com/watch?v=hUA-LEuo_XI
https://www.azlyrics.com/lyrics/frankturner/theslowtrain.html

1 Bethlem Royal, the Hood Unit: Robert Hobson
2 Fulbourn. David Clark: Malcolm Heron
3 Claybury. Dennis Martin: Elisabeth Shoenberg
4 Birmingham. The John Connolly: John Yerburgh, John Tibbitts
5 Gloucester and Oxford: Bertram Mandelbrote
6 Goodmayes: Raymond Gledhill, Dianne Lefevre
7 Leicester: George Spaul
8 Manchester: The Wilton: Barbara Dick
9 Paddington Day: Julian Goodburn
10 Shrodells: Alan Edwards, Philip Evans, Meg Sharpe
11 St Bernard's: Harold Bourne, Bob Hinshelwood
12 Kensington and Chelsea: Raymond Blake

We can still go to Cassel, Henderson, Frances Dickson Lodge, Ingrebourne and Grendon. There are new openings, in Reading with Rex Haigh and Jane Knowles and in Oxford with Geoff Pullen. The Association of Therapeutic Communities has its journal and its training scheme; Cassel and Henderson are providing us with splendid research data and their future, not so long ago in doubt, is now secure. Maxwell Jones, a founding father of the therapeutic community movement, could look with some optimism on the present and future situation of the therapeutic community concept, which undoubtedly will survive into the next millennium. I look forward to future Maxwell Jones lectures, which may fill in some of the unwritten history of the therapeutic community concept and movement.

Notes

1 This paper was given on 26 June 1998 as the Maxwell Jones Lecture for 1998 at the Henderson Hospital in Sutton. This is an edited version of the paper as published in 1999 in the *International Journal of Therapeutic Communities* 20 (1): 23–42. Acknowledgements are made to the editor of the journal for consent to its publication here. (Ed.)

2 We do not know if Foulkes was at all aware of Aichhorn's work in Vienna during the time when he was there doing his training, but though I have not traced any reference to Aichhorn in Foulkes's writings, there must have been overlap. This vignette will give a glimpse of Aichhorn's style. Introducing one of his delinquents

to an American visitor, he said: 'This one is a scamp! If he keeps it up, he is going to be a pimp in the Kaerntnerstrasse'. To which the man, in a comfortable relationship with Aichhorn, replied: 'But I am already a pimp in the Kaerntnerstrasse'. In the UK, Aichhorn's influence came through Anna Freud, F. C. Lenhoff (a fellow Viennese refugee educator) and Otto Shaw at Red Hill School, and his work certainly influenced Marjorie Franklin, David Wills and the planned environmental therapy movement (Mohr 1966). (MP)

3 This section was drafted for the paper's presentation in 1998, but unfortunately other commitments stood in the way of its publication. I am delighted to report that in 2017, Edi and Giorgio Pertegato brought out their excellent account of the life and work of Burrow, and I honour their fine contribution to the understanding of this otherwise *almost* forgotten pioneer. (MP)

4 In 1949 Burrow wrote: 'Harry Stack Sullivan helped himself lavishly to my material. I knew him at Johns Hopkins and he received throughout the years all my reprints' (Letter to T. Sancton, 28 September 1949, in Burrow 1958: 584).

5 In an interval at a theatre, A. A. Brill introduced him to Freud and Jung. A few months later, encouraged by Meyer, Burrow went to Zurich for a year of psychoanalytic study with Jung. (MP)

6 He was the first native-born analyst in America, the second after A. A. Brill – who was Austrian by birth – to train in Europe. (MP)

7 This anticipates the work of Mahler on separation/individuation and of Kohut with his notion of the self object, functions performed by the environment that are necessary to the infant's sense of well-being. Similar ideas are later to be found in the writings of Georg Groddeck and Ian Suttie. Another anticipation of Kohut is Burrow's assertion that the sexual drive, which Freud considered to be biological and basic, is a breakdown product of the psychology and physiology of the isolated individual. The sexual instinct seeks out a physiological and psychological continuity between the organism of one individual and another. Pursuit of sexual contact is the pursuit of the confirmation of social image rather than seeking for the completion of one's self through intercourse with the other. (MP)

8 The Champernownes were an ancient Devonian family who owned the Dartington Estate before selling it to the Elmhursts at the end of the 1920s, who then built up Dartington School. (MP)

9 Schumacher College, where 'small is beautiful' teaching is carried on, is also in nearby Dartington, another interesting confluence. (MP)

10 By his experience at Bethlem, Hobson felt that the personal cost to himself and to other members of the staff was too high, with serious psychological breakdowns, scapegoating developing to extrude from the community patients carrying the burden of unconscious acting out by the remainder of the community. 'One, amongst many other less obvious but perhaps more serious effects, is a chronic state: a narrowing of the lives of staff members as well as long-stay patients, who become devoured by the dragon unit. Then, they remain relatively out of touch with the rest of the world in the state of what can be termed an "exclusive incestuous regression"' (Hobson 1979: 232). (MP)

11 Another strange coincidence is that the administrator who tried to preserve the community but whose influence led to its closure in the end was a Major Foulkes! (MP)

12 Dr Marjorie Franklin (1887–1975) came from a leading upper-middle-class Jewish family. After training as a teacher at a forward-looking educational college, she qualified in medicine and turned to psychoanalysis, having worked with Adolf Meyer in America. Ferenczi was her analyst, from whom she went to Budapest, though after that, Ernest Jones seemed to doubt her mental stability in the early 1920s. She joined the British Psychoanalytical Society in 1926 and very soon applied herself to penology and delinquency. She was active in the Howard

League for Penal Reform and was amongst the initiators of the Institute for Scientific Treatment of Delinquency and the Portman Clinic. She was also an honorary consultant to the British Hospital for Functional Nervous Diseases. Soon she became convinced that in small therapeutic communities based on what she called environmental methods 'fundamental progress could be made'. Much to her surprise, she was appointed to the Research Committee of the British Psychoanalytical Society, where she took part in a discussion group on psychopathology and psychotherapy. There she met Lawrence Kubie, a future great figure in American psychoanalysis, and Dennis Carroll. Carroll was another psychoanalyst who, in collaboration with Edward Glover, pioneered psychoanalytic work with delinquents. Franklin and Carroll remained in close collaboration until his early death at the age of fifty-five. Franklin also seems to have collaborated with Anna Freud's associate Kate Freedlander, as well as with Melanie Klein's protégé, Paula Heimann, and with Klein's errant daughter, Melitta Schmideberg. Donald Winnicott also appears in the correspondence in the 1940s as an adviser on environmental therapy. (MP)

Section III

Development of method and technique in group-analytic psychotherapy

5 Aims of a wandering psychotherapist – Interpretation, dialogue, response

Changes in psychoanalytic theory and technique[1]

I am grateful for the opportunity to review changes in my own views on this subject. My paper could be subtitled 'Aims of a wandering psychotherapist', and I shall chart my course over many years of practice in both individual and group psychoanalytic psychotherapy. I hope to show that this dual experience is mutually enriching. A psychoanalytic psychotherapist as group conductor is a participant-spectator in the 'natural experiment' of persons engaged in free-floating discussion and is privileged to witness the unfolding of remarkable capacities for enquiry and understanding. He obtains an abiding respect for that part of the mind, the preconscious, that can be brought to consciousness through self-reflection and self-enquiry. My three areas of work – individual, group and therapeutic community – widen and deepen experience and contribute to what Mikhael Bakhtin has called a 'surplus of vision' (Holquist 1990: 241). By this he means that each vision occupies a unique position in time and space and offsets the limitations of the other. With a personal vision we can bestow on one another: my vision is not yours, yours is not mine. Together, our combined vision will extend our always limited grasp of reality.

Psychoanalytic psychotherapy in a new 'thought community' – and its history

During my psychoanalytic training, and for many years after, there was no forum in the British Psychoanalytical Society for the discussion of psychoanalytic psychotherapy. The divisions were firmly etched: Freudian, Kleinian, independent. Within the Psychoanalytical Society, most people wanted to practice full-time psychoanalysis. Michael Balint, who had been the president of the society and had wide influence in its thinking and practice, led a focal therapy workshop in a National Health System setting to give some of us the opportunity to form a 'thought community' – a kind of workshop. We did not need to question our psychoanalytic heritage and training but could question our practice and try to open new ways of seeing and hearing. We recorded our sessions on agreed lines, evolving new questions as our

DOI: 10.4324/9781003494713-8

experience grew: dynamic diagnosis; desirable outcome; change to be evaluated according to whether a shift in the underlying dynamic conflict had been achieved; true or false resolution; and final, careful follow-up. We kept each other on our toes. Balint was a hard taskmaster and questioned everything. What interpretations had we thought of and not given? Negative findings were to be reported, as was the aim of the therapist's intervention and how its effect could be assessed. The fruits of our endeavours in the early 1960s are well described in Malan's (1963) definitive book.

In the background was the influence of Franz Alexander, whose controversial book on psychoanalytic psychotherapy had pioneered brief psychoanalytic psychotherapy. Behind him stood the figures of Sándor Ferenczi and Otto Rank, whose early advance of revised principles in technique put them at odds with Freud. Alexander, who came originally from Budapest, led a team of skilled Chicago psychoanalysts who introduced the controversial concept of the 'corrective emotional experience' (Alexander and French 1946). This involves the deliberate adoption of an attitude towards the patient that might significantly affect the transference and the course of the therapy. Alexander's novel approach running through this work aroused a stormy protest in the American psychoanalytic community. Their protest was that Alexander's ideas sullied the purity of the transference neurosis. The 'orthodox' in the psychoanalytic community believed that the beneficial insights offered by psychoanalysis would arise – and arrive naturally – in response to the psychoanalyst's *correct* technique. This technique was seen to rest on the neutral, abstinent analyst giving their primary attention to the systematic analysis of the patient's defences whilst adhering strictly to the psychoanalytic setting.

But thanks to the changes introduced by the line of innovators described here, analysts can now openly reconsider elements of the psychoanalytic situation in themselves that may contribute to or reduce its therapeutic agency. The new constants are found in the constancy, availability and reliability of the therapist 'being there' and 'being for' the patient in the particular way each of us evolves from our own character, personality and experience. At seventy, I am different from the rather stiff, apprehensive, 'correct' therapist that I was in my thirties. I can well understand why some of my patients walked out on me, and I console myself by thinking that is what Dora did to Freud and that the analytic climate is experiencing some global warming. I have tried to teach my trainees how not to repeat my errors, to be more comfortable with themselves in the psychotherapeutic situation, and to offer a friendlier, less antagonistic stance to the patient, who is the anxious person who seeks our help.

Availability: Our main gift to the patient

Therapists in training and after can be over-occupied with the self-imposed task of presenting a 'correct' attitude and just looking for the traps the patient is laying for them. The person seeking help has a story to tell which they want to recount to this authoritative stranger. Our interest in listening, in making ourselves available to help the self-revelation that is the essence of the psychotherapeutic enterprise, is our main gift to the patient. It requires thoughtful listening, a listening out for the meaning of what is being said or not said. We try to feel something of the patient's psychic world, to feel our way into their situation, to determine what the underlying factors are that bring them forward for therapy now – and to formulate the problem in ways we can communicate back to the patient. The aim of the initial encounter is to offer the opportunity to know oneself more deeply and more openly, to create a coherent life story from what is already known and from what is yet to be known. The therapist-stranger can help in this through their interest and curiosity. The freedom to enquire, to offer a climate of enquiry, does to some extent distinguish psychoanalytic psychotherapy from psychoanalysis proper, where we can follow the recumbent patients' streams of consciousness, where thoughtful silence rather than a question may be a better contribution to the patients' self-explorations.

Herbert Schlesinger (1988) defined psychoanalytic psychotherapy as a treatment based on psychoanalytic principles that differs from psychoanalysis in some necessary but non-essential respects. He states that psychoanalytic theory takes a circular, not a linear course. We circle around the same issues, rediscovering therapeutic factors anew, but differing in our emphases on insight, experience, relationship and attachment. Where insight then was, relationship now appears: we listen again to Ferenczi, who returns from the exile to which Ernest Jones had sentenced him and who asserts, to Winnicott and Kohut, what we consider the essential qualities in the therapeutic relationship. It is essential to our understanding of a therapeutic action of psychoanalytic psychotherapy that we link the relationship factor to the interpretive process.

I return now to my formative experience in the short-term workshop where we aimed not to extend therapy beyond thirty sessions, though I valued the discipline and the necessity to think carefully about aims, intents, methods and results. After some years I did not feel as committed to that model. This was partly because I was no longer in a research team with its companionable support and challenge and partly because I was evolving my own style. Style, expression of the person in their work, is something we grow into through experience and, hopefully, maturity. Patients sense the offer we make - that we are available for this type of special and deep conversation, both compassionate and companionable, that is psychotherapy.

Maturity as a goal of therapy

Hans Loewald (1988) writes of the implicit factors in therapeutic action: therapeutic authority, based on aspects of the conduct of a good parent, teacher, educator or lover. The patient places us in these positions, as a matter not solely of transference to be resolved but of deeply felt needs and hopes for loving guidance, a guide in self-understanding. A therapist's self-understanding matures into compassionate objective understanding that goes beyond the patient's self-understanding and self-tolerance. Maturity, writes Loewald, has to do with adversities that have been met without becoming crippled or too damaged and with life experience that has been digested and metabolised.

I went through many stages to find my own style and I found it enlightening to look beyond the Kleinian/non-Kleinian debate. For a while I was impressed by Robert Lang's microanalytic study of the communication between analyst and patient, but eventually I found it somewhat obsessive and oppressive. I lived through the rise of the Kernbergian and Kohutian empires and learned from both. Kernberg (1975), who integrates British (mostly Kleinian) notions with American ego psychology, describes the early defence mechanisms of borderline and narcissistic personalities. I appreciated his clear delineation of the dynamics and structural analysis of the different forms of neuroses and personality disorders. I saw it as an extension of the work we had begun with Balint and Malan (Malan 1963). But in Kohut, I found something new to which I had an empathic surge: 'self psychology' has stimulated psychoanalysts to think and feel intersubjectively, and I found resonances in his work with Winnicott and Foulkes (Kohut 1984; 1985; Wolf 2002).

North American literature

In North American literature, I listened to the voices of Erik Erikson (1950), Heinz Lichtenstein (1977), especially Hans Loewald (1988; 1989), to René Spitz (Brody 1956) and Margaret Mahler (1968; Mahler et al. 1975). They were enlarging and deepening the field of psychoanalysis, using concepts of identity, self and the continuity of personal development throughout the life cycle. They were caught up neither in American ego psychology – the doctrine according to Heinz Hartmann (1958), Ernst Kris (1977) and Rudolph Loewenstein (1966) – nor in the British Manichaean struggle between good and evil objects in Kleinian theory. They began to link the psychoanalytic situation with the developmental situation of childhood and to see the links between good parenting and psychoanalysis.

Mentality, personhood

Our knowledge of what makes for good parenting is now so much greater and deeper through the work of John Bowlby and the school he fostered. Colwyn Trevarthen (Malloch and Trevarthen 2010) has led the research into intersubjectivity, and now we have Anthony Bateman, Peter Fonagy and Peter Hobson who lead us into the fascinating arena of how we human beings come to grasp the reality of our mentality and personhood and how we recognise these in others (Fonagy et al. 2002; Fonagy and Bateman 2004). What, you may ask, is the relevance of all this research? Firstly, a psychoanalytic psychotherapist has to be aware of and integrate the new information about the nature and growth of mind. Our job is to recognise the structure and dynamics of our patients' minds, to interact with them and to understand how we can facilitate the growth potentialities inherent in the psychotherapeutic situation.

Another area that has come into focus, belatedly but importantly, is the affective side of our nature. Psychoanalysis had bequeathed a limited concept of affects as the products of drive discharge, but now we know of the repertoire of emotions that are inborn and that form the 'anlage' from which our capacity for living rich emotional lives evolve and which we have to learn to manage. Joseph Jones, writing about affects, argues that two of the goals of the therapeutic process are very specific: (1) to help the patient expand, in both breadth and depth, his affective range, and (2) to help the patient develop the ability to think, culminating in the achievement of a certain type of mindfulness that leads to a deeply felt appreciation of life, including its tragic aspects. He comments on what a subtle art is the ability to think well – it can be one of an individual's proudest achievements. Helping the patient learn *how* to think is radically different from directing him *what* to think. The notion of the therapist as neutral or non-directive is, he suggests, a somewhat clumsy attempt to draw this distinction. If the analyst, in his heart, truly values the individual mind of the patient, then the technique will probably follow; if he doesn't then no amount of silence can possibly hide the fact and salvage the analysis (Jones 1995). Jones's writings resemble those of Hans Loewald (1988), who led a quiet revolution in our views on the aims of therapy.

Loewald and the psychic field

Of transference neurosis, Loewald states that if the patient can dare to take the plunge into the regressive crisis of the transference neurosis, bringing him face to face again with his childhood anxieties and conflicts, if he can hold on to the potentiality of a new object relationship, represented by the analyst, then this new discovery of objects (not the discovery of new objects) allows rediscovery of the early part of object development that can lead to a new way of relating to those objects, as well as of becoming and relating to oneself (Loewald 1988; 1989).

As analysis progresses, so patient and therapist constitute a psychic field and gradually come together from their respective polarities in the 'ego-activity' of scientifically guided self-scrutiny. This requires an objectivity and neutrality, the essence of which is love and respect of the individual and individual development. Loewald emphasises that the analyst's vision, as that of the parent, is directed to the possibilities of development that are latent and inherent but that can be reached through the organising understanding provided by the analyst. Thus, the analyst functions as a representative of a higher state of organisation and mediates this to the patient. Loewald calls analysis that kind of organising, restructuring interaction between patient and therapist that is predominantly formed on the level of language communication through which buried emotions can be unearthed and explored. But analysis does not consist only of verbal interpretations and Loewald makes mention of tact, as Poland does when describing how tact, basic rapport and its fluctuations, the analyst's breadth of life experience and imagination, the manner in which intercurrent events in the patient's life, incidents before, during and after the analytic hour, are handled—all these and other factors are significant ingredients of the therapeutic action. He describes this as the actual medium without which the most correct interpretations are likely to remain unconvincing and ineffective (Poland 1975).

A clear statement of the aims of psychoanalytic psychotherapy can be found in the work of the Mount Zion Research Group, directed by Joseph Weiss and Harold Sampson in San Francisco (Weiss et al. 1986). They believe, with research to support their thesis, that patients unconsciously seek to test the therapist in an effort to disconfirm pathogenic beliefs. Living a life determined by danger avoidance, unconsciously assuming that he would be endangered by awareness of warded-off mental contents, these unconscious defences can be lifted when the patient decides unconsciously that it has become safe to experience these contents. Pathogenic beliefs date from early childhood – for example, the belief that by challenging parents you risk punishment or humiliation, or that either dependence or independence is burdensome or worrying to parents – and these beliefs are transferred into current life experiences and to the therapeutic situation. The original twist of their approach is that, though suffering from pathogenic beliefs, the patient is unconsciously highly motivated to disprove them. The patient seeks the analyst's help in his efforts to disconfirm these pathogenic beliefs, and in essence, the therapeutic process is the way in which the patient does this.

The patient tests his pathogenic beliefs with the analyst, carrying out trial actions in the hope that the analyst will not behave as the beliefs predict. We know this through the way in which patients will test out the limits of an analyst's ability to understand or tolerate their actions, in the way that they court rejection or become seductive or overdependent in order to prove that the analyst/parent needs to possess and exploit them. Through the analyst not responding in a way that reinforces these pathogenic beliefs, and through the therapist's explanations and interpretations, beliefs move from unconscious to preconscious levels and can now be seen as restrictive and maladaptive. The patient has to transfer new knowledge into life actions, and the analyst tries to help the patient feel secure enough to face the dangers foretold by the beliefs. A process begins: patients begin to develop a more robust, realistic sense of safety and develop insights of their own unassisted by interpretation. Interpretation does remain an essential technique because it enables patients to retain insights in explicit verbal form, helping focus attention on insights and increase the ability to use them.

The underlying model is of collaboration rather than opposition and resistance; patients unconsciously wish therapists to help them to disconfirm pathogenic beliefs and therefore unconsciously bring crucial issues to therapy, efforts to solve problems. Seeing the patient as a person who is basically collaborating in the therapeutic process, as Loewald sensitively expresses, does help create a more positive attitude for the therapeutic enterprise than selectively concentrating on unconscious efforts to wreck therapy. We come back to the notion of therapy as a corrective emotional experience but an experience that evolves naturally in the course of therapy, in contrast to Alexander's experiments at modifying the analyst's attitude in order to provide those experiences. Tolpin (1983) has introduced the concept of the 'corrective developmental dialogue' in the interactions between infants and caregivers and between patients and therapists, which I find an attractive concept. It gives us the opportunity to look forwards and not exclusively backwards and to bring movement rather than petrification to the patient's experience in therapy.

In my work with patients who have come for further therapy or analysis after a painfully negative experience in therapy or a stalemate, therapeutic movement and change can occur when the therapist adopts this forward-looking stance and seeks out developmental opportunities that did not occur in the previous therapy.

I refer again to psychoanalytic tact and to 'therapist shame', which sensitises the therapist to the impact of their approach – to style, ambience, verbal and nonverbal interventions – the effect of which may not be taken into account and can relate to some unrecognised empathic failures. Greater awareness of the presence and power of the shame that the patient brings to therapy and to the shaming power of the therapist would make negative results less likely. Shame is overshadowed by guilt in much of our theorising, and a greater awareness of shame as the Cinderella of the unpleasant emotions – as described by Rycroft (1968) – can help us to understand many dark corners of the mind. Feelings of shame and narcissism are closely entwined, for shame represents the loss of an idealised self-image which itself serves as a defence against an unconscious self-image and body image. Shame attacks the self for being dirty, greedy, dependent, out of control, defeated and deficient. The management of shame is intimately connected to the regulation of self-esteem, to identity formation, and to the social image of the self. Rycroft says that if a person is unable to tolerate shame, he cannot acknowledge a defective self-image, and unless a person can acknowledge a defective self-image and a defective body, he cannot experience shame. Inability to experience any sense of limitation or deficiency goes hand in hand with inability to experience the affect of shame. Harbouring a denied defective self-image requires the continual effort of defence. It also precludes a person's learning from life's failures. Instead, each failure is experienced unconsciously by the person as confirmation of his self-representation as defective and must be warded off (Rycroft 1968).

If we are able to tolerate blows to self-esteem and can experience shame without significant ego regression, then we are able to modulate and contain the affect of shame and use it as a signal. Those who are unable to tolerate shame are overwhelmed by it and tend to respond to shame with ego regression, defensive grandiosity and impaired reality testing. Their self-esteem depends on a grandiose personality structure, behind which are defective self-representations, self-contempt and a lack of self-empathy.

Such powerful shame experiences interfere with emotional growth and the development of autonomy, whereas the capacity to experience shame without severe humiliation helps with the recognition of realistic limitations and helps to confirm one's sense of identity. If we help patients to be more in touch with feelings of shame and develop more capacity to tolerate them, this in turn enables the patient increasingly to acknowledge more shame-laden issues.

Shame and the countertransference

As analysts who are human beings, we may react to patients who feel ashamed by feeling ashamed ourselves, just as shame is evoked in those who witness the shame of another. This can tell us when we need to handle the patient very sensitively and must recognise how therapy can represent a painful invasion of privacy. The development of the capacity for shame brings with it the inner conviction of a good self despite imperfections. The person then has the capacity to develop a sense of self as unique and autonomous and love his/her imperfect self. I think that Hans Loewald would be very much in agreement with this description of the therapeutic process.

My final reference to shame is to quote Francis Broucek (1982: 369), who wrote that 'shame is to self psychology what anxiety is to ego psychology—the keystone affect! It is the basic form of unpleasure in disturbances of narcissism'.

Empathy

I turn now to empathy which – Freud (1921: 66) wrote – 'plays the largest part in our understanding of what is inherently foreign to our ego in other people'. Through empathy, we 'feel into' the experience of the other, an act which Kohut considers the essential and unique psychoanalytic activity – prolonged vicarious introspection into the patient's mental life, which can lead on to understanding and explanation.

Poland raised the question of why empathy, which Alex Strachey said was 'a vile word, elephantine, for a subtle process' has become such a feature in contemporary psychoanalysis (quoted in Margulies 1989: xi). He places this in an historical context (Poland 1975). In the early days of analysis, the question of what the analyst was to himself was, 'What do I know that I can interpret?' He drew on a stock of knowledge that the observer, the possessor of secure knowledge, could impart to the less knowledgeable one, the analysand. But this situation is no longer tenable, because we understand that analyst and patient create a dynamic field in which both are participants, though within that field each is different; the therapist bringing capacities developed through training. Now the analyst has to search within himself to discover the sources of his own knowledge, rather than relying on estab lished knowledge. He has to ask the question, 'How do I know what I know to interpret?' rather than 'What do I know that I can interpret?' And once we know what it is that we want to interpret, how do we convey this? Poland emphasises 'tact as a psychoanalytical function'. That follows empathy as the way we can use information gained via empathy to reach a patient through interpretations. Empathy is at the sensory end of the analyst's activities and tact at the motor end: 'We learn with empathy and understanding, and we interpret with tact' (Poland 1975: 156). Empathy involves some sort of a merger between self and other, analyst and patient; tact derives from separation. Having understood, we withdraw, become separate, and then re-establish contact verbally. Therapists' verbal tact has some of the qualities of a caregiver's soothing touch, bringing about union through touching while acknowledging the essential separateness between the parties. The concept of 'therapist's shame' describes the way in which a therapist, by sensitivity to the possibility of shaming the other, would himself be ashamed by doing so. A sensitive awareness of shame, of over-exposure to unfeeling probing and touching, can be a good guide to a therapist's activity.

Robert Emde (1990) outlines what he considers to be the ways in which the empathic process plays a significant role in psychotherapy. They are:

1 The caregiving role: 'developmental empathy'
2 The affirmative role: 'affirmative empathy'
3 The availability of the therapist: 'empathic responsiveness'

Through the caregiving of *developmental empathy*, the therapist gives opportunity for and aids the patient to discover potentialities, as good enough parents and caregivers do. They attribute intentionality to their charges, and the recognition of the intentionality that is latent in the child can become purposive. Here, empathy is a creative act within the therapeutic relationship. It can be playful and involve positive affects.

Affirmative empathy has to do with the way the therapist can enable the person to put together a sense of continuity and coherency of life, an affirmative sense of life pattern and direction, helping to knit together past and present, to have empathy for the self of the past and the self of the present. This comes about because of the shared affective field of therapist and patient, within which the patient can experience common humanity with the therapist but also his unique participation, personality and individuality.

The therapist's availability can foster trust, confidence and consistency of expectation, through the therapist's ability to regulate events within the shared affective field. Through regulation of affect, the therapist can handle and help the patient to understand their own feeling states and to make them manageable. Making them understandable involves interpretation or, as Kohut (1984) prefers to call it, explanation. Good interpretations encourage exploration and anticipate direction; within their shared affective field, the patient can use what the therapist has offered – consistency and availability – to take in that understanding and make it part of the self.

Emde (1983; 1990) asserts that these therapeutic functions of empathy repeat for the adult some fundamental motivational aspects of childhood development. We have inherent capacities for self-regulation, for 'social-fit' for affective monitoring. Self-regulation enables the child to feel in control of their 'social-fit', to understand, accept and integrate with the social world. Affective monitoring means to understand one's feelings and to understand the feelings of others. These capacities need emotionally available adults and can lead to:

1 Consolidation of an affective core as the early stage of self-development.
2 Having this, the infant self develops a sense of reciprocity, understanding of rules and empathy, understanding of others and an understanding of oneself, leading to a world of shared meanings and early moral internalisations, a sense of right and wrong, fairness and unfairness.
3 The next stage Emde (1983; 1990) calls the 'executive we': the child in a world of shared meaning, knowing with others, sharing in the knowledge, strength and capacities of the other: two together making one. This 'executive we' is both cognitive and affective, feeling in tune with and understanding the other. This sense of a sharing, the use of the self-object in Kohutian terms, is essential to the background of safety (Sandler 1987) for separation and individuation to occur. Mahler (Mahler et al. 1975) called this a stage where the adult becomes a 'beacon of orientation', shedding light on the world and being a safe place to retreat to.

A relationship with this powerful other in childhood, in adult love and in psychotherapy, leads to moments of intense feelings of togetherness and shared meaning, a sense of confidence, the power to cope with uncertainty and painful affects. Emde (1990) concludes that therapeutic action can be viewed as both a corrective emotional experience and as a corrective empathic experience if offered with sensitivity, tact and appropriate timing.

Self-empathy, empathy with oneself

An aspect of empathy less frequently referred to is self-empathy. Empathy with oneself implies that in the observing, judging, controlling and understanding parts of the self - the superego - the early introjects are able to receive and understand, accept and care for the anxieties, pains, fears and conflicts that the person experiences. Much psychopathology arises from the rejection persons feel themselves subject to, in their own inner worlds.

For Grotstein (1985), people become patients because of a breakdown or failure of self-empathy, and this incapacity follows on parental empathic failures. The process of learning from experience has to do with the interaction between knowing an experience and empathising with the self that is having the experience. Grotstein postulates, as do Joseph and Anne Marie Sandler (1987), the necessity for a background object of safety, built up in early development, that enables us to contain our own experiences.

Kohut and the self psychologists have emphasised the functions of self-objects needed for healthy development: to be soothed, protected, stimulated, educated and nurtured. These experiences awaken correspondence and responsiveness. They develop what Brazelton et al. (1979) called the 'reciprocity envelope', which holds the developing infant together within the interpersonal matrix. Skin-to-skin bonding, eye-to-eye gazing, speaking and listening all contribute to the building of this reciprocity envelope. Gaps in this envelope lead to distortions of homeostasis and are experienced as persecutions.

Through secure attachment, confidence in separateness develops; with separateness, empathy begins. The human condition of attachment and separateness from birth onwards is the dual track forming the core of the developing self. Confidence is built up in many ways: through positive and negative experiences, through complaints, if the infant's rage is understood and appropriately responded to. 'Complaining to the caregiver', a process with which we are all too familiar in psychotherapy, can build up confidence in the effectiveness of unreasonable complaints to bring about understanding and change.

Empathy enables two to experience the pain of the one and allows an infant to gain the experience of reciprocity and a sense of self. Failure to achieve this through failure of caregiver empathy can lead to shame, helplessness and ineffectuality, to defences that can lead to profound states of withdrawal and encapsulation. Grotstein (1985) outlines the development of 'perverse objects', which have a quality of hardness and continuity, and can maintain an everlasting presence. In the presence of these objects, the person experiences neither empathy nor kindness, neither understanding nor warmth. But this 'perverse object belief system' does provide a relationship, it gives continuity and eliminates doubts. In the presence of such internal hardness, it is forbidden to feel justified in feeling sorry for oneself; it is contemptuously disregarded as a shameful form of self-pity.

Feeling sorry for oneself is a natural function that enables us to preserve the sense of self in the face of pain and disappointment, for then we can soothe, contain, hold ourselves and eventually recover from distress in the way that the other, the self-object, had helped before.

Empathy betokens a state of faith in the relationship to an object, a sense of its protection, its nurture and stimulation. Empathic failure leads to a sense of autistic encapsulation, withdrawal, confusion and loss of coherency. Empathy gives a memory of having been contained, of being in relationship with a mother and a father who were able to bear the infant's pain without shattering, thus making the pain endurable.

Interpretation

My final words are about interpretation, an essential psychoanalytic act which I think of as the insertion of oneself through dialogue into the mental life of the other. Glover (1931) wrote an early paper on 'The therapeutic effect of inexact interpretation' that introduces the suggestive contaminant into the purity of psychoanalysis. A significant change in attitudes to interpretation is illustrated by comparing Glover's early paper with the recent observation by Ivri Kumin that psychoanalytic interpretations arise out of uncertainty. An analyst cannot know precisely in advance either the accuracy or the effect of his other interpretations because interpretations are conjectures about the unconscious (Kumin 1996). The effect of inevitable therapist errors can be experienced as a disillusionment, a small-scale repetition of misunderstandings, or of need failures in past relationships. Self psychologists have focused attention on these repetitive empathic failures, disruptions that reveal the therapist's transference significance to the patient and, along with this, some countertransference attitudes to the therapists that have led to the disruption. Disruptions promote self-reflections in both parties and, with that, a better chance for preconscious material to enter consciousness (Ornstein 1988).

Kumin (1996) proposes that the patient relates to interpretations on the basis of early developmental processes of phase-adequate holding, mirroring and affect attunement. I agree with Kumin that interpretations are in some senses a shared creation of analyst and patient, a transitional object within a transitional space, an object to be created and used, to find oneself in and eventually discard. Loewald (1988; 1989) describes the effects of good interpretations as an internal form of translation, enabling an intrapsychic mutual connection between unconscious and conscious mental life, whereby rational and irrational life mutually enlighten and enrich each other. Our therapeutic language can facilitate its own intrapsychic communication by establishing interpersonal communication. Our words and sentences – Bakhtin (1981) calls them utterances – have the potential of awakening memories and fantasies that bring back to life the persons or things they name, a symbolic summoning function. The primitive magic of words is in their 'calling' power, for to name an object is to call it into our presence. No one has expressed this better than Bakhtin, whose last written words are:

> There is neither a first word nor a last word. The contexts of dialogue are without limit. They extend into the deepest past and the most distant future. Even meanings born in dialogues of the remotest past will never be finally grasped once and for all, for they will always be renewed in later dialogue. At any present moment of the dialogue, there are great masses of forgotten meanings, but these will be recalled again at a given moment in the dialogue's later course when it will be given new life. For nothing is absolutely dead: every meaning will someday have its homecoming festival.
>
> (Holquist 1990: 39)

Note

1 This paper was presented to an unknown audience in 1996 and has not been published previously. (Ed.)

6 Dialogue and selfhood

Discovering connections[1]

Introduction: Dialogue, self and group matrix

Selfhood emerges from the matrix of primary relationships through the infant-caregiver dialogues. Current knowledge of early development clarifies the nature of these dialogues and confirms their significance. The group-analytic situation is based on dialogical exchanges, and in these situations it is possible to recognise and work with those dialogues and exchanges that are disturbed. By its very nature, group analysis has considerable power to facilitate the restoration of more sensitive and creative exchanges that can lead to the reemergence and transformation of self and self-identity.

The words 'dialogue', 'self' and 'group matrix' are at the growing edge of new developments in group analysis and also in psychoanalysis. The concept of dialogue has always been central to group analysis through S. H. Foulkes's (Foulkes and Anthony 1957/1965/1983) emphasis on *communication*, working towards an ever more articulate form of communication. These are the individuals' minds, the links between the members and their relationship to the group as a whole and to the conductor. All these links represent that network of communication that forms the dynamic group matrix. Foulkes takes the social nature of humankind as his starting point. Because we are all social, communication is central, vital to our development. Therefore, how communication becomes dialogue, how dialogue appears in the group, is central to group-analytic work. It is also central to the growing edge of the study of personality development in the earliest mother-infant relationships, work that also uses the concept of Self as a central essential notion, replacing earlier ideas based on instinct theory, where the 'other' is the object of instinctual drives or of massive projections from the inner world. These newer theories underlie notions of *mutuality* and *complementarity*.

The concept central for a *communicative* mode of psychotherapy is the self-other relationship from the very earliest days of life. It is from this self-other relationship that dialogue develops. When dialogue is halted, broken or derailed, positions of personal isolation develop and parts of the self become encapsulated, lost to mature development. The ways in

DOI: 10.4324/9781003494713-9

which these isolated parts develop and the ways they are coped with lead to problems of personality, neurosis and, in the extreme, psychosis. Psychosis has been defined as that situation in which there is no other with which the self can engage. The whole experienced world becomes self, a desperate denial of, as well as a desperate search for, the other.

Foulkes conceived of the group as a natural arena for therapy because he viewed the very mind of the individual as a group. We are born into a group, develop intricate and close relationships with others in our basic group unit of family and clan. We learn to speak the same language and these constant complex interactions become our mind. Though we may regard our mind as the most precious and personal aspect of ourselves and hence attempt to guard it from change through interaction with others, our own mind is, in essence, a group matrix. 'Just as the individual's mind is a complex of interacting processes (personal matrix), mental processes interact in the concept of the group (group matrix)' (Foulkes 1975: 130). Thus, in the group what is reproduced is basically the matrix of evolving personality.

Foulkes postulated two levels to the matrix of a small group. First is the foundation matrix, which represents the basic culture in which we are born and which we hold in common with all humanity; this must involve our genetic structure. Erik Erikson (1950/1995) said that humans are born with an instinctual capacity to adapt to that segment of nature that has personal meaning – that is, the relationship with mother. Mother is not an isolate; she is part of the reproductive pair which itself is part of the social group. Foulkes wrote:

> Group psychotherapy uses the group and its power for therapeutic purposes . . . but does not treat the group for the group's sake, to improve its working efficiency, in the way . . . a team might be treated. The group is treated for the sake of its individual members, and for no other reason. All psychotherapy is, in the last resort, treatment of the individual.
>
> (Foulkes and Anthony 1957/1983: 32–33)

Then there is the dynamic matrix which is an organised system formed, maintained and changed by the flow of meaningful information – communication – between its members. This is the dynamic matrix in which communication channels link and join members into a whole.

We fully grasp the nature of the matrix by recognising that complex, living, open systems are not described in terms of energy but through meaningful information. Human behaviour is described and explained through meaning, not through causes, through information, and not through energy alone. Seeking meaning is related to pattern recognition and information is communicated through modulation in the energy carrier, as Ernest Hutten (1983) emphasised. It is the wave pattern of the electrical impulse that gives information that can be read, not the electrical impulse itself.

Developmental theory

I now outline the model of self-development that evolves from the group-analytic approach which dovetails with the most recent of child development studies, such as those of Daniel Stern, Louis Sander, Robert Kegan and Colwyn Trevarthen. These workers have shown how rich and active is the very early field of experience, the exchange between infant and mother. They form an interactive, open, communicative system in which communications are at their highest when the system is at its most open. For instance, in terms of infant feeding, it is when the infant's hunger has been satisfied that there is a rich exchange of signals between infant and caretaker. This involves some sense of mutuality and reciprocity that leads to the beginning of a sense of intersubjectivity. These very basic exchanges between self and other take the form of a rhythm, 'now you, now I', as described by Leal (1983). These have been termed 'proto-conversations' and are initiated in the context of participation in a caring partnership. Attachment between infant and caretaker will only occur securely and helpfully if these basic exchanges have taken place plentifully and satisfactorily. It evolves to become an externalisation of an effectively established communication system serving as a protective shield for the developing child.

Contingency, the experience of actions and reactions initiated by oneself, is a vital point to consider. It is the basis for the games that infants enjoy from very early in life. There is a pleasure in seeking out and finding responses contingent on the infant's own initiative. People become important to the infant because they 'play the game' with the infant – infants are genetically equipped for the game of reciprocal feedback. Humans are equipped for the experience of two-sided modifications of behaviour with implications of mutuality and expectations that another will complete one's own actions. Self-other is again the basic paradigm. In this game between self and other, there is always a place for the pause: my action, a pause, your reaction; your action, a pause, my response. The place for the pause, so clearly pointed out by Donald Winnicott with his spatula game, is the place and time for the *between* to develop, and it is in this 'in-between' space that communication, growth and differentiation all take place (Winnicott 1973: 75–76) and dialogue develops (Winnicott 1967/1971; 1968). If the pause is not accepted or respected, the infant becomes anxious and withdraws. Secure attachment takes place on the basis of these earlier proto-conversational actions. Where they have been properly established, attachment takes place healthily; where they have not, attachment takes place on the basis of a false self, on anxious dependency, on a one-sided appeal to seduce or coerce the caretaker into providing safety for the basically insecure infant. 'The world then seems a dangerous seducer and novel things appear as threats to the baby's dependency needs' (Leal 1983: 193).

Secure attachment is the basis for further developments within the infant-mother relationship. Emergence from that relationship occurs by the differentiation of self from other. This is mediated through the development of the third area of mind, that which develops in relationship to the toy, the 'transitive other' that appears in transitional space. The infant now is able to look for responses in the world outside that are represented by the mother. As the infant finds the toy that responds to play, the infant also finds himself or herself as an active agent. Beyond the toy, the infant finds his or her father and siblings.

The basic rhythm of discovery of self in search of the other, and by obtaining the responses of the other differentiating the other from self, is the basic rhythm of human development. Kegan (1983) speaks of the lessons we can learn by watching unselfconscious therapy taking place in nature – that is, the natural and healthy responses of caretakers to their infants. What we see the mother offering is a culture of embeddedness, shown visually and auditorily by her recognition of her infant through gaze interaction and echoing – by all her holding capacities, as emphasised by Winnicott (1965/1985) in his account of 'the maturational process and the facilitating environment'. The mother also terminates the embeddedness by allowing and fostering bridges from herself to the toys and to other people. Winnicott (1968) spoke of the mother progressively failing the infant, leaving the infant to develop his or her own capacities and to do without the mother continuing to minister to his or her omnipotence.

The contribution from self psychology

All that I have briefly outlined is fully compatible with the basic approaches of both group analysis and self psychology. The latter has drawn the attention of the psychoanalytic community to the self-other developmental paradigm. This paradigm has been developed by other psychologies but, within psychoanalysis, we have lost sight of it (in both the classical and the Kleinian schools); though you will remember that Ronald Fairbairn (1949) asserted that we do not grow out of dependency, but rather, we move from immature to mature dependency. Kegan (1983) writes that the communal culture of embeddedness throughout the life cycle in different forms is determined by the levels of the relationships between our self and other, and Heinz Kohut (1971) describes how we never give up our self-object relationships. They are always with us, and we are always embedded and intertwined in a matrix of self-object relations. Throughout life, we struggle for individuality and for meaningful belonging, and this is the paradox in which the human being is forever immersed. It is the recognition of this paradox that informs the group analyst in his or her therapeutic stance and technique.

The essence of the group-analytic process can be described as the presentation of oneself: the losing and re-finding of oneself; the differentiation of oneself from others and from the group as an entity; the embedding and emergence of oneself in the group matrix, which the individual himself or herself has helped to create and to modify. Mirror reactions and resonance are of the essence in these group-analytic processes.

Ego training in action

Foulkes (Foulkes and Anthony 1957/1965/1983) uses the term 'conductor' for the therapist in the group, which leads directly to a consideration of the music and rhythm of the group. There is a rhythm in the creation of meaning, of mourning for loss and the discovery of meaning for oneself, within the group situation. Foulkes described these processes as 'ego training in action' (Brown 1994/2000). The self is faced with the complexity of a group of selves, of others. We are faced with discrepancies that we have to struggle to resolve, and at each stage in which we have resolved these discrepancies we are able to move on to deal with greater complexities and to make sense out of the ever-changing realities of the group. Rhythm, empathy, attunement – the rhythm of individuality and belongingness are ever constant in the group. This is a situation that cannot appear in dyadic therapy unless the situation becomes one of 'encounter' as described by Martin Buber (1958/2000). The latter is far removed from the formal psychoanalytical situation, though closer to the client-counsellor relationship of Carl Rogers. It is likely that Buber's conception of the subjective nature of the 'I-Thou' relationship influenced the climate of thinking and practice in Frankfurt, where he and Foulkes shared common origins.

Group-analytic theory has insisted on communication as the therapeutic factor par excellence. In group-analytic theory, symptoms represent blocks both in communication and in relationships that can be resolved through verbal exchanges under group-analytic conditions. What are these conditions, and how do these changes come about? These issues are now addressed and consideration is given to some fundamental aspects of human personality formation that have their basis in dialogue and in communication.

The contribution from Mikhail Bakhtin: Communication, monoglossia and heteroglossia

In the theory and technique of group analysis, communication is privileged as the major therapeutic force, above that of interpretation. The theory of group analysis itself is based on dialogue: a dialogue between psychoanalytical psychology (a one-and-two-body psychology) and social psychology (a three-and-more-body psychology), both set against the background of an historical psychology that interweaves society and the individual as society itself evolved.

Because there is a dialogue between these different voices, individual, social and historical psychologies, group analysis escapes becoming a dogma, a condition called a 'monoglossia' by the Russian savant Mikhail Bakhtin. In contrast to a monoglossia is a 'heteroglossia', a condition where several languages are in dialogue, which gives the possibility for the growth and change blocked by dogma. Bakhtin, an explorer of psychology and language who lived and worked in Soviet Russia under conditions that made him very sensitive to such situations, wrote that each culturally predominant group strives to legislate its dialect as *the language*. Whilst it is in reality only one dialect among many, its social prestige turns other dialects into implicit forms of cultural opposition (Morson 1986).

Bakhtin even extended this model to the language of psychoanalysis. Taking the psychoanalytic concept of consciousness and unconsciousness, he regarded unconsciousness as representing language that is both suppressed and repressed, while consciousness represents language that is officially sanctioned. Thus, both consciousness and unconsciousness represent states that are determined by personal and social forces. Bakhtin took issue with psychoanalysis and its fundamental distinction between primary and secondary processes. He argued that at a particular moment in time – the end of the nineteenth century – psychoanalysis had biologised language through the influence of Freud. The language of primary process, of the id and of the instinctual drives was relegated to biology, as drives were seen to originate in bodily processes. According to Bakhtin this rendered the human being an abstract biological organism outside of history. For Freud (1913), the human drives were outside history (other than for his Lamarckian speculations about the inheritance of acquired characteristics). Take, for instance, Freud's theory of group formation: the murder of the father by the sons leads to the totemic brotherhood, which is the origin of group formation. For Freud, groups do not exist as a natural and primary form; they are secondary to the vicissitudes of individual drive and individual narcissism.

But when we take history into account, we have to accept Bakhtin's challenge and account for the emergence of psychoanalysis at that particular time, at the end of the nineteenth century in Western society. That is, we have to develop an historical psychology, not a biological one. Group analysts should here remember that Kurt Goldstein, who had a powerful influence on Foulkes, was a philosopher of biology. Goldstein (1939/2000) escaped from this psychoanalytic dilemma because, by his use of Gestalt psychology, he took into account the fundamental fact that the organism constantly attempts to adapt as well as it possibly can, to its ever-changing environment. This environment is both the external environment and the organism's own internal environment. The external environment is cultural, the internal environment is developmental. As regards the external environment, as pointed out by Norbert Elias (2000), contemporary Western men and women have to adapt to a very different social situation than their ancestors of 500 years ago. Society has taken over the regulation of violence, and individuals have to internalise the control that society exerts over the individual's aggressive tendencies, in exchange for which the individual is protected from the violence of others. Thus, the very drives that might otherwise be seen as internal and external are always subject to the 'colossal forces of society' that penetrate the individual through and through. These changes in society profoundly affect the culture of the family in its child-rearing practices, and this is reflected in the cultural differences between communities.

Group-analytic theory

Group analysis preceded modern psychoanalytic object-relations theory by taking communication and dialogue as its basis: dialogue between self and other, between self and society and by discounting the supremacy of the biology of drives. Intrinsic to such concepts as self and other, of *alterity*, are concepts of response, reciprocity, interplay, shared experiences in a shared dynamic field bounded by space, time and circumstance. Let us take a closer look at the word *circumstance*, meaning that which stands around us. As we work within a group circle, in which each one derives meaning in relationship to those who stand around us, such a word is central to our theoretical framework. We bring persons together into a group of which we ourselves are an intrinsic part, and we accept to work out together with the group members our individual and collective destinies. It was the Spanish philosopher José Ortega y Gasset (1963: 45) who answered the question, 'Who am I?' with the answer, 'I am myself plus my circumstances'. Circumstances are both human and nonhuman, thus again the individual is profoundly influenced by the environment. It follows also that 'myself' is both an 'I' and a 'you', a 'we' and an 'us', formed as we are through the circumstances into which we are born and within which we are raised. To ourselves, we are both subject and object; with others, we are also both subject and object.

What connects us to other persons? Basically, it is our emotions, our intuitive appraisals of the relationships that we have with others and of our significance to them as well as their significance to us. Emotions, which are both physical and mental, connect us to ourselves, to inner worlds of sensation and experience, of body and imagination, and emotions connect us to the worlds of others, a world of other bodies, other feelings, fantasies and experiences. We have moved theoretically beyond conceptualising emotions and affects as isolated drives. Emotions are connectors to consciousness, to community, to cooperation, and in the fields of groups to such concepts as group cohesion and group coherence. Emotions drive us towards and away from others, those others who are both present in the external world and as internalised representations in the inner world. The experience of being driven may have led Freud to his concepts of the biological drives, but as George Klein pointed out, our experience of being driven does not logically lead to conceiving of drives as entities. There are indeed peremptory forces, which exert pressures upon us to act, but there are more adequate ways of conceptualising our experience of being driven than to ascribe them to hypothetical drives, which, in themselves, have no explanatory value (Klein 1976; Reppen 1980).

The concept of drives in psychoanalysis belongs to the realm of the one-body psychology (Rickman 1957a; 1957b; Schlapobersky 2016). All the words I have used that begin with 'co-' indicate how we are intrinsically linked to each other. Consciousness means 'knowing with others', so knowledge belongs to the realm of thought, which derives from the experience of language. Before verbal language, there is the pre-language of gesture, interplay, attunement and state-sharing, as modern infant observation and research clearly shows. Here we can recall how the Russian psychologist Lev Vygotsky (1962/2012) insisted that the social precedes the personal, as the person develops from exposure to social processes such as language.

Dialogue as the basis of human development

Each one of us is unique, an entity existing in our own experience of space, time and personal history. No other person can occupy the time and space I occupy, and conversely, I cannot occupy the space and time of any other person. Each one of us has a viewpoint that is not available to any other but that can complement and fill out the viewpoint of the other. For this, Bakhtin used the phrase 'a surplus of seeing' (Holquist 1990: 35–37). What is meant by this? Physically, I cannot see behind me, cannot see the back of my head or my trunk, therefore my own body image is incomplete. I need a mirror, or two mirrors, to complete my own picture of my physical body. The mirror adds to my capacity to see. The surplus of seeing that each one of us has lies in the fact that I can complete the viewpoint of the other. I can see what the other cannot see, just as he or she can see what I cannot see. There can never be an identity between persons of what they conceive and perceive. Thus, for completion of my own self, to see myself 'in the round', I need the viewpoint of the other, just as the other needs me to complete his or her own self-perception. But this completion is always incomplete: there is never a final completion, neither to myself nor to the other; the self remains an unfinished project. This leaves Bakhtin to state: 'The other is in the deepest sense my friend. It is only from the other that I can get myself' (Holquist 1990: 149–151). For this notion of the building of the self through actions we undertake with others, Bakhtin uses the term 'architectonic', a term for the construction, the building, the architecture of the self.

In his concept of the social construction of the self, we can see the basis for this powerful observation that 'What the self is answerable *to* is the social situation; what the self is answerable *for* is the authorship of its responses'. Thus, we are always adapting to the pressures and demands of the external environment, our context. How we respond is our responsibility. In this context, the self is figure against the ground of the context.

Dialogue of therapist and patient, of group conductor and group members

I now turn to the dialogue of therapist and patient, of group conductor and group members. An important aspect of this dialogue is represented by the therapist's attempts to grasp relevant aspects of what is happening in the therapy situation and to offer these in his or her own words to the listeners, the other group members. This brings us into the realm of interpretation and of the many meanings of the word *interpretation*. The ones I want to concentrate on here are:

- An interpreter offers an understanding to speakers of different languages that they can share, thereby helping to connect them. In the therapy group, each group member brings a different personal language of response to the situation, and the therapist tries to understand these different languages and make them understandable amongst others.
- Interpretation is a term used for a performance and therefore has an artistic and aesthetic connotation. To my mind, the therapist's interpretative act is the insertion of himself or herself through dialogue into the mental life of the other, whether individual or the group.
- Interpretation is a speech act that seeks a response. In some ways, interpretation is an act of revelation, an attempt to gain access to what is hidden, but to be effective it must be a cooperative act; the other, the patient, the group members, must be in a position that enables them to release, to reveal, to offer up hidden aspects of the self to the interpreter and to each other.
- Conversely, the speech acts of our patients are directed to us for our hearing and for our response. An interpretation, therefore, is an offer to the other of a possibility of recognition and understanding, an offer of the human response; at its best, it is a creative and aesthetic act.

Bakhtin wrote of the human situation, of the speech that seeks a response, as an *utterance* (Holquist 1990: 59–63). An utterance means that the words are spoken forth into the world, into a social context – every utterance has a context and seeks a response. His final words on dialogue are given at the end of Chapter 5, and here again I will call on some of his most resonant language: 'There is neither a first word nor a last word. The contexts of dialogue are without limit. They extend into the deepest past and the most distant future. . . . Nothing is absolutely dead: every meaning will someday have its homecoming festival' (Holquist 1990: 39).

To return to the group situation and the relationship between group analysis and self psychology: we can understand that the group represents a very basic, maternal entity from which the individual has become separated in the course of development. We can see it now as functioning in one or the other aspect of the way stations of narcissistic development as they are described by Kohut (1971) – that is, as either the mirroring parental object or the idealised, grandiose parental object. Through the mirroring function of the group, confirmation of weak areas of self-identity occurs, leading to a sense of empathic understanding and tension reduction. The group as the idealised object enables the individual to share his or her own narcissistic self-investment with that of the group, experienced as comforting, powerful and wise. And these are not mere illusions, for the group is, indeed, much wiser than the individual, and the group does in reality confirm and support the person through anxious and depressed stages of existence. The group also provides the opportunity for what Kohut increasingly came to recognize as important in human development: the opportunity for twinships and partnering, here following the path that had been laid out by Harry Stack Sullivan (1964). He showed the importance of pals and friendship in the development of the latency and of the early pubertal child. Indeed, one of the vital areas of human development that has not been properly recognised in psychoanalysis is the nature and function of friendship. This is not surprising, because friendship is not desired or recognised in psychoanalysis; we talk about therapeutic alliances, splitting of egos, but the asymmetry of the analytic situation scarcely allows for the development of friendship. And yet the psychic strengthening that comes from the establishment of secure friendship is undeniable (Kohut 1971).

I return to a further consideration of friendship later. Now I want to draw your attention to some further structural-dynamic processes inherent in the group-analytic situation.

Dialogue

Group analysis develops a culture of acceptance and understanding, of safety, support, confrontation, participation and ever-increasing communication. The therapist establishes a stable structure within which this can occur and, in doing so, accepts and fulfils the function that Foulkes (Foulkes and Anthony 1957/1965/1983) called the 'dynamic administrator'. The therapist is the executive of the group; he or she is vested with power and authority by society and this is *not* transferable to group members. In this sense, the therapist retains the ultimate authority. However, at the same time, in functioning as the conductor of the group, the therapist uses the very structure he or she has created, using power and authority in the service of the therapeutic aim, which is the facilitation and increase of communication and understanding, the furtherance of psychological growth. This is a transferable function that increasingly becomes the property of the group itself as the agent of change. Foulkes described this in terms of the crescendo in the authority of the group, which allows for a decrescendo in the authority of the therapist as the group develops. This is an essential paradox of group analysis.

Another essential paradox is that there are two ever-ongoing principal functions in a group situation: *holding* and *containment*, which maintain the earliest and most vital conditions for psychological needs, the maternal functions emphasised by Winnicott (1958a, 1958b, 1960, 1965) and W. R. Bion (1962). At the same time, the culture is based on *analysis* and *translation* – that is, the higher mental functions of adult life.

Thus, there are inherent contradictions in the group situation - a delicate, stable, yet unstable balance that has constantly to be monitored and managed. Each therapist develops a personal style of management and of conductorship in which he or she attempts to enhance the group's authority over itself yet respecting the therapist's managerial authority. This will be tested out again and again. Foulkes talked of this as the move from being leader *of* the group to being leader *in* the group. The therapist's style of management arises from their inner world, inner authority relationships, their own assembly of rules, controls, and boundary functions based on his or her personal development.

These earliest functions of containment were developed by Bion (1962), though long after he had ceased to work with groups. Intolerable tensions and pains of the infant's experience are transmitted to the mother through projective identification. The mother responds intuitively, transforms what is intolerable into that which can be tolerated and this then allows for the development of mind, for thought and for curiosity. Failure of containment by the mother leads to breaks in relationships and to breaks in intrapsychic experience, interference with thought and with curiosity. In extreme cases it can lead to a hatred of emotion projected onto external reality and to attempts to destroy the capacity for perception and for thought. This results in the fragmentation and massive projective identification of psychosis.

The group-analytic situation, which develops a culture of acceptance and understanding, reenacts these early developmental processes. The members learn to contain and tolerate the painful, they learn to be able to think in the face of pain and learn to tolerate their thoughts.

Against the background of this growing capacity to contain, there will be many instances of excessive projective identification, as when, for instance, a person gets put into a role that serves to carry unwanted emotions or experiences for the rest of the group. The person becomes isolated, possibly scapegoated. The therapist, verbalising the question of how the person gets into such a situation, why he or she needs to be there and why the group needs this person to be there and begins to put into words what has happened silently and unconsciously. This is a fostering of dialogue, a verbalisation of inner feelings, wondering aloud about feelings that take people over. It is by identifying with the therapist who speaks about the unspeakable that the members' capacity to hold and recognise their own feelings grows.

From patient to self in the group

I now consider some essences of patienthood and selfhood and how the move from patient to self in the group context may be conceptualised. To be a patient in an analytic setting is to face the task of self-revelation before another who does not reciprocate with a corresponding act. The patient is uncovered; the therapist remains covered. Another way of describing the therapeutic setting is to say the patient talks about what is most *private* to a person who is professional, therefore a *public* figure.

Leon Wurmser (1981), a masterly writer on shame, observes that analysis is a situation of almost ruthless exposure and intrusion into privacy, a shameless procedure he describes as the art of self-revelation, met by disciplined respect; yet shame is its unavoidable companion. James Anthony (1978) also describes analysis as 'an arena of shame'.

How, then, can a person evolve, mature, become more himself or herself in this arena of shame? In early human development, as I have indicated, growth takes place in an arena of mutual responsiveness where shame may be said to be absent or minimal. Some of the answer is to be found in the exercise of analytic tact, of empathy, of sharing in an accepting and fundamentally supportive environment. What constitutes this support?

Gaston Bachelard (1992) said that human beings are 'half-open beings', always partly exposed, partly covered. The nature of our covering and the respect we show for this need lies in the recognition of the *protective* function of shame. To be ashamed is to be uncovered before oneself or before others, inappropriately, suddenly, painfully. The nature of tact – a word that derives from the Latin *tangere*, 'to touch' – is to touch gently, sensitively, inoffensively. We cannot expect a group of patients always to exhibit such tact. Indeed, frequently patients will be insensitive, hurtful, provocative. Yet with the maturation of a group over time, as people grow in their capacity to empathise, and to see aspects of themselves in others and to accept that others are aware of them on reciprocal terms, the sensitivity and depth of understanding grows. This leads to that extension of the range of articulation and communication that Foulkes saw as the essence of the therapeutic process.

For the therapist, we should remember the imperative need for 'therapist shame', which will guide him or her to acting tactfully. In the Dora case, Freud (1905) painfully learned that this therapeutic task was not boldly and unashamedly to uncover what was hidden from his patient's self-knowledge, to bring to light what human beings keep hidden within them. When Dora no longer disputed Freud's interpretation about her hidden sexual wishes for Herr K., she opened the next session with the words: 'Do you know that I am here for the last time today?' (Freud 1905: 105). And at the end of that hour, despite Freud's continued attempts to show her *his* truth about her, she said goodbye and came no more.

We can recall here what Foulkes (1964; 1975) said about avoiding 'plunging' interpretations, which do not respect the need for balance between surface and depth and for recognising the sensitivity of the interplay between private and public domains. Correct interpretations are not necessarily good interpretations. They can be experienced as attacks and humiliations. Truth is not objective and impartial; it is always *personal*. It is only in the development of trusting personal relationships that people can reach to and speak out their truths, that speech will reveal more than it conceals.

This brings me back to the point of departure of these comments, to the nature and importance of friendship. In friendships we can be intimate with ourselves through the opportunity of intimacy with others. This is why our patients value the group and why they need and use it, despite their fears about the stresses and pains that are inseparable from the group experience. And that is how they, and we, inch our way along the difficult path from patient to self in the group context.

Note

1 This paper was presented to an unknown audience in 1996 and is an edited version of the paper published in 1996 in *Group Analysis* 29 (3): 327–341. (Ed.)

7 The self as a group

The group as a self[1]

The notion of 'the group as a self' is challenging. Is there any point in linking an individualistic notion such as the self with the plurality of a group? The rationale for doing so becomes more evident when we consider in the first place 'the self as a group'. For if there is an essential element of 'group' in the constitution of the individual, as indeed group analysis affirms, then it becomes more possible to consider that there is value in regarding 'the group as a self'.

Indeed, group analysis gives primacy to the social. The individual is conceived of as being born into and constituted out of a network of other persons and gains a sense of personal identity from the possibilities offered by the nature of the network. The horizontal or lateral dimension of social organisations, therefore – notions of culture, politics, religion, economical and historical circumstances – have to be considered as constituents of the individual self. Norbert Elias uses the term 'figuration' to indicate our fundamental connectedness. This is in contradiction to the notion of the individual as a monad, standing alone amidst a multitude of others, connected through instinctual needs or for self-preservation: the vertical dimension. The notion of a plurality of selves, rather than a single unitary self that constitutes the person is closer to psychological reality and is gaining recognition. Thus, the idea of 'multiple selves' does not relate only to pathology, as in the concept of 'multiple personality disorder', but is representative of the multifaceted complex structure of each one of us.

Modern Western society released individuals from the grip of compelling religious ideologies but has left us with the problems of constructing our own individual identities. One of the pioneers of Western psychology facing the question of personal identity was the great American psychologist and philosopher William James. He distinguished between the 'I' and the 'me', between the physical, material and spiritual aspects of self, and he tried to deal with the question of how a sense of personal identity is created and maintained against the background of the constantly changing, flowing level of consciousness. Edward Sandford Martin (1882) elegantly epitomised this problem in his poem 'Mixed':

DOI: 10.4324/9781003494713-10

Within my earthly temple there's a crowd:
There's one of us that's humble, one that's proud;
There's one that's broken-hearted for his sins,
And one who, unrepentant, sits and grins;
There's one who loves his neighbor as himself,
And one who cares for naught but fame and pelf.
From much corroding care I should be free,
If once I could determine which is Me.

The individual identity of each one of us is constituted by intrapsychic, interpersonal and transpersonal processes; the boundaries of the individual extend far beyond those of the corporeal self. Along the dimensions of selflessness to selfishness there is a wide range of human behaviour. All of us contain and manifest traits of selfishness and selflessness. Sometimes our self-interests dominate, related to our personal concerns which, as William James (1890/2017) pointed out, can extend to those persons and things that represent parts of ourselves, our family, children, prized possessions. Selflessness at its extreme leads to acts in which persons willingly give up their lives in the service of others, as when a father or mother will risk death to save their children, or comrades will endanger themselves to aid others, to situations where people give up their lives for symbolic causes, for nation, religion or politics.

If we grasp the complexity of the individual both constituted from and functioning as a group, it becomes less problematic to look at the contrasting notions of 'the group as self'.

The cultural anthropologist Clifford Geertz (1973) defines a person as a bounded, unique, more or less integrated centre of awareness, emotions, judgement and action organised into a distinctive whole and set contrastingly both against other such wholes and against its social and natural background. This concept of the person is holistic, bringing together consciousness, affect and conation within a bounded entity, set as figure on ground, against its social and natural background and contrasting with other such bounded entities, other persons. Could this description not also apply to certain types of groups? It could apply to a family, to a group held together by a common history and by powerful bonds of attachment, a group which allows differentiation but still retains a distinctive wholeness. This is the notion of a group-analytic group.

The theory of group analysis derives from social psychology, from Gestalt psychology, individual psychology, primarily psychoanalysis and from a sociohistorical viewpoint on the nature of human personality. This makes it imperative to set the notion of 'the individual' against the sociohistorical background of family, society and culture. Norbert Elias coined the term 'figuration' to illustrate how an individual can only be understood as part of a connected set of relationships, a figuration. In group-analytic theory and the practice of face-to-face therapy in the group circle, we rely on Foulkes's concept of the *matrix* which develops from the web of interrelationships occurring in the group situation, the *dynamic matrix*, set against the *foundation matrix*, based on the biological and on the sociohistorical cultural setting from which individuals derive fundamental aspects of their personality (Roberts 1982). Amongst these, one of the strongest factors is the sharing of a common language, as language is the filter through which we perceive and apprehend both external and internal realities. I want now to consider the notion of 'the group as self' in relation to our concept of the matrix.

The matrix is the shared common history of the group, the conscious and unconscious repository of all events. The group analyst's faith, belief in the matrix concept, enables him or her to offer this to the group members from the moment of conception of the group in the mind of the therapist. By offering a group-analytic situation to the individual seeking therapy, there is already in mind a field of interaction, a social space that is somewhat, though not completely, empty. It is to be filled by the evolving history of the group, through which each group member brings to this new potential space their own personal matrix drawn from their family and life experience. The resultant matrix is derived from the intermeshing of all these personal matrices within the setting offered by the group analyst. The therapist offers and maintains the boundaries of time, space and the search for meaning, which shapes the dynamics of interaction of the individual members. The therapist maintains a belief that it is possible to understand 'the group as a whole' and attempts to see the dynamic interactions within the group matrix, as figures against ground of the evolving group history. Thus, the group offers both a *culture of embeddedness* and a *culture of enquiry*.

The culture of embeddedness enables each person to develop a strong attachment to the group situation, to the other group members and to the group conductor. The culture of enquiry offers group members the opportunity to investigate the nature of their own self and the natures of their group neighbours. This culture of enquiry both enables and requires persons to look at and listen to others, to themselves, and consider, perhaps accept, the viewpoint of others. This is an opportunity to see ourselves 'in the round', to see those invisible and hidden dimensions which constitute our individual selves, for just as we cannot see our physical selves without reflections from mirrors, so we cannot perceive ourselves as social persons without the seeing and hearing of the responses of others to us and considering, if not always accepting, the ways in which we are experienced by others.

The Russian philosopher/psychologist Mikhail Bakhtin described the human situation as one of 'alterity' (Holquist 1990). By this he means that we gain ourselves only through our dialectical relationships with others. We need the other to aid in the creation and completion of ourselves, through the vision the other bestows upon us. Each one of us has a 'surplus of vision', as compared with any other person, for each one of us lives in a unique space-time dimension which Bakhtin termed the chronotope. What we see can be seen by no other person; others can thereby give us aspects of the world that cannot be ours. The other person is ultimately my friend, the person through whom I gain myself; the other can therefore be a cause for celebration rather than frustration and conflict.

Healthy human beings grow within a *culture of embeddedness* where others provide reciprocity, gratification and impetus for continued growth. Within the culture of embeddedness provided by good-enough caregivers to infants, the vital developmental processes of attachment and relatedness develop. From attachment and relatedness develop both autonomy and connectedness, the psychological double helix of human life. The thrust of research into early human development exemplified in the work of Daniel Stern (1998), Robert Emde (1980; 1981; 1983; 1988; 1990; 1992a; 1992b), Beatrice Beebe and Frank M. Lachmann (1992), Alan Fogel (1993), Colwyn Trevarthen (1979, 1993a, 1993b) and Hanuš Papoušek, Uwe Jürgens and Mechtild Papoušek (1992), amongst others, points to the central reciprocity of human relationships. Rita Leal (1968, 1983) in her papers on group analysis and early infant development, defines *reciprocity* as an 'inborn organized capacity for initiating, maintaining and terminating social interactions'. 'Turn taking' – action, pause, response, interaction – is the basic rhythm of human life as pointed out many years ago by Margaret Mahler (1968; 1975). Through this turn taking of gesture, and later on through language between infants and caregivers, the basis is formed for fundamental procedures of communication through language, whereby the person enters not only into the cultural system but also into the moral systems of society. Reciprocity implies a sense of fairness, of good-enough exchanges between persons that leave both partners satisfied. From this fundamental biologically rooted sense of reciprocity leading to a sense of fairness develops the drive to 'get it right' and to get satisfaction from doing so. Getting things right means also putting things right when they have gone wrong; that is, the drive for reparation and the origins of the sense of 'getting things wrong' from which comes the sense of human guilt, without which human relationships become impossibly destructive. Thus, the human infant and its caregivers are 'prosocial' beings, biologically programmed to turn towards and care for others. The very early smile of the newborn infant, appearing at only two weeks, is a prosocial gesture that increases the bonding between itself and its caregivers.

The school of self psychology (Kohut 1971) has added the concept of the 'selfobject' to the psychoanalytic vision of object relationships. This fundamentally refers to the functional relationships caregivers provide so that the infant's developing sense of self is affirmed, strengthened and repaired through the vicissitudes of the early years. The well-known functions of mirroring, idealisation and twinship, to which now can be added the idea of friendly opposition, are essential to the infant's developing sense of self. What needs, however, to be added to the self psychological vision is that of the active interaction between selves, the self of the infant and the selves of the caregivers. The infant seeks out and receives the active responses of the caregivers, seeking in particular a sense of completion of its own actions. By the response of the other the infant begins to derive a sense of efficacy, of closure, of contingency, of acting in the world in such a way that the world begins to take on a satisfying sense of shape and meaning. The infant's cries obtain appropriate responses, its physical gestures elicit reciprocal gestures, its cries and gestures are interwoven into narratives and plays, and the infant begins to enter human culture. What is important is the acquisition of 'mentality', the sense of possessing a mind of one's own in a world where meaningful contact can be made with other minds. This is the world of intersubjectivity, not simply of other relations.

To elaborate upon this, object relation theory is grounded in a system of categorisation, that of subject and object, inner and outer, which centres primarily upon the psychic life of the subject. There is much reliance on projection, drives, fantasies and a belief that the psychological precedes the social. The group-analytic viewpoint is complementary to this. Here the social precedes the psychological, internalisation precedes projection, the categories of subject and object, inner and outer, are not taken as constituents to the early sense of reality. Foulkes stressed that the social is so deeply within the individual that one cannot begin to say where the social ends and the personal begins. Where is the boundary between inner and outer? Is reality not more like the Moebius strip, where the same surface endlessly turns both inwards and outwards (Foulkes 1964)?

Another contribution from early development to 'the self as a group' comes from recognition of the essential 'we-ness' of human beings. No one of us survives and develops outside a nexus of relationships. George Klein (1976) put it many years ago that psychoanalysis lacks the concept of the 'we-go' to complement that of the single ego. Now Emde (Emde et al. 1991) offers the concept of the 'exclusive we', the sense that the infant discovers, enjoys and utilises the capacities of the caregivers to act in concert, to achieve a sense of power and effectiveness in the world. We help the child to grasp, to walk, to talk, and in this we freely share our executive powers. Freud (1923) wrote of the ego as being the rider on the horse of the id. But how can we fail to think of the child riding on the back of the parent or of the older sibling secure in sharing in the power of that greater entity of which it feels itself to be a part? Emde describes the 'executive we' as creating a sense of togetherness, bestowing a sense of power and control for guiding behaviour and for resisting temptation! This approach combines well with the approach of Vygotsky, who through his 'law of proximal development' showed that the potentiality of any individual, particularly a child, can only be estimated properly when it is in the proximity of and in relationship to a more developed other (Wertsch 1991). The child will succeed much more successfully, whatever task it is set, when aided by or in the company of another person who will help it to get it right. This is the basic nature of the human condition and one which we draw on freely in the group-analytic orbit – that of human beings who are trying to understand and to help themselves and each other.

Note

1 This is an edited version of a paper first published in 1996 in *Group Analysis* 29 (2): 183–190. It was then issued in *Self Experiences in Group* (eds. I. Harwood and M. Pines), Jessica Kingsley, pp. 24–29. Grateful thanks are extended to the editor of *Group Analysis* for permission to reproduce it here. (Ed.)

8 The contribution of mirroring and resonance to psychoanalytic and group-analytic dialogue[1]

Psychoanalysis is a form of communication that occurs in a privileged setting where, uninterrupted, the therapist facilitates for the patient a new internal communication that widens and deepens the person's self-experience. This sonorous process, the exchange of meanings, is many-layered. The desired aim is to reach a phase of free association for the analysand and of free-floating attention for the analyst.

In this paper, written about therapeutic communication and conversations in the group-analytic setting, I shall concentrate on two specific processes that arise in group-analytic groups: mirroring and resonance. I will look at how they arise in groups conducted by a trained group conductor in a secure setting with selected patients and a group composition that aims to put together a group with a reasonably good work capacity.

> Mirror reactions are characteristically brought out when a number of persons meet and interact. The person sees himself, or part of himself – often a repressed part of himself - reflected in the interactions of other group members. He sees them reacting in the way he does himself, or in contrast to his own behaviour. He also gets to know himself – and this is a fundamental process in ego development – by the effect he has on others and the picture they form of him.
>
> (Foulkes 1964: 110)

Foulkes also writes of the child's emergence from narcissism through the greater awareness of the self, evoked by reflection coming from outside, which helps him to differentiate between what he is and what he is not (Foulkes and Anthony 1965/1983).

These clear, simple descriptions could only be made after Foulkes observed groups in action. His account acknowledges that our capacity for self-knowledge is always limited and can be enlarged through observation of others. We all have parts that are known to ourselves, yet knowable to others; if we accept to be in an open relationship to those observing others, we will see ourselves more in the round, more in depth. Experience confirms that explorations, exchanges of insights and outsights, are therapeutic and

DOI: 10.4324/9781003494713-11

that under the right conditions, group members can be helpful, both to themselves and to others. Foulkes called the underlying change instrument 'ego training in action' (Foulkes and Anthony 1965/1983) and this was later elaborated by Brown as 'self-development through subjective interaction' (Brown 1994/2000). As knowledge of child development extends, so we recognise the crucial role of factors such as empathy, sensitive responsiveness, contingency and agency, and proto-conversations (Schore 1994). These events unfold in the group-analytic situation.

Mirroring, procedural and semantic memory

I have gathered these processes under the concept of mirroring and tried to link them with current research into the vital process of visual exchanges in early childhood. These have confirmed and extended our knowledge of early development. Infants are visibly active from birth, seeking visual intercourse, and are able to imitate adult facial expressions. Equally, adults are programmed to provide 'biological mirroring', which is an essential step in the birth of intersubjectivity: to provide the infant with the dawning awareness that outside and beyond themselves, someone else is there. A possible link with events in psychotherapy has been suggested involving the mind neuron structure. The mirror neuron system stores and encodes unconscious, non-reflective behaviour patterns, patterns of responses that are called *procedural memory* (Stern et al. 1998). This is the unconscious memory of how things are done – riding a bicycle, playing a musical instrument – as opposed to *semantic memory*, which is a conscious verbal recall. If responses to trauma are encoded thus, they will be unconscious defensive actions to prevent re-traumatisation, but these very actions block any possibility of change. However, we know that being with another during frightening situations, another who remains calm, caring and friendly, can protect against traumatisation. Anna Freud and her colleagues at the Hampstead Nurseries showed this through their work during the Blitz with children in London under bombing (Midgley 2007). Similarly, being with a therapist who remains calm and understanding, who shows compassion and caring when a patient is reliving a traumatic situation, brings about a corrective emotional experience. This can be seen as a form of mirroring that signals safety, a non-interpretative, yet significant, component of change in psychotherapy.

Mirroring between infants and caregivers

As I have described in an earlier paper on the subject (Pines 1997), mothers begin to connect with their babies visually from the very earliest days; they look into their babies' eyes, looking for contact and recognition, for interaction, for the play of the eyes. The infant and the mother who look into each other's eyes are looking into the central nervous system of the other as the eye, the retina, is the extension of the brain. Indeed, the wider the pupil, the more intimate the exchanges (Hess 1958). The pupils dilate in states of pleasure and communicate interest. Babies prefer to look at people whose pupils are dilated, and the babies' own large pupils release caregiver behaviour. A mother's animated facial expression, looking joyfully at her infant, is like a searchlight that evokes brightness in the infant's eyes – the interplay of eyes.

Thereby, infants and caregivers tune in to shared affect states, which leads to the beginning of intersubjectivity, the knowledge that there is another out there who is like me and who understands me. In these mirroring transactions, the mother expresses her joy, which stimulates the baby's vitality affects, enhancing the feelings of strength, vigour and agency. These experiences further the attachment bonds between infants and caregivers. Shared attentional states, shared interest in objects looked at together, such as the toy in the baby's or the mother's hand that is played with, is a way of sharing mental states. The mirror neuron system can be said to be activated in such play.

How infants learn about their own affect states through parental mirroring responses

What we call parental mirroring is of course radically different from self-observation in the physical mirror. Between one to two years, infants are very interested in their mirror reflections and discover that the mirrored actions are identical with their own. But parental mirroring is always different: we smile, laugh, talk, commiserate, interact. The question of what the infant learns from parental mirroring was raised by Gergely and Watson (1996): how does the infant begin to feel that its affects belong to the self? How do parental actions contribute to that learning? And how do we begin to link inner and outer?

We want the baby to know that our displays are responses to and *markers* of the infant's feelings: I know that you are hungry, upset, cross, happy; I want you to know that I know, that we understand each other; I want you – baby – to know that I am responding to, mirroring, your experience. We do this by producing exaggerated versions of realistic emotional expressions, a process which has been termed *marking,* as in pretend, 'as if' play (Gergely and Watson 1996). The baby can find out that this *pretend* version of emotional expression belongs to the parent but corresponds to the feeling state of the child. Gergely and Watson called this process *a social feedback model* of affect mirroring. Fonagy describes 'a complex biosocial system in which the infant is instinctually driven to express the dynamic changes in his internal affect status behaviorally, while the mother is instinctively driven to reflect the infant's state-expressive behaviors in a marked form' (Fonagy et al. 2002: 190).

Two developmental functions are derived. First, the mirroring environment helps in regulating the infant's affective state changes, and second, it provides a kind of 'teaching' or 'scaffolding' environment that results in the internalisation of maternal affect-regulative function as the infant begins to recognise its own emotional states (Vygotsky 1962/2012). The mother's ability to adaptively 'mirror', 'echo' or 'match' the infant's affective states is a significant central mechanism underlying the early development of self. Here we can refer to Bion, Mahler, Kohut, Stern and of course Winnicott, who suggested that the infant looking at the mother who is looking at it sees itself in her face. This, says Winnicott (1967/1971: 131), is because when 'the mother is looking at the baby *what she looks like is related to what she sees there*' (emphasis original).

If, however, the parent does not reflect a baby's anger but expresses his/her own anger, the parental response will not help the baby to regulate or modulate its own state of anger. Instead of a negative feedback situation, a positive feedback results that escalates the affect and can result in trauma. This can lead to states of confusion or to projective identification, in which the infant is no longer able to locate its own feelings within itself but either experiences the mother's anger as if it were its own, or misattributes its own anger to the other. A further possible misattribution is when a parent responds 'wrongly' to the infant's affect display. If the parent misunderstands the infant's erotically coloured excitement about physical contact, inducing anxiety and defensive anger in the mother due to her own conflicts in relation to bodily tenderness, she will respond to the infant as if it were displaying aggression rather than joyful excitement. These processes can lead to distorted self-representations.

These considerations can influence our mode of relating to patients, especially to children, who have not become secure in 'pretend play' and therefore become locked and frightened of the affect states of their instinctive drives. It is here again that therapeutic mirroring can help to normalise distorted early mirroring pathologies.

Conclusion: Mirroring responses in positive and negative states

The Narcissus story in Greek mythology continues to hold our attention down the centuries, and our fascination with its narrative is closely related to our subject today. In conclusion I will relate this mythological figure to a story that we have from Hans Christian Andersen (1983) – the story of the ugly duckling.

Narcissus had rejected all human approaches and had no experience of the benefits that come from exchange with others. His sole companion was the maiden Echo, and she could only repeat his words. Thus, he had no experience of otherness, the otherness which makes for change and difference. This story stands at the opening of our enquiry into the developmental stages of mirroring responses. In the very earliest stages, when mirroring represents predominantly the active response of the other in a dyadic relationship (mother-infant), love is only a potentiality. The infant is, as it were, a pupil, seeing himself in the mirror of the mother's eye, bathed in her vision, feeling her love and satisfaction expressed through her holding and caretaking. Her responses to his gestures give meaning and intentionality to his developing self-concept; when he experiences disapproval, disapprobation, it is within the overall context of the positive relationship; her positive mirroring serves to contain the negative. Hope predominates and the ugly duckling will discover that he is a swan – mirroring is predominantly benign and reflective.

However, when the mirroring response is more negative, the infant's early experiences are of one who is not a *subject* but an *object* to the other, who does not predominantly give and receive pleasure in rhythmic responses with the mothering person. He is prematurely objectified to himself and with sometimes tragic consequences, the ugly duckling remains as he is, never to discover that he is a swan.

Note

1 This paper was given to an unknown audience, we believe in 2000, and has not been published previously. (Ed.)

9 Changing times, changing realities

A group-analytic perspective on the history of psychotherapy[1]

I shall first look at the birth time of group analysis, which was during the third decade of the last century. A change in the zeitgeist of psychotherapy was emerging, a shift in consciousness towards the social. Social and industrial psychologists were examining groups and organisations in the Hawthorne experiments to better understand how persons behave when grouped together in both large and small groups (Wickström and Bendix 2000). Pioneers of what later became the therapeutic community movement – self-governing communities that were first established for rebellious adolescents (Eichhorn in Austria, Homer Lane in England) – were then extended to other populations. The movement included Kurt Lewin's research in field theory that led to the recognition that there were benefits in democratic organisations, when compared to authoritarian or laissez-faire regimes. Many aspects of these developments have already been discussed in Chapter 4 above, 'Forgotten pioneers: An unwritten history of the therapeutic community'. In this chapter I will relate some of these developments specifically to psychiatry and psychotherapy in the UK today.

In psychiatry, the pioneers included Jacob Moreno (1932), Louis Wender (1936) and Paul Schilder (1938). An anlage was being laid down for what, under the pressure of war conditions, led to the first Northfield experiment of Wilfred Bion and John Rickman, followed by the second experiment led by Tom Main who brought in S. H. Foulkes, Harold Bridger and others. Maxwell Jones's exploration was parallel and was more socio-psychological than psychodynamic. Fired with enthusiasm at these new approaches to treatment and rehabilitation of war-stressed and neurotic soldiers, psychiatrists and psychologists created new organisations within psychiatry. They included outpatient clinics for group therapy of neuroses and personality disorders and inpatient settings for sociopathic patients, as at Maxwell Jones's Henderson Hospital. Main's Cassel Hospital developed inpatient psychoanalytic psychotherapy with a combination of individual and group techniques, all set in the context of a therapeutic community. Chronicity in mental hospitals was challenged by introducing new dynamic methods of patient management.

All this was over half a century ago, and for over forty years now I have been part of the group-analytic movement. I will give you some reflections

DOI: 10.4324/9781003494713-12

and perspectives on the development of group analysis over this time and a glimpse of its possible future. Enthusiasm lights the flames and leads to action; action has to be organised into theory and practice that can be transmitted to teaching; and eventually, practice has to obtain the sanction and support of the wider community.

Developments along these lines show trends of very specific kinds in different parts of the world. North and South America have different histories, though we should note here the work of the pioneer Swiss Argentinian psychoanalyst Enrique Pichon-Rivière (1971; 1995), whose work with 'operative groups' has had a powerful impact in Latin America. Quite independently of Europeans, his work has striking convergences with group analysis. Beyond this, I will confine myself to developments within Europe.

In England, the two great group traditions are connected with Wilfred Bion and S. H. Foulkes. Bion's became known as the Tavistock approach and Foulkes's as the group-analytic approach. Bion's basic assumption theory has been very influential through his writings, principally his *Experiences in Groups* (1961/1998). This book has an everlasting appeal for, on reading it, we are in contact with a powerful and creative mind, one who has the gift of seeing group phenomena in an entirely new way.

While we continue to reap a rich harvest from Bion, his later work on the epistemology of thought and its destruction in psychosis has had less influence on group analysis than his earlier work on the basic assumptions. I am in the process of editing, together with Robert Lipgar, a book that we have called *Building on Bion*, which will to a considerable extent focus on this later work (Lipgar and Pines 2003a; 2003b). Bion's work has not yet been developed into a widely accepted clinical tradition but has found its niche in the study of organisations, the training of people to work in them, and the study of large groups.

The major clinical school in group therapy has been that of Foulkes. His work has been at the core of the teaching at the Institute of Group Analysis in England and has been central to group-analytic work in Scandinavia, Germany, Croatia and Slovenia, and latterly throughout Europe. Here in Italy, it is well-represented in Turin, Rome, Bologna and Palermo.

A critical reappraisal of Foulkes is underway by group analysts, who find some insufficiencies and inconsistencies in his work. This is a healthy and desirable development, without which a work will stagnate into sterile repetition. The field has recently had two significant challenges, one from Morris Nitsun (1996), with his anti-group concept, and the other from Farhad Dalal (1998), who differentiates orthodox Foulkes from radical Foulkes.

Nitsun's basic thesis is that Foulkes overemphasised the potential benefits of group analysis and underplayed the negative forces inevitably unleashed in the group. These forces are beyond resistances; they are intended – unconsciously – to destroy the possibilities of progress and change. Though I do not altogether agree with Nitsun's thesis, he has raised our awareness of these powerful, unconscious negative forces.

Dalal's differentiation between orthodox and radical Foulkes is based on his research into the influence on Foulkes of the sociologist Norbert Elias. The two were friends and colleagues from their time together in Frankfurt, a city where, in the 1930s, psychoanalysis and Marxist social theory were brought into close contact. Foulkes and Elias continued to meet in England, where Elias at one time thought of becoming a group analyst. Fortunately, he did not, for we would have lost his invaluable contribution to sociological theory. He gave us the model of 'homo apertus' as contrasted to 'homo clausus' in which he emphasised that human beings can never be seen as separate entities: we are connected in 'figurations', chains of interdependency (Elias 2000). Foulkes's thesis certainly corresponds to these fundamental features of Elias. According to Foulkes, each of us is a nodal point in the psychic network (Foulkes 1948; 1964; 1975; Foulkes and Anthony 1965/1983). Here he was adapting the thesis of his teacher, the neurologist Kurt Goldstein (2000), that the functioning central nervous system is always a synaptic network. Only when damage occurs does part of the network become isolated, thereby causing symptoms. For Foulkes, this is the position of the emotionally disturbed person who ceases to be part of a well-functioning psychic network. The strength of the therapeutic or experiential group situation is that it creates a network in which the person can once again become a functional part. Dalal asserts that Foulkes was trying to live in two camps – that of psychoanalysis on the one hand and that of group analysis on the other – and could not fully commit to the latter. In making this assertion, Dalal has brought the work of Elias from background to foreground (Dalal 1998).

Now I want to widen the focus. Group analysis is essentially an open system, incomplete in itself and influenced by developments in the neighbouring fields of psychology and developmental psychology, in particular attachment theory, evolutionary genetics and scientific models such as complexity theory. Relational psychoanalysis is a development within psychoanalysis that argues for the primacy of complex interpersonal and intersubjective experiences in the construction of personality. Self psychology, originating in the work of Heinz Kohut but now a much wider discipline, also argues that we should take self-experience as the centre of our psychology and to a large extent gives up psychoanalytic structural theory and ego psychology. Influenced by self psychology, I have offered the thesis in Chapter 7 that as the Self is a Group, so the Group can be seen as a Self, a unit made from diversity.

I propose now to look at the current world of psychotherapy in the United Kingdom, but I am sure that our experience is in many ways similar to other European countries. We have a comprehensive National Health Service, which most persons seeking psychological assistance have to turn to. Seriously underfunded for many years, the system fails to meet the needs of the public. Biological psychiatry is what is predominantly funded, taught and researched. Evidence-based medicine is in fashion, and psychotherapy is challenged to provide evidence of its own efficacy. These evidence-based models do not fit well with psychotherapy, but nevertheless the demand has stimulated significant research projects, some of which I will now present. They mostly concentrate on the treatment of personality disorders, as it is widely accepted that these are not amenable to pharmacotherapy, other than for the reduction of acute symptoms.

I am impressed by advances in the psychological theory of personality disorders. Recently, I attended the Fourth European Congress on Personality Disorders, 'New Trends in Personality Disorders', held in Paris. Much attention was given to severe personality disorders, principally borderline personalities, and it is to research in this area that I now turn. We have known for a long time that some borderline patients can well be helped in group-analytic groups. We have advocated that only one or two borderline personalities can be contained and helped in a well-functioning group-analytic group, but serious research in this area is recent.

I will begin with the clear exposition on the nature of borderline personality and the essentials of treatment by British psychiatrist Jeremy Holmes (2004). He gives guidelines as to how these persons can be helped in non-specialised psychiatric services. Patients with severe personality disorder are in general poorly served by non-specialised psychiatric units. The disturbed interpersonal dynamics typical of such disorder manifest themselves in the relationship with mental health workers, leading to friction, stereotyping, manic enthusiasm or despair. Psychodynamic concepts that may help relieve these negative consequences include understanding the deficient mirroring and excessive use of splitting, projection and dissociation that are characteristic of severe personality disorder. Insecure attachment and inability to self-soothe are also typical. Psychodynamically informed management needs to recognise these features and to use an approach that identifies those who are suitable for intensive psychotherapy, those for whom a supportive approach is best, and those who need to be kept out of the mental health services altogether. Psychotherapeutic treatment involves providing a secure base, limit-setting, responsiveness, and training in self-soothing and realism. For inpatient settings, group sessions are essential, as they allow disruptive behaviour to be acknowledged, contained, understood and resolved or worked through. This contributes to the inpatient experience as a 'living-learning' experience, to use the phrase from Maxwell Jones (2013).

I will continue to refer to some writing of Holmes (2004), a general psychiatrist working in the National Health Service who has played a leading part in the integration of psychotherapy and general psychiatry. He has written a foreword to an excellent book, *An Introduction to Group Work: A Group-Analytic Perspective* (Barnes et al., 1999) where he writes that group analysis has an invaluable part to play in the running of organisations such as psychiatric units. Group analysts, psychiatrists and non-medical colleagues work within complex bureaucratic structures created to give the appearance that something is being done. Psychiatric work is regulated –

over-regulated – by governmental policies, some of which are helpful by indicating the standards that should be aimed at, while others are hindrances. There is a danger that institutional defences are put into place, giving the impression that if only the correct procedures are followed, there will be satisfactory outcomes to clinical work (Menzies Lyth 1960). Hidden beneath organisational procedures, paperwork and hierarchical structures are the mental pain and emotional distress of both patients and staff. Paperwork can become a substitute for mental work of the group – the work of containing fears and anxieties on a collective basis, of facing inadequacy, the partial successes that are often the best that can be hoped for, the inevitable relapses and failures.

The more a group can admit to fears and failures, the less likely it is for failure to occur. Staff groups that aim at open communication of feelings aroused by the work have to overcome group defences of splitting, projection, denial and scapegoating, and therefore need skilled leadership. Beyond the staff who are engaged in the clinical work, and their own management groups and structures, they need leadership from 'outside' or 'above' – dynamic groups that can open the culture to review – but it is all too often just not there. Management regularly regard staff groups set up for consultancy or support with suspicion, viewing them as indulgent time-wasting procedures. It is notoriously difficult, but essential, to hold management and clinicians together for the organisation to be able to carry out its primary task of dealing with mental distress.

Other workers have produced impressive evidence of the efficacy of specialised centres such as the Cassel Hospital, where the research department is headed by Dr Marco Chiesa. His paper 'A combined in-patient/out-patient programme for severe personality disorders' (Chiesa 1997) describes the two-stage programme at the Cassel Hospital: six months of inpatient psychotherapy, followed by one year of twice-weekly group-analytic groups on an outpatient basis. The programme has been devised to meet the needs of former inpatients for support to deal with life problems, which they meet after hospitalisation. The group therapy, which is held in another hospital to demarcate the difference in the inpatient and the outpatient setting, is conducted with an orientation largely influenced by Bion. The aim is to contain and interpret primitive emotional experience and attacks on such experiences, to show the patients how unconsciously they act out using defences of splitting and projective identification.

This programme reduces the period of hospitalisation, thereby lowering costs and increasing turnover. Knowing that continuing group therapy is going to be available has the effect of raising the patients' optimism and tolerance of uncertainty and provides a sense of continuity. Also, the shorter period of hospitalisation reduces some of the anxiety connected with the sense of entrapment that the hospital can engender.

An alternative model has been described by Anthony Bateman (Bateman and Fonagy 1999; 2000). They describe the programme at St Anne's

Hospital where there is an inpatient period of up to eighteen months followed by outpatient groups for three to four years, again on a basis of two meetings per week. While in the hospital, the patients attend a small group three times a week and a large group twice a week. The therapists are specially trained nurses. The patients also have one individual session a week, the aim of which is to stimulate reflection on their experiences and to enhance mentalisation.

What these programmes provide, either as inpatient or outpatient programmes, is a secure base for treatment. The ingredients of the secure base must include consistency and reliability, the capacity to deal with aggression and protest without retaliation, and the ability to offer appropriate mirroring and empathic responsiveness. These features can be offered in well-conducted group therapy. Groups represent a potential space in which aspects of the inner world can be projected. The inner worlds of these patients are characterised by fears of annihilation, emptiness and boredom, which stimulate anxiety, panics and self-destructiveness. In a well-selected and conducted group, the patients under the leadership of the therapist create this secure base for themselves. The group becomes an emotional bank to which they all contribute and in which they are all shareholders. They invest in building up the group as a reliable, consistent base for the expression of emotions and attitudes. It is there for them to draw upon when needed to meet their many different needs, for support, understanding and working through problematic relationships. The group leader or conductor has the task of ensuring the survival of the group through attention to limit setting, to boundary maintenance, and to representing and maintaining the search for meaning, the culture of enquiry and meaning attribution that characterises the psychotherapeutic enterprise.

In the institution the therapeutic team has to work together to understand the behaviour of the patients and to guard against those projections that lead towards splitting and the creation of conflict in the team. These patients with severe personality disorders lack the internal experience of a good parental couple who would be able to care reliably for their children. Over time, this is what the team can become, which allows for the internalisation of the relationship to the therapeutic environment and the release of patients from their fear of inner emptiness. Slowly, patients come to recognize that they are 'held in mind' by the therapeutic team, which begins to reduce the unconscious fear of emptiness and annihilation that haunts patients with severe personality disorders.

Bateman and Fonagy summarise very well the essential ingredients of the psychotherapeutic enterprise for these patients. Individuals with personality disorders derive benefits from treatment through carefully considered, well-structured and coherent interpersonal endeavour. This allows them to internalize a thoughtfully developed structure – to understand the interrelationship of different reliably identifiable components, the causal interdependence of specific ideas and actions and the constructive interactions with professionals.

They benefit above all through the experience of being the subject of reliable, coherent and rational thinking (Bateman and Fonagy 2000).

Silvia Corbella (2003) presented her work in Paris to the French meeting on Personality Disorders. She states that group work enables patients to confront their experiences of separation and individuation, which have led to pathological object relations. The group setting sets up a space of acceptance, listening and thought, where through shared and shareable memory history can be built. This allows for the awareness of self and other as objects of value, enhancing the capacity for symbolisation and thus to think in a responsible and adult way. The members learn to endure the frustrating time of waiting and of risk, to overcome pathological splitting and dichotomous logic, and to face the complexity of ambivalence and life.

The National Health Service is funding two further Henderson Hospitals, having been persuaded of their clinical efficacy and economic benefits. The future seems bright with regard to personality disorders. However, the future is not so bright as far as psychosis is concerned. The Scandinavian model of the psychosis team, which treats the outbreak of a psychotic disorder with the urgency that is given to acute physical illness, scarcely exists outside the Nordic countries. However, the evidence of this rapid teamwork being efficacious is so good that in time the model will be more widely adopted.

Group analysis is gaining ground in the field of chronic mental illness. Recent books by Walter Stone (1996) and Nick Kanas (1996) show how psychotic illnesses can be understood and managed in group therapy. My co-editor Victor Schermer and I have produced a major book on the psychotherapy of psychoses, *Group Psychotherapy of the Psychoses* (Pines and Schermer 1994; 1999), and an Italian translation is being planned.

Forensic group therapy is gaining ground. There is a well-known prison in England, Grendon Underwood, where all the therapy is on a group basis and the prison staff have been trained to do this work. Broadmoor, the high-security prison hospital in Berkshire, has a psychotherapy department and outpatient forensic psychotherapy is well established. I have described this range of developments in more detail in an earlier paper (pp 42–51).

What more of the future? Consumer demand for much more psychological help is growing. This demand to some extent can be met by group-analytic therapy, short- and long-term. There may be a place for medium and large groups as well as for small groups. Internet groups are already here, and further developments in that area are bound to come.

The efficacy and relative economy of group therapy when compared to individual therapy is well-established. We can hope that this message will be listened to by those who fund therapy services. This makes it all the more imperative that good training opportunities be available to those many persons in different professional areas who wish to conduct therapeutic groups.

It is vital to provide more evidence for the efficacy and economy of group psychotherapy. That group therapy is as effective as individual therapy in a variety of psychiatric disorders is already demonstrated through several studies. The September 2000 issue of *Group Analysis* presents several empirical studies, and more will appear. An extensive survey from Germany shows that the cost of group treatment is quickly returned to the community by the reduction in demands subsequently made on medical and social services, as well as a reduction in time taken off for illness (Heinzel et al. 2000). The quality of life is reported as being improved. The cost of individual therapy for the community is far, far higher than that for group therapy, in a ratio of more than ten to one, and the improvement in quality of life is no greater.

I will end with some thoughts about why I assert that group analysis will gain ground in our twenty-first century. Over and above, and below, the great advances of biological psychiatry, the community of patients and therapists has a need to talk, to talk separately and to talk together, and to talk about the painful issues that life presents to all.

Some years ago I wrote that psychoanalysis and group analysis are both stepchildren of Vienna (Pines 1986). Beginning with Freud, psychoanalysis is the more Apollonian, the aloof one, *la voix du père*. It carries authority, and the psychoanalytic movement is highly organised and somewhat authoritarian. Group analysis is more Dionysian, beginning with Jacob Moreno's psychodrama. In group analysis, there is a multitude of voices and the therapist's voice is one amongst many. The group analyst must retain authority over the setting and is accountable to the community for his/her work, but effective group-analytic work arises from a gradually evolving collaboration between the members of the group, between the patients, and between them and the therapist. Slowly, the group accumulates social and emotional capital, founded on trust in the truth qualities of the enterprise. The more the patients emotionally invest in their group, the more they have emotional capital to draw from. The more society invests in group analysis, in training and making groups available, the more society can profit. Group analysis in the twenty-first century can help to hold back the rising tide of mental illnesses.

Note

1 This paper was given as a Keynote Lecture to the European Symposium in Group Analysis, Bologna 2000, and has not been published previously. (Ed.)

10 Resonance as a factor in the development of intimacy[1]

The group-analytic situation is one in which intimacy is privileged: there is an opportunity for developing intimate relationships and thereby reaching deeply to the inner world of self and of others. In group analysis, we hope to achieve this through the processes of communication, through recognition and sharing of attitudes and of emotions and through becoming part of the group or group matrix with its transformational potential. I shall be looking at some factors that favour the development of intimacy and those that stand in its way. I shall also discuss levels of accessibility and non-accessibility in our patients.

First of all, what is intimacy? Intimate relationships involve sharing desires, fantasies, opinions, preferences – a wide range of biographical facts that are hidden from practically everyone else. Further, a partner to intimacy is allowed to hear, see and touch in ways barred to outsiders. The exclusive character of this privileged access provides it with its special, intimate character. The potentiality for intimacy is given to human beings and allows for attachment and bonding, and it is equally true to say that attachment and bonding lay down the essential groundwork for the development of intimacy. Our affects connect us to other persons and to ourselves, to inner worlds of sensation and experience, to body and to imagination. Emotions connect us to the worlds of others, other bodies, other feelings, other minds. Emotions are connectors; they connect us to community and to consciousness. The dialogic processes of human development consist of the interplay between self and others, between ego and alter, and the principles of alterity. Vygotsky (1962/2012; 1981) and Bakhtin (1981; Holquist 1990) show us that to a very large extent we gain ourselves through the actions, feelings and responses of others: the other is in the deepest sense my friend. It is only from the other that I can get myself. Thus, the gaining of a self means becoming accessible to the actions of others, those others representing 'self objects' in the Kohutian sense (Ornstein 1978). The resources of others are experienced as belonging to the self, a process that is at its highest in infancy and childhood and yet continues throughout the life cycle.

In group analysis we can follow this process through the capacity or incapacity of the person to move from monologue to dialogue, from isolation

DOI: 10.4324/9781003494713-13

to exchange, and we can recognise the self in the other and the other in the self. Bion (1990) called this the movement from narcissism to socialism. We can understand in this, his sense of 'us-ness', of 'we-ness', that modifies the experience of being on one's own, the opening and closing of the boundaries between ourselves and others, the intrapsychic boundaries that separate areas of one's own self – a vital process in group analysis. Unfortunately, the clinical material from my practice that illustrates this cannot be included here.

Resonance is the prolongation of sound by the response of another system. I am trying to differentiate between those forms of resonance that are either sympathetic or empathetic and those that involve mere echoing. In an echo, what is returned does not add another dimension to what has been emitted or uttered: an echo returns the sound to its source without any significant difference. Later, I shall refer briefly to Narcissus and Echo, the non-dialogical, non-resonating couple who can also be seen as isolated systems within the one person – an absence of coenesthesia.

The developmental studies of infancy show how vital the qualities of mirroring and resonance are for the development of mind and for the recognition that one exists in a world of similar others. Empathy is registered through state-sharing, attunement, reciprocity and the development of mutuality. This is the way in which the infant 'mentalises' – that is, recognises that there is a person, another self who is sufficiently similar to but also somewhat different from the infant's own self. Smiling, verbalising and playing are all parts of this process. Sight and sound give the infant its sense of being embodied. They help establish the boundaries between self and other, and an awareness of the bridgeable space that is between persons. In resonance, we recognise that the other has a place in our own cognitive and affective selves and that we simultaneously have a place in theirs. In echoing, there is no mutual recognition, no state-sharing, no amplification of understanding. Resonance belongs to the sphere of the 'I-Thou' relationship, the state of intersubjectivity (Buber 1958/2000). In echoing, the other is the hard rock, the 'it', and equally the self is a hard surface to the approach of the other, not allowing for an opening of the self and for a creative response. To echo is to react; to resonate is to respond. In the therapy groups we conduct we come across people who can be described as hyper-resonant (acutely sensitive) or as hypo-resonant (avoidant or insensitive) who pose particular challenges for the progress of their own therapy and sometimes for the progress of others. The conductor's special responsibility is for work with the group as a whole that ensures the safety of individual members at either of these extreme positions and the progressive resolution of their difficulties.

The most extensive work on the concept of resonance I have found is by John Watkins, an analyst, a professor of psychology and an expert on hypnotherapy. He describes resonance as 'a key tool of the effective therapist' (Watkins 1978: 230). Psychological resonance is an experience of which all people are capable, although some more than others. In the psychotherapeutic situation, it is 'that inner experience within the therapist during which he co-feels, (co-enjoys, co-suffers) and co-understands with his patient, though in mini form' (Watkins 1978: 234). He replicates within one state of his own ego (his own, experienced ego) and senses it by its impact on another through an observing part (the observational ego of the 'self'), that is also called the executive ego state. Watkins draws extensively on Paul Federn's (1952) analysis of the ego and its boundaries.

During resonance a part or state of the self incorporates the impressions that come from an external object (another person) and infuses these with selfness (ego cathexis). They then become a part of the experienced ego. When these contents impact on an experiencing or observing ego state, they interpret it as one's own thoughts and feelings. Accordingly, the therapist's self *at the moment* is capable of experiencing a patient in two different ways: directly, by the impact of the other on the external boundary of the therapist's executive ego state, and simultaneously or alternately through a facsimile of the other as an introject. This introject is invested with ego cathexis (self energy) and therefore experienced as self. That is, the other's feelings, behaviour and thoughts are felt as one's own. This is recognised as emanating from within but experienced as thought, not as perception. This is the process Watkins (1978) called resonance. It may be cognitive, affective, or both. The self now is capable of comparing the data it receives about the external object from two different sources: the direct sensory impressions of the individual (objectivity) and the apprehended inner replication (resonance). Resonance increases as the intensity of an interpersonal relationship grows, and resonance can extend, as William James (1978) originally pointed out, to inanimate objects as well as to humans and animals. An attack or criticism directed against one's private possessions is reacted to as if it were an attack on the person of the owner. The self that has never learned to resonate is filled only with objects devoted to its own immediate survival and first-hand pleasure. Stimulation comes almost entirely from without, and it is therefore the pawn of its environment.

Watkins (1978) differentiates resonance from 'accurate empathy' as described by Carl Rogers (1951). He says that Rogers emphasises the *understanding* of the feelings of another, not necessarily *experiencing* the feelings. The latter would be identification, not empathy. Resonance is a type of identification that is temporary and is true resonance only if the resonating one is himself actually experiencing inwardly the same feelings as the other, even though in a derivative, mini-form. The understanding is derived from the replication of the inner affective or cognitive experience happening at that time to the other. It is a temporary and partial identification in a common feeling state and an understanding derived by participation in such a state.

Watkins differentiates resonance and countertransference. In countertransference, the patient is an object to the therapist; in resonance, he is a subject. Countertransference is an 'againstness' between therapist and patient; resonance is 'withness' between them. Countertransference feelings are towards the client; in resonance, the feelings are with him and directed towards some person or aspect of life significant to him. In resonance, the therapist takes over a feeling state from the patient temporarily and internalises it for the purposes of understanding by experiencing it personally within his own self. Watkins emphasises the 'withness', the co-feeling, co-suffering and co-enjoying. He has engaged in some research to identify the therapist's capacity for resonance and to see whether that capacity can be enhanced by training, and it seems to have shown that this indeed is so.

He asserts that for the therapist to have a 'therapeutic self', he or she has to have sensitive capacity for resonance. Resonance occurs when an individual temporarily identifies with another and experiences the other as his or her own self first; this other is an object, and if permanently internalised becomes an introject. However, this object may be changed into a part of the self through the process of identification or by investing it with ego cathexis, so then it becomes subject and is termed an 'identofact'. The feelings of the other are now experienced within oneself and the ideas of the other felt as one's own thoughts. One has duplicated in mini-form the existential world of the other. It is through such resonance that one lives in the experiential world of the other. Experienced from the inside, the other is understood differently than when sensed from the outside. Both ways of knowing about another are valid and represent different viewpoints, but together they are superior to either one alone.

The therapeutic self is one who can understand his or her patient from both the objective and the resonant points of view, either simultaneously or in alternation. Through therapeutic resonance, a 'we-ness' is established that encourages the patient into a reciprocal quid pro quo. When the therapist understands and accepts the patient's pathology, the patient identifies (resonates) increasingly with the integrated self of the therapist. Resistances are lowered, interpretations become more palatable, and insights are achieved sooner. Through resonance, the therapist can experience the patient's defences as protection rather than as resistance, allowing for a different approach to the patient which is more akin to that of self psychology.

Two of the essential features of resonance in therapeutic interaction are differentiation and integration. The separate self of the therapist enables objective perception to take place, but by integrating, he or she temporarily gives up the separateness and resonates. The integration of self and other can be likened to Robert Emde's (1992a; 1992b) concept of the 'executive-we', and it thus extends to the relationships between adults in a therapeutic situation, the essential part of healthy human development between infant and caregivers.

Note

1 This paper was presented to an unknown audience soon after the year 2000 and has not been published previously. (Ed.)

11 Listening and the sonorous self[1]

Tonight I will address, from a somewhat different angle, the speaking and listening that is the hallmark of the psychoanalytic situation. As psychoanalysts, we spend most of our lives listening. We listen, then speak, listen again, to hear how what we have said has been heard, which we gauge by our patient's response. The patient's task is speaking and learning about themselves through what they hear themselves say. They also are listeners who listen to themselves and to us. Together, as a pair, we relate and communicate most evidently through speech, though here I discount nothing of the other powerful forces within the analytic situation that are not verbal. For the moment, I want to look with you at the sound elements of analysis which of course must include the silences.

The spoken dialogue of analysis

I have been drawn to a greater interest in the spoken dialogue of analysis for various reasons. First, because spoken words are our craft, we are known through what we say. We open and reveal ourselves through our words, and through our words we enter directly into the mental life of our patients, intending thereby to offer understanding and to help bring about change. The great body of literature on interpretation is indeed concerned with what we say but to a much lesser extent with how this should be said and, to a lesser degree still, with the significance of sound and dialogue. Maranhão (1990) points to this in emphasising the centrality of dialogue itself as the primary subject for interpretation – not so much the monologue of the patient on the couch, not even the product of the analyst's introspective scrutiny offered as a countertransference construction but, rather, the dialogue between them. Schlapobersky (1995/2000) also explores the spoken word at work in his account of monologue, dialogue and discourse in group analysis. His study of the language of the group begins with a paper with this title – the language of the group – and the work is continuing (Schlapobersky 2016: chapter 4).

As a supervisor, I have often asked therapists to reflect on how what they say, or intend to say, is likely to be heard by the patient. Often the therapist then realises that his therapeutic intent, the wish to convey understanding,

DOI: 10.4324/9781003494713-14

will not be heard. Rather, it may convey unnecessary detachment and judgement, theoretical preoccupation or unwarranted projection. But relatively few therapists seem to concern themselves as to how they might be heard – or indeed, whether they will be heard at all! Once or twice a day, my own listening hours are also shared with others in psychoanalytic groups. Here, eight persons converse under group-analytic conditions of free-floating discussion, which involve associations, resonances, mirroring, interpretations and so on. In these situations, I am constantly reminded and impressed by the skills of listening and speaking that develop in such groups, natural skills that often surprise me by their insight or by the sensitivity of the responses. In these groups, I learn of the great potential resources of sensitive responsiveness that we humans are capable of. What I learn constantly of the natural, latent resources possessed by many of our patients has formed the basis of my own writing (Pines 1984a; 1984b; 1984c; 1987a; 1989; 1990).

Contributions from self psychology

In recent years, my own way of listening has been influenced by the school of self psychology. Theories of human development from this school have led adherents to devise a language of responsiveness to patients that enables patients more quickly to feel understood and thereby held in the psychoanalytic situation, as I have found myself (Kohut 1977). The self psychologists seem to me to have found ways of a finer tuning in to warded off affective states, which helps to bring about the conditions of safety required for analytic work to proceed. In this connection, for some years, I have taken particular interest in the affect of shame, and a greater familiarity and confidence with the phenomenon of shame has led, I believe, to a significant development in my ability to listen sensitively and for my patients to feel accepted and understood (Pines 1987a).

To introduce myself further to you, I should say that my own training was with the Anna Freud group in London at a time when the split with Kleinian colleagues was sharp and intense. We were scarcely able to listen and to understand each other, but fortunately, the situation now is less extreme, and both groups have adopted something of the language of the other. I believe that the work of the Hampstead group, though overshadowed for many years by the Kleinian group, has a sounder base in observation and practice and will form a more fundamental base, which can be integrated with the newer studies of child development to which I will be referring later on. But I have always been strongly influenced by aspects of Donald Winnicott's (1951; 1958a; 1958b; 1965/1985) work which, to my mind, resembles aspects of the self-psychological approach. In my account here I will call especially on his ideas about transitional phenomena – just one from among his many original contributions – to illustrate the 'space between' infant and mother (Winnicott 1951). Also, my work with groups as well as with individuals has made me very aware of the power of the therapeutic setting with its resources of holding and containment. Yet another source of analytic wisdom I have found is in the writings of Hans Loewald. He has found a comprehensive and elegant way of integrating object relations and drive theory and relating these to the psychoanalytic situation and the changes that can occur there (Loewald 1989).

There are some more influences I want to reflect on – some negative, others positive. I can still react quite strongly against some colleagues' ways of speaking with and about their patients. I hear of patients who are plunged suddenly and traumatically into a transference situation that emphasises both the primitive and the negative, and I have seen many patients who have not been helped; indeed, they have been traumatised by such experiences. I believe that the negative and the primitive will find their natural place as therapy unfolds and that the impact is all the stronger for that. Then, in my own development, I have moved away from earlier attempts to be very accurate and 'correct' in my listening and speaking – I shall explain this later – and am more engaged now in seeking for what seems to me to be 'the appropriate response' to the patient's material, rather than always thinking about what is 'the correct interpretation'. By the way, I rather dislike the word 'material', for do we deal in *matter* or in *what matters*? Material is easily rendered inert, a substance to be delved into and poured over, whereas 'what matters' is that which is carried across the analytic space through sound and to which we find ourselves responding.

Contributions from child development

Then, in child development, I have been much influenced by work such as that of Robert Emde (1980; 1981; 1983; 1988; 1990; 1992a; 1992b) and Daniel Stern (1998), research that now shows us how vital is the dialogue that develops between infant and caregivers. This dialogue between self and self-object, later self and other, needs to be present for the infant's potentials to develop. Current work guides us away from the model of the arising mind of the infant as an isolated monad and towards models of intersubjectivity, mutuality, exchange and reciprocity, which biologically and psychologically make good sense for survival and for the unfolding of human nature.

Closed neurotic systems lead to repetitions of internal object relations through the familiar mechanisms of transference and countertransference, powered by projective identification and other mechanisms. The psychoanalytic situation re-presents patients with a situation where such dialogues can recur. This sets in motion essential conditions for psychic explorations, leading to possible change. The term 'sonorous being' is found in Merleau-Ponty (1968), who combined a phenomenological and psychoanalytical vision in an illuminating manner. He emphasised how the body is deeply involved in perception, in being in the world, and each sense contributes in its own fashion to a mode of experience of being in the world. His analysis of the difference between vision and hearing draws on those of others, who have considered this issue. Some of this analysis comes from philosophy rather than from psychoanalysis, which is regrettable because it is an analysis that touches on fundamental issues for our theory and technique; perhaps this goes some way to accounting for the neglect of our sonorities.

Looking and hearing

Looking and hearing are built into the development of the psychoanalytic situation. In his discovery of free association, Freud abandoned looking for hearing; even so, the significance of this shift in modality is not yet fully reflected in psychoanalytic theory. Recently, Anzieu (1989) and Fiumara (1990) have begun to explore this area, but the most illuminating and accessible position I have found is that of a Chicago philosopher, David Michael Levin (1989), in *The Listening Self.* He begins with Hannah Arendt, who writes that

> each . . . [mental activity] . . . draws its metaphors from a different bodily sense. . . . Thus, from the very outset, in formal philosophy, thinking has been thought of in terms of *seeing*. The predominance of sight is so deeply embedded in Greek speech, and therefore in our conceptual language, that we seldom find any consideration bestowed on it, as though it belonged to things too obvious to be noticed. . . . [But] if one considers how easy it is for sight, unlike the other senses, to shut out the outside world, and if one examines the notion of the blind bard, whose stories are being listened to, one may wonder why hearing did not develop into the guiding metaphor for thinking.
>
> (Arendt 1971, quoted by Levin 1989: xiv)

What, then, of hearing? John Dewey (1954: 234) has put it succinctly and beautifully: 'Vision is a spectator; hearing is a participation'. Why is this so? Perhaps because we cannot shut out sounds by closing our ears in the way we can shut out sights by closing our eyes. Our ears can be closed only to the meaning and to the appeal of the sounds. Sound is deeply affecting from the moment of the infant's cry that follows the mother's moment of triumph and pain, the sounds of childbirth. Sounds are transitory, hard to catch and retain in the mind, and less amenable to abstraction for those of us who are not musicians. Ordinarily, we possess less of the world through sound than we do through sight, though in analysis we come again to recognise how much of the world is represented for us through hearing. It is hand and eye that work together to make tools to master the world. Yet it is through sound, hearing and utterance, that human beings become themselves and are able to enter into dialogue.

Levin (1989) outlines, in a psychological and philosophical account of the place of hearing in human society, how nature's gift of the potential, the capacity for hearing, represents an unfinished task, a social task. For language is a social institution, and therefore verbal language and the pre-languages, the proto-conversations of gesture, gaze, the interplay of infant and caretaker, are all involved in the development of the capacity for hearing.

What characteristic differences do we need to hold in mind between vision and hearing? The eye best sees what is in front of it; the eye measures distance. Vision can grasp an object in space, retain an image in the absence of an object. We can turn away from an object yet retain a certain power over it through retaining the image in the mind, as is easily seen in the magical beliefs that surround the image of an object. Vision can focus narrowly and discriminate finely. Vision leads to abstraction, to speculative thinking, to a recognition of the separateness of self and object. The vision of the rational world of the Enlightenment, here a significant visual term, has been the predominant mode of the Western world for centuries. Yet, with the scientific mastery of the world that this vision has given us, there comes also an imprisonment of the human being within his visual horizon – a small concentric circle of the personal horizon.

I believe our understanding of early development has been greatly increased in the past decade by such researchers as Emde (1992a, 1992b), Stern (1998), Sander (2008), Malloch and Trevarthen (2010) and others. Their frame of reference and of observation is the couple: infant/mother. Their observations are of the dialogue that develops from very early on, after birth. It seems that natural, good enough parenting leads to what is termed 'biological mirroring', the intuitive and natural capacities for looking, touching, speaking, responding physically, verbally and affectively to infants. Infants begin to experience their humanness by immersion into the dynamic processes, the affective offerings and responses of caregivers. Over and above the familiar notions of holding and containment are such experiences as state-sharing. Through these experiences, infants begin to recognise themselves through the responses of the other and to become an other who is separate but yet part of the other. The infant seems to learn to be apart through the experience of being a cherished part of the other. Thus, the self-object concept of the self psychologists begins to give a set of concepts and language to be compared with the language of part and whole objects.

They may well be complementary languages, as Grotstein (1993) has suggested with his dual track theory. Working with the self-object language gives us the opportunity to better recognise and produce some of the skills of good enough parenting, as an important part of early development is to learn the skills of listening.

A developmental line for listening

Levin (1989) has proposed a schema akin to a developmental line for listening:

1 As hearers, we begin with the primordial gift of nature, which is the capacity to hear. Our ability to respond becomes our response-ability, but it is one that needs to be fostered before we can take that

responsibility for ourselves. Infants seem to listen with their whole bodies. Merleau-Ponty (1968) says that I echo the vibration of the sound with my whole body. We know that infants quickly learn to discriminate sounds such as mother's voice and the sounds of nursing. Quite quickly a more discriminating, ego-based activity of hearing develops which is more object-directed from a self now experienced as object to oneself. Yet this capacity for the early, undiscriminating hearing is always latent and can be aroused through aesthetic and religious experiences and through poetry, and as Kohut pointed out in his early papers, through music and rhythm (Ornstein 1978). He dealt with the soothing and arousing qualities of music and emphasised how important it is for a person to develop that capacity for self-soothing that originally came from the early care-givers, that emerged through the transitional phenomenon of infantile babbling, that then lends itself to vocalisation and is retained in the singing voice.

2 Throughout childhood and early adolescence, we have to learn to hear in the ways that society lays down, which is to listen, to obey, to listen practically, to fashion a listening suited to the everyday. Much of this listening becomes internalised as a morality. This practical listening occupies most of childhood and adolescence, but it is interesting to observe that the listening that requires obedience, part of the socialisation process, also has another meaning. The Latin word for 'obey' is *oboedīre*, which means 'to listen with obedience, to "give ear" by paying attention' in a relationship of respectful understanding. Similarly, the word 'understand' literally means 'to stand in the midst of', to stand in a position from which we can share what it is to be another person.

3 The third stage of listening takes us into more complex areas. We can learn to listen both to ourselves and to others in ways that will make us more responsive to the inter-relatedness and commonality of all sonorous beings. As this awareness grows, so do processes of reversibility – the I in the other, and the other in me. This reversibility can allow for reciprocity, and out of reciprocity a sense of rightness and of justice can emerge. This natural process is greatly enhanced by the experiences of individual and group therapy. The group situation by its very nature offers more opportunities for the exploration of reciprocity, reversibility and the discovery of human commonality.

4 There is a fourth stage where we may even be able to go beyond the mature adult to return to the child's ability to hear in a less discriminating manner, to unfocus, to let go of auditory discrimination and thereby to listen to the harmony that lies behind disharmony. In the words of the poet Blake, to go beyond 'The Ear, a little shell in small volutions shutting out / All melodies & comprehending only Discord and Harmony' (quoted in Erdman 1988: 99).

The listening process

I am inviting us to look at what we might learn through taking a deeper look at the listening process in human life and to see whether, in doing so, we find issues that relate to the psychoanalytic situation. Listening and being listened to are fundamental for the condition of our humanity. We are immersed in a sonorous world in uterine and postnatal life onwards. We are creatures of culture and history, transmitted through language for which there is no better reminder than that of the dramatic story of the wolf boy of Aveyron, a feral child found at the age of nine who, being without language, could not be socialised. The patient care that he was given and the learning derived from this experience brought him only part of the way into a human condition, and this episode changed the face and nature of remedial education (Montessori 1948/1986). We are social beings who are formed of sound and biological mirroring. Visual and auditory features involving intuitive motor actions can awaken and elicit pro-social exchanges. Gazing and echoing are shared activities that bring infants and caregivers into reciprocal actions and thereby to the experience of a shared world, a communion inscribed in the body.

Good enough caring involves understanding and giving respectful attention and recognition to the needs of infants and children as expressed through their sounds, and there is a good and a bad listening. There is a listening that responds to a child's needs and also leads a child on to develop its own autonomy, hopefully an autonomy that will also recognise the autonomy of others. Through this good enough listening, the child gets to hear, to know and to recognise itself. It gets to know, both consciously and unconsciously, that it is always immersed in an intersubjective world where, between 'us-ness' and 'we-ness', the us is always the ground for the I, for the ego.

I would like to share with you a quotation from Aristotle:

> Of these faculties, for the mere necessities of life and in itself, sight is the more important; but for the mind [*nous*] and indirectly [*kata symbebēkos*] hearing is the more important. . . . [It] makes the largest contribution to wisdom. For discourse, which is the cause of learning, is so because it is audible; but it is audible not in itself but indirectly, because speech is composed of words.
>
> (Quoted in Arendt 1978: 227)

Arendt (1978: 227) comments drily, 'The point of the matter is that Aristotle never seems to have remembered this observation when he wrote philosophy'.

Didier Anzieu and the sound bath of the infant

Anzieu's (1989) concept of psychic envelopes, originally based on the skin as the first sense of body limit and boundary, was later extended to include sound. In his chapter on the sound envelope, he suggests that a rudimentary, sensory unity and identity can arise from the infant's own experience of both sound and respiration, which gives a sense of volume emptying and refilling. On the mythological level, this is represented by caves and caverns, which are the home of the primitive, but whence also originates culture, symbolised by the rough, primitive god, Pan. Anzieu points out that it is through sound, through crying and the maternal response, that the infant experiences a vital, circular reaction, a to and fro of sound that elaborates into communication and mentation, and this circular reaction is significantly different to the more one-way process of feeding and elimination.

Also, the infant experiences itself in the 'sound mirror' provided by the environment. Its own sounds are responded to in this way and the resonance is returned all the time – the infant is immersed in a bath of sound, all the noises of the human environment. So the self begins to form a sound envelope through all these sonorous experiences, an envelope that, Janus-like, faces two ways: inwards towards the sounds of one's own body, outwards towards the world. Is this not the essence of a psychoanalytic situation, where recumbent on the couch and freely associating, the person listens to their own sounds and listens for the response of the analyst? McDougall (1989) speaks of 'one body for two persons' when describing a patient who moves from chair to couch and hears her tummy rumble in every session. She remarks to her analyst that her tummy is singing to her. She is embarrassed yet intrigued. McDougall describes the level of symbolic fusion in which it falls to the analyst to understand for her patient what it is that her body is expressing and to pass this on in digestible form.

This patient does not yet own her own mental or imaginative capacities, as she grew up singularly unimaginative, always close to an arthritic mother who needed her child to enter into her own adult, mental space and console her for her affliction. The child knew little of play, and the mother did not encourage her individuation and physical and mental entity. She says of their relationship, 'we were joined at the hip'.

According to Anzieu (1989) and in line with all nursing experience, babies need to be stimulated to make sounds, through being immersed in a bath of sounds, talk, melody, responses to the infant's vocalisations; this is the repertoire of biological mirroring already referred to. The absence of such a sound bath is again mythologised in the story of Narcissus, to which I will return in the last two chapters of this collection. Before Narcissus rejected the male lover for which he was punished by having to fall in love with his own unattainable image, he had already rejected the nymph Echo. Her words and cries echoing his own grief were the only sounds that reached him as he lay dying – Echo, whose body turned into the inorganic rock that surrounded the fatal pool. Thus, sound is given precedence over vision in the legend, and sound is given a feminine quality.

Anzieu writes of the pathology of the sound mirror, of when the sound bath or silences make the infant feel that he means nothing to the mother.

Her sonorous responses may be discordant, out of tune, untimely, impersonal – again, all the potential pathologies of the analytic situation, of being out of touch, intrusive, untimely, impersonally distant, or experience-distant, to use Kohut's words (Ornstein 1978). This is over and beyond any countertransference issues that can be understood and worked through as unconscious communication from the patient. These are issues that can arise from an analyst's own personality or from his/her ideas of what represents good technique.

Edith Lecourt (1990) is an analyst who works with music and has elaborated Anzieu's ideas. She points out that the sound envelope has two different aspects. There is the verbal, which develops towards the outside through speech that becomes linear, univocal, a visible thread in the texture of language, emphasising articulation and abstraction. This is the differentiated individual, the 'I' part of the self. The other component is the musical: woven into the texture of sound, the plurivocal, vibrating and resonating in the body, directed inwards and yet connecting with other sonorous beings in music and chant. This is the part of the self that holds the knowledge of undifferentiation and knows of the 'we', the 'us', that integrates both inner and outer groups.

This move towards recognising and valuing the us, the 'we two together making one', is at the forefront of psychoanalytic infant observation, which takes the pair as the unit of research that began with Winnicott's work and is now described by Emde (1990), Stern (1998) and others. They both study how the infant comes to acquire a sense of self through experiences with caregivers that convey a sense of being in a shared world of affect through such responses as attunement, state-sharing and intersubjectivity. The rhythm of a child's psychic development is better and more adequately described as taking place through games of turn-taking and circular reactions, more adequately than through more linear models of needs, frustrations and gratifications. Pleasure is indeed a better teacher than pain, though no analyst can discount the task of understanding and dealing with infantile pain and frustration.

Language as dialogue: The enduring contribution from Vygotsky and Bakhtin

When Stern (1998) comes to describing the acquisition of a sense of a verbal self, he uses the term 'dialogism'. With this he refers to the Russian psychologist Vygotsky (1962/2012), who showed that language emerged from shared experiences, a view that stands in contrast to Piaget's linear view (Piaget and Inhelder 1967). The social act precedes and makes possible the personal act. Language acquisition is another step in the experience of mother and child being with each other in an intersubjective world in which they create together verbal symbols and share mutually created meanings about personal experiences. This applies, of course, to all the sonorous expressions and exchanges that precede words. Language acquisition can thus also be understood as a transitional phenomenon, a process of giving words to what already exists as thought in the mind. The word is in the transitional space between the infant's subjectivity and the mother's objectivity.

Language acquisition also faces two ways and brings the pair together at a higher level of development, described by Vygotsky as the zone of proximal development. The child can discover that its own personal, experiential knowledge is understood and is indeed part of a language culture, which it is joining. But we must also recognise that language can never re-create or express the original force and wholeness of experience, though poetry and music lead us towards or back towards such intimations of immortality.

Stern (1998) does not mention the prime figure behind the concept of language as dialogue – the Russian savant Bakhtin, for whom the question of who we are is being constantly formed through the language of the other, which tells us who we are for them. The self is always an unfinished project and, therefore, I need the other to complete the work of becoming myself (Bakhtin 1981; Holquist 1981; 1990). Thus, the other is indeed my friend, whom I need for my own project, not someone who alienates me from myself but someone who gives myself to me. This is again a reciprocal relationship because the other needs me to give them their sense of completion. Thus, as unfinished souls, we are always immersed in this world of dialogue, each of us carrying that 'surplus of seeing' for the other that is needed to be more fully and wholly oneself. And is not the psychoanalytic situation the most profound example that we have of the power of dialogue? The much greater acceptance of countertransference, as part of the analytic process, takes us part of the way towards a more complete acceptance of dialogue within psychoanalysis. And yet, I believe, we still have a long way to go.

Bakhtin describes the process of formation of the self as 'architectonic', constantly being built through the experience of oneself as a living entity immersed in dialogue with the other, through whom one builds one's self. I do not take this to be an endorsement of the Lacanian linguistic approach to psychoanalysis and the unconscious. I cite it more as evidence for the dialogic principle, both in child development and in the process by which we open our minds and ourselves to the thoughts of others.

In conclusion: A fairy tale

I will tell you a story about sonority that I believe delicately expresses a range of experience that we can reach and express through this newer understanding of openness to sound, to the psychology of the self and to dialogue. The story is Hans Christian Andersen's (1983) 'The Nightingale', which I learnt about from the Californian therapist Lawrence Hedges to whom I make acknowledgement (Hedges 1983). It begins in the emperor's palace, a vast building filled with beautiful and costly things that are so fragile that one must be cautious in touching them, lest they break. The grounds surrounding the palace are so enormous that it is difficult to tell where they end and where the world outside begins. This seems to be a delicate evocation of the fragile nature of grandiosity, which is so vulnerable to the touch. This can lead to a loss of the sense of reality, so the person does not know where their limits are.

Only beyond the palace grounds is the kingdom's most spectacular treasure to be found. It is the nightingale in the forest – free, available to everybody and superior to anything else in the kingdom by virtue of its song. The emperor, hearing of the bird's beautiful song, wishes to possess it, for his envy has been aroused. However, none of the courtiers who surround him have any knowledge of this bird or where it is to be found. The only person in the whole court who knows about the bird is a little kitchen maid who passes it in the forest whenever she goes to visit her sick mother. She tells the emperor that the effect of hearing the nightingale's song is the same as receiving a kiss from mother.

This little kitchen maid takes the courtiers to the forests and points the nightingale out to them, but the courtiers cannot hear the song. 'Is it a frog's croak or a cow's bellow?' they ask, and they are disappointed when they find that the nightingale is only a plain, little brown bird. Their grandiose wishes separate them from an appreciation of simple beauty, represented both by the bird and the little kitchen maid.

The nightingale says that she will be glad to sing for the emperor and goes with them to court. On first hearing the nightingale's song, the emperor is moved to tears. We can hear this as the creation of an empathic bond, the arousal of the experience of a caring relationship, a good introject. Further, the emperor now needs to possess the nightingale, and to make sure of his possession, he imprisons it in a cage and proudly exhibits it to his visitors. Thus, the bird has been incorporated into his own grandiose self.

One day the emperor is sent a gift. It is a beautiful, artificial bird encrusted with jewels, and one of the songs that the mechanical bird can sing is that of the nightingale. Everyone agrees that it can sing just as well as the nightingale and that, in addition, it is much prettier to look at. While they are making these comparisons between the artificial bird and the live bird, the nightingale takes the opportunity to fly out of the window. The courtiers agree that the mechanical bird is superior to the nightingale because with the real bird, you never know what you are going to hear, but in the artificial bird, everything is decided beforehand. This illustrates the omnipotent, narcissistic merger with the object, possession rendering it predictable and furthering the sense that it is a product of man's omnipotence.

The real nightingale is therefore branded as an ungrateful creature and banished from the kingdom. It cannot be valued because it can be replaced by the mechanical bird. Only those people who live outside the palace are aware that something is missing in the song of the artificial bird, but within the palace, all are content and admire its songs. The emperor is pleased with his new bird for it is always with him. Thus, he is now in possession of an object which can soothe him at his command and thereby gives him the illusion that he has the capacity for self-soothing.

One evening while the emperor is listening to the mechanical bird, the music suddenly stops: a spring has broken in its mechanism. First, the emperor sends for his physicians, as if the bird was suffering from an illness that could be cured, but they tell him that they cannot help and that he should send for a watchmaker. The watchmaker is able to repair the mechanical bird, but he cautions the emperor – now that the mechanism is wearing out, it should only be played once a year and the tune it plays may not always sound the same.

A few years pass during which the emperor has the bird sing to him once each year, as he was advised by the watchmaker. And then the emperor becomes very sick. He lies in his bed, weak, pale and cold, and he is not expected to live much longer. Lying in his bed, he feels a heavy weight on his chest. He opens his eyes to find Death sitting on his chest. Death is wearing the emperor's crown and holds his royal regalia, his sword and his banner. The emperor sees himself surrounded by faces, which seem to him to represent his good and his bad deeds. He is very frightened and wants to drown out the faces with music, but he is no longer strong enough to wind up the mechanical bird. Thus, we see the consequences of the failure of infantile omnipotence with the subsequent release of states of confusion, splitting into good and bad, near-psychotic regression and fears of annihilation.

Just at this point, the nightingale returns from the forest beyond and begins to sing. As she sings, the faces become fainter, and colour and life begin returning to the emperor. Even Death asks the nightingale to continue her song, and she agrees to do so if Death will return to the emperor his royal insignia. Death returns the objects to the emperor and is so moved by the nightingale's song about mourning and how the mourner's tears can bring a new growth that he slips silently away. The emperor is grateful to the nightingale, and he asks her why she returned after he had banished her from his kingdom. The nightingale reminds him that he had shed tears when he first heard her song and that those tears had created a bond between them. The emperor says he will destroy the artificial bird. The nightingale says he should not do so, for the mechanical bird did its best and should be appreciated and not destroyed.

The emperor now wants to keep the bird with him but, recognising that she is a separate object, asks if she will be willing to stay with him and to sing only when she wants to do so. The bird declines, saying that she prefers the forest as her home and wants to be able to travel freely. But she reassures the emperor she will come and sing to him frequently. She tells him that now she will sing songs that are not only songs of joy but songs of suffering, of both good and evil.

And so, we hear of the passing through of the regressive crisis, reaching the depression, the attainment of an object of constancy and the acceptance of ambivalence. The emperor and the nightingale are now separate persons.

Both become centres of autonomy and initiative, both are free to come and go and both are free to stay in relation to one another, when either one is absent or present. That is what we hope to see in the outcome of the work we do with some of our patients, aided by imagination and the capacity for creative listening.

Note

1 This lecture was given to an unknown audience in about 2000 and has not been published previously. (Ed.)

12 More about listening[1]

The essence of the therapist's listening act is to put himself into a position to hear sensitively and deeply what the patient is saying, then to find that communication to which he wishes to respond, and then to respond from his 'therapist self'. This is the act of an unfocused listening, which widens the frame of reference to make use of a knowledge of human nature, self and others. This knowledge can be integrated with what the therapist knows about the nature and development of human mentality, derived from their own development and the study of psychology and other sources.

There are many conditions needed by a therapist to attain this mental state and to be able to preserve it in the midst of the turmoil and pressures which naked contact with another human being, often in distress, will produce. What is essential is that the therapist should have his or her own inner time and space – time in which to reflect and to respond to his patients – and an inner therapeutic space to gather and reflect on the experiences that he or she is having in the room with his or her patient.

All observations and responses in our work as therapists filter through our perceptions and are received by and absorbed into our therapist self. That therapist self is formed, as I have said, by our life experiences, personalities and temperaments, and by our training. I should really prefer to use the word 'education' rather than 'training', for education brings things out from a person, whereas training has rather the connotation of holding things in. Our therapeutic education is within one or another of the schools of psychodynamic psychology, and within those schools, there are cleavages and divisions. There are different claims for priority, for correctness and for the most appropriate way in which to hear and respond to our patients, to their situations and our relationships with them.

Reflecting on such debates as the 'controversial discussions' held in the 1940s during the war between the Kleinian and Freudian groups of the London Institute of Psychoanalysis, where rival parties drew up their confrontations, their lines of attack and defence and zealously presented and defended their positions, one is impressed with the strength of the arguments and counterarguments (King and Steiner 1992). Yet at the same time, from the perspective of fifty years on, I find myself, and possibly you do as well,

DOI: 10.4324/9781003494713-15

regarding this as all somewhat anachronistic. The anachronism derives from our changing concepts of what represents truth and the nature of knowledge. It is the question of epistemology and of scientific philosophy. When opponents contest against each other with arguments, the implications of which are that one must be right and the other wrong, they are setting up their situations in an ideological world whose basic assumptions are that truths are incontestable and that our goals must be to demonstrate the truth or falsity of one or another of the propositions set forth. The background to such arguments is provided by the model of a universe where finite measurable forces, such as Newton demonstrated, can be searched for and found in the area of psychological concepts. The current position, in contrast, is that we use various models that may often seem contradictory as vehicles for thought and for the construction of our understanding of the universe. The prime examples of this are the contesting yet complementary wave and particle theories of light, seemingly contradictory and yet both necessary for the explanation of the observed phenomena.

The nineteenth-century metaphor for scientific research, for exploring the deeper aspects of nature, including human nature, was geological. The great discoveries of geology demonstrated incontestably that the earth was not created in 4004 BCE, as had been claimed by James Ussher, the archbishop of Armagh and primate of all Ireland, a view that dominated the Victorian world. The fascinating layering of strata discovered by geologists established that the earth was veritably millions of years old. The uncovering of facts, therefore, was like the uncovering of solid material. We know that Freud was fascinated by archaeology and that he thought to reconstruct the archaeology of individual childhood through exploration. Similarly, his hero, Heinrich Schliemann, had established the historicity of places mentioned in the works of Homer through archaeological excavation of Hisarlik – now presumed to be the site of Troy – and the sites of Mycenae and Tiryns in the Peloponnese. So Freud uncovered the early residues of childhood development and felt that he had established a new archaeology that went back through stratified layers of the mind to the infantile sources of neurotic difficulty (Gay 1989). When the generation of female analysts began to explore female sexuality and when the first generations of child analysts explored the actual living child's mind, Freud responded with astonishment that new layers of totally unsuspected civilisations had appeared and had to be accounted for. For Freud, the pre-Oedipal levels of development were like the Minoan-Mycenaean layers of civilisation uncovered by Schliemann, which had radically altered all previous knowledge of Greek civilisation.

Our own current model of psychological reality is the discovery of the way in which we create our truths – that we create our histories, the histories of our families and the histories of our distant childhoods. We recognise that reality and truth are elusive, generally unknown and unknowable, and that there are a variety of ways of interacting with what is termed truth or reality, often by inventing or creating ideas about how things are or once were. In this seemingly fluctuating and unpredictable world of ideas, we can, however, take a position in which:

1 We define and limit what we want to look at.
2 We find which perspective gives us the best vantage points over the area that we wish to survey.
3 We construct a vocabulary that will give us the clarity we need for communication with others who are working and toiling in the same vineyards.

This is why we need to belong to 'schools' of psychotherapy and why we constantly need to review and clarify the basic frameworks within which we operate. To have a shared consciousness of our notions of reality, we need to understand the metaphors we use.

In *Listening Perspectives in Psychotherapy*, the psychotherapist Lawrence Hedges (1983) offers the following way of viewing what he calls the 'listening perspective':

1 Listening in psychotherapy is the act of comprehending the private experience of others.
2 People feel a benefit from having their words and actions understood. What the listener is prepared to hear is determined by his or her subjective frame of reference.
3 Different schools of psychotherapy can be defined in terms of what features of our private experience are consistently discernible and worthy of attention – that is, through our listening perspectives or vectors.
4 Each school of psychotherapy has successfully defined those features of private experience that it deems useful, calling on concepts and techniques that encourage the elaboration of personal meaning along subjectively helpful lines. These are particular vectors through which experience can be conceptualised and abstracted. Therapists are having to make choices as to how to use these perspectives and how to understand the nature of the experiences that are revealed by their use. They have to be aware of the methods and parameters involved in those particular types of listening experiences. Thus, to Jung and his schools we owe the understanding of the mythical aspects of human nature, the enrichment that the individual life experience has, when linked up with collective experience (Jung 1991; Storr 1986). To him we also owe the introduction into Western epistemology of aspects of Eastern wisdom that emphasise the importance of balance between the different psychic functions and the notion of life as a constant inner journey of exploration and discovery. To the Adlerians we owe the recognition of the social nature of mankind: our constant strivings to maintain and acquire self-esteem and the constant danger of losing self-esteem, the struggle between feelings of superiority and inferiority, and an early understanding of the battle between the sexes (Adler 1925/2011).

Recently, interesting links have been shown to exist between this early psychology of Adler and the much later self psychology of Kohut and the Chicago school. The latter have so refreshingly brought back into psychotherapy concepts relating to the central experience of self within the framework of self and other (Ornstein 1978). To Adler we owe the early introduction of the importance of aggression and rivalry in basic human experience.

5 These varied approaches focus on different aspects of human experience, and we have different, competing theories about the nature of human development, the stages through which we pass, and the timetable of such events. Erikson (1950) greatly enriched Freud's biological timetable of the development of the libidinal zones by bringing to this psychosexual model the very necessary psychosocial dimension. Piaget brought his great contributions to the understanding of cognitive development, and a flourishing school of neo-Piagetian psychologists, including Kegan (1983), have begun to bring together a rich and illuminating vista of an integrated emotional-cognitive developmental perspective.

6 As knowledge accumulates, the dominant models change. Freud's early topographic theory gave way to his structural theory. Later, Anna Freud's (1989) concept of developmental lines and Margaret Mahler's (Mahler et al. 1975) individuation-separation schema have been of enormous value in helping us to clarify the richness of the experience of human bonding and separateness. Melanie Klein brought into the very early stages of human development the vital concepts of the paranoid and the depressive positions. How, then, are we to relate the richness of these theoretical approaches to our actual listening experiences with our patients?

We can now more clearly outline four different stages of human development and see if these fit in with distinctive clinical entities, then see whether the recognition of these clinical entities and their links with those developmental stages can bring about differences in the way in which we listen and respond to our patients. The four developmental stages are:

1 The earliest stages of human life are now recognised as being concerned with the very origins and emergence of the subjective sense of self out of the primal self of a matrix. Current research does not confirm Freud's (1917) hypothesis of primary narcissism, that the infant has no relationship to others in its earliest stages, nor does it support Mahler's (Mahler et al. 1975) very earliest of all stages, that of symbiosis. Current research shows us that the child from birth onwards, and very likely while still in utero, actively explores and responds to those features of the environment that are crucially important to it and that arouse interest. From the start, there is a busy traffic of experience between the infant, its mother and its other caretakers, who are biologically primed for adaptation and for survival.

2 The next stage is concerned with the emergence of contrasting experience of others and the construction of the representation of self and of others out of the common matrix of early experiences. According to this model, the Self arises in relationship to Other and by virtue of experiences, contrasts and transactions with others becomes a new emergent. This is a central tenet of the British school of object relations theory, of the Chicago school of self psychology, of some aspects of the Lacanian school, and certainly of that branch of social psychology known as symbolic interactionism, based primarily on the work of George Herbert Mead (1934). It is also the working model for the neo-Piagetian school, well-represented by Kegan (1983).

3 The next recognisable stage of development is the differentiation and integration of the affective aspects of self and other experience, now as related to features of the real world. This world has been clearly mapped by Otto Kernberg (1981/2012), with models of the way the child has to integrate what were separate experiences of loving and hating affective links with others. These links gradually come to mesh and be enclosed within the growing sense of reality that enables the child to recognise that loving and hating experiences both belong to the one-self and to the one-other. This leads to the experiences of ambivalence, of the unity of self and of the unity of other. It further leads to that great step forward in social reality: the sense of destiny and of fate that descends on us in early childhood when we have to begin to come to terms with the reality of the world and where the shadows of shame and of guilt add to the richness of our perceptual and conceptual fields.

4 The stage is now set, given the unity of the personality, for entry into and recognition of the triangular experiences of one child with two parents that leads to that basic cornerstone of human adult experience, the Oedipal situation.

Varied models are offered for these successive stages of development, and if we have a firm grasp of their sequences and their distinctive characteristics, we have maps that will enable us to chart our way through our therapeutic encounters. This is what our theories are– maps and charts of psychic life. They are our ways of making the invisible visible and the abstract tangible and of harnessing the enormous powers of psychic forces.

How, then, do these maps and charts help us in our encounters with patients who live predominantly at one or another of these different levels of experience?

1 First, consider the person whose mental life is not yet organised distinctly and clearly within the primary setting of the self-other matrix. These psychotic patients live in a world in which parts of themselves and parts of others seem to act and interact in chaotic, mysterious and uncontrollable contexts. To enter into and understand this form of

psychic existence, we need reliable guides provided by some of the Kleinian analysts, such as Herbert Rosenfeld (1965), Henri Rey (1994), Salomon Resnik (1995) and others. Different but also reliable charts have come from other such centres as Chestnut Lodge, which was home to Harold Searles (1986/2018), and others.

2 The next recognisable level is the one we associate with borderline patients. Work with these patients is long, arduous, intensive and usually exhausting. The therapist feels invaded and threatened by the power of the other person's capacities for projection, projective and introjective identification, and the almost total demands that they make on the therapist for merger. So, much of the work for these patients has to be done with the therapist himself or herself. You cannot rely on the patient as a separate entity who can continue with the work of thinking, imagining, holding, containing and working through others' conflict, and containing his or her own experience. The therapist and the framework of therapy have to be the container, and we have to accept the patient as part of our content. Much of the work consists of gradually enabling the patients to become the container of their own experiences and to give up both the wished for and the feared state of symbolic oneness with the other that they seek. Eventually, they come to recognise and accept their own oneness, and their need to integrate within their own mental and emotional world. They come to recognise those apparently incompatible aspects of love and hate towards their primary objects, which have remained split off or have become split off under the impact of powerful regression and comfort, for consolidation of a sense of self that should be as available to the self as should be any part of the person's own body. The person has not yet developed the capacity to soothe, repair and restore states of disequilibrium, of tension and fluctuations of self-esteem. Indeed, the very nature of self-esteem is still related to idealisation of the object. By a relationship to the object, that esteem becomes claimed or felt to be a part of the self. Others are experienced as parts of a grandiose self and are idealised for the way in which they serve to complete the sense of self. Much of the focus of work in therapy is on the way in which a tension-relieving self object is experienced and on the need for the empathic understanding that only the self object can provide. These needs do entail a different listening perspective on the part of the therapist, and it was by altering his listening perspective that Kohut was able to explore the nature of this world of the patient, whose narcissistic needs predominate and can be recognised and met appropriately within the therapeutic framework.

3 Beyond this developmental line, we come to the situation of work with the many patients who recognise us as being separate from themselves, and we experience them as separate persons. Separate persons are the centre of their own initiative, volition and motivation. They are separate from us, and we are separate from them. We co-exist as separate entities

in space and time, and we are differentiated by individual boundaries. We are also linked with each other by virtue of those boundaries, by the opening, closing and alterations of these boundary functions in good relationships. Boundaries are not barriers to communication. In this world of continuing entities, entities that have continuity in space and in time, persons who have attained self-constancy and object-constancy, and threats of fragmentation and loss of self are remote. They will only be experienced through the threat of really great external trauma.

4 At the level of self and object constancy, we experience the necessity to form close and intimate relationships with others. Inevitably, we become involved at the Oedipal level and then have to bear the consequences of the strivings to deal with erotic and aggressive feelings that complicate all our triangulated relationships. It is a challenge to understand what the patients at earlier levels of development are experiencing constantly, daily and nightly: fragmentation, dissolution, the loss of self, the loss of cohesion.

These four levels are linked respectively, therefore, with neurotic, narcissistic, borderline and psychotic symptomatologies and nosology. I would like to illustrate something of the differences between what we aim to achieve, which is a form of creative listening, and the more mechanical listening, which we very often find ourselves doing and which, if we can listen to our patients, they will help us recognise and correct. It has been my experience over and over again, both within my own practice and through supervising others, that patients will very often refuse to accept and make use of an interpretation that comes from a therapist situated outside the realm of their own experience. The therapist 'targets' an aspect of their mental functioning in a way that seems more designed to meet the therapist's needs to be active, to demonstrate his understanding of psychodynamics and to use the patient as an example of his knowledge. The patient will feel vivisected by such an approach, and if he has the courage and the capacity to resist will do so actively. By contrast, when the patient is offered an interpretation that says to the patient 'this is something that involves you and I together', then the response is quite different.

Note

1 This lecture was given to an unknown audience, we believe in 2002, and has not been published previously. (Ed.)

Section IV

Metapsychology, philosophy, mind/body

13 The 'in-between'[1]

The journey from West to East is a mental journey, and in our gathering where we now meet to explore the cultural zone created by our meeting, we have a potential space for novelty and creativity. I shall speak of some Western ideas related to the concept of the space between people which is the space for therapy – where people act with and upon each other in dyadic and group situations.

The 'in-between'

When I speak about what is meant by 'in-between' people, I become aware of how much my vocabulary is based on imagery and metaphor. 'In-between' conjures up the image of bodied, bounded entities separated in space, the space of the 'between'. Words for describing how persons are interconnected include 'relate', 'communicate', 'like' or 'dislike', 'attract' or 'repel' and so forth. Some of these terms originate from physics, from the forces of attraction and repulsion that entered into the Western mind with the discovery of physical and magnetic forces. The underlying premise of this kind of mechanistic thinking is that people can be regarded in the same way as we regard non-human physical objects. This was not always the case, and we can see how the idea of the closed person, 'homo clausus', appears in European thought over centuries (Mennell 2001). In this, we can distinguish at least two processes: the concept of individuality and the concept of how the human organism functions.

In Western society, psychological individuality can be traced back at least to the twelfth century, before the Renaissance. In religious writings, in history, in personal memoirs and letters, in literature and portraiture, distinct individual creatures begin to appear. We hear the voices of men and women who introspect, who begin to become self-conscious, who discover that their minds are not only reflections of religious teachings and accepted authority but are precious for, in and of themselves. It may seem strange that such a mentality takes so long to emerge, for nowadays, at least in some sectors of Western society, individuality is taken for granted (Elias 2000; 1991/2001). A great deal of historical, sociological, psychological and literary writing is

DOI: 10.4324/9781003494713-17

devoted to tracing this development. Each generation is able to look back on its predecessors and see the culture in which people were then embedded, to see what those people themselves could not see of the great economic, social and religious forces that moulded them. Our vision of the present is always partial.

The psychology of the Western individual is, in many ways, a child of the Enlightenment, the seventeenth- and eighteenth-century drive to bring rational scientific thought into the forefront of society, replacing religion, magic, myth and superstition. In the nineteenth century, psychology begins to differentiate from philosophy and, with the founding of the first psychology laboratory in Europe by Wilhelm Wundt, psychology becomes an experimental science (Wundt 1911/2019). There are forgotten aspects to Wundt to which I shall later return.

From the individual to the mind

The most powerful model of the mind became that of a mechanism, a Newtonian clock whose parts could be assembled and disassembled. It was thought that each part could be studied separately in the laboratory and each person could be studied as a separate entity. These changes brought about the loss of the religious sentiments that held the Christian worldview together. As the Protestant ethic took place during the Reformation, each individual was seen to have a place on earth and, by their own personal conduct here, could find assurance of a place in Heaven, in an afterlife that was elsewhere. This view stands in contrast with other worldviews, like those here in the East, in which the departed have a continuing presence amongst their loved ones. Western man and woman become more single and solitary; they became more self-enclosed within a personal horizon that was apparently freed from religious, military or aristocratic control but was now enclosed within the 'iron cage' of modern industrial and capitalist society.

As part of the great Western process of secularisation, psychology grew into the conceptual space left by the decline in religious belief. This psychology was not only to do with the rational and the conscious. Freud (1900) propounded a psychology of the unconscious that was also a way of filling the empty space left after the loss of religious belief – a way of trying to understand the soul, the spirit and the mind. But even as he set about discovering the hidden depths of the unseen person, forming a new model of the individual governed by inner conflicts between ego, id and superego, Freud (1900) relied for his account on the idea of mental mechanisms, a Newtonian concept that returns us to clockwork. He was not only a positivist man of science, though: he was also a speculator, an explorer of dark spaces and an inheritor of German Romanticism, which was the antithesis of German and French Enlightenment rationalism. His depth psychology takes the individual as given, as already in existence as a psychic entity, which is true in part but in a far different sense to what he originally thought. There is a vertical layering in the psychoanalytical model of the person. In *The Ego and the Id*, the depth of the psyche is located in the primitive forces of the id. The ego is seen to mediate between the id and its drives and the superego, which is the internalised outside world (Freud 1923). But whilst he was developing this structural theory, he was also turning to social psychology through works that had their inception in the 1920s. At a relatively late point in his development, then, these perspectives became an increasingly important part of his oeuvre. They include *Group Psychology and the Analysis of the Ego* (Freud 1921), *The Future of an Illusion* (Freud 1927), *Civilisation and Its Discontents* (Freud 1930) and *Moses and Monotheism* (Freud 1939). However, the social groundwork of his psychology is always written from the position that culture and the individual are basically in opposition. He gave little attention to the 'in-between' beyond stating that the space between two persons is mysterious and uncomfortable, offering the analogy of two porcupines settling down to be as comfortable in their closeness as is possible, without penetrating each other with their spines. You may think that there is not much of melting warmth, loving closeness, or eager openness in this image (Ginsburg 1985).[2]

To return to Wundt (1911/2019), the originator of experimental psychology, there is a neglected side to him which is his great interest in what he called *Volk* psychology. This involves the study of language, mythology, customs, all the forces that impinge on the individual, which mould personality and the ways of life of a whole community, a *Volk*. Wundt regarded this 'supra-individual' psychology as far more important than laboratory psychology, where the isolated individual, an abstract entity, is a fish out of the social water. It is to this that I now turn, the concept of the person as intrinsically developed from and immersed within culture and society, interpenetrated and interconnected to the very core by social processes. My mentor, Foulkes, likened the individual to one of the Japanese flowers that were popular in his childhood, a small dull object which, when immersed in water, flowers into resplendent beauty (Foulkes 1964: 100). So, the individual outside society is a theoretic abstract; he can only develop in society, and unfortunately, he often does so on distorted and damaged terms.

Foulkes's work is situated within a conceptual model that we call holistic or organismic. At the turn of the twentieth century, psychologists began the study of larger entities – not the notes of a tune but its melody. Our capacity to recognise the same melody or harmony in different guises shows in how we grasp the world through our perceptions, in how patterns of sense data are imposed on the brain and in how we see Gestalts, whole figures, often before we can see their elements. The organismic psychology that emerged is one where the organism, in our case the person, is inseparable from its environment, which it constantly struggles to adapt to and master. Organism and environment are as figure to ground, inseparable and reversible. The intrinsic interconnectedness between organism and environment must be the starting point for any proper study of psychology or psychotherapy.

Organism and environment interconnected intrinsically and responsively; life takes the form of an unending dialogue. And here we can begin to connect with psychotherapy which – in all its forms – can be seen as aspects of a dialogue that takes place in the 'in-between'.

Psychotherapists have not yet fully grappled with the importance of dialogue as a developmental and therapeutic factor. A survey of infant and child development clearly shows that we are on the way to this. We understand much better the way in which human infants, born into an intensely social world, develop and unfold as does the Japanese flower in water. They survive because their needs are recognised and more or less adequately met by adult caregivers who are biologically and culturally equipped for this. The dialogue of infants and caregivers can be called 'proto-conversations', which exist long before the infant develops the capacity for speech. In this language of gestures, we can see the responsive actions of participants in subtle and sensitive interactions. These can be studied minutely in the natural situation of caring, feeding, playing, soothing, sleeping – all the situations where participants in the infant's life have to demonstrate a capacity for understanding and responding to each unique infant's mode of living and adapting. There are new words in the vocabulary of infant development and psychotherapy, words such as 'attunement', 'intersubjectivity' and 'state-sharing'. These words show how the enterprise of understanding human development is now concerned with following the ways in which infants begin to recognise themselves as human beings, how they begin to recognise that they are both alike to and different from other human beings through interaction, through dialogue. These are momentous developments in an infant's life, discovering that out there beyond the boundaries of its own body and its own developing sense of self is an other who is both other and yet similar. We can begin to see how we give infants the opportunity to discover who they are, both for themselves and for us, through the way in which we interact with them. Gaze, sound, handling, holding and playing are all inseparable from this process. We interpret infants' gestures as meaningful to ourselves, and by responding to them we make them meaningful to the infants who discover that their gestures make an impact on the world.

The Russian writer Mikhail Bakhtin (1981; Holquist 1981; 1990) is the originator of 'dialogism', a key construct in Russian psychology in which Lev Vygotsky (1962/2012) is another principal figure. This psychology integrates the psychological and the social. The 'personal' and 'social' are indivisible; the social fact 'precedes the psychological fact', for we take into ourselves (we internalise) the processes and results of our interactions with others. Thus, for Bakhtin, language and its precursors are always an utterance, a speaking out into the world that seeks response. An action is never complete until it has been answered by the utterance, the response or gesture of the Other. The basic human act is between one person and the other, a dialogue. Another word for this is 'alterity', a recognition of the fact that we become ourselves through the alter, the other, for the other can give me to myself by their regard, their response to me. They thereby give me a sense both of who I am and of who they are. And if we take this concept of alterity, of dialogue, as our start, then so many aspects of psychotherapy fall naturally into place. Without actually having to seek out and make conscious such early processes of human development, in the interpersonal situation of the dyad in the therapeutic group we retrace these early developmental paths.

Lateral depth

Human life takes place in the 'in-between'. Love-hate, cooperation-rivalry, understanding-misunderstanding – all these acts, mental and physical, involve the movements of approach and withdrawal, the opening and closing of ourselves, of our mental, emotional and physical boundaries to another or others. Emotions drive us to act; the word itself implies motion, movement.

We live in fascinating times in which we are increasing our understanding of human life. As group psychotherapists, we need to inform ourselves of significant research in emotional and mental development and be open in applying this to our theories and practice when there is relevance. You will already, I am sure, know about the trend of research in infant-caregiver processes. Research methods show with beautiful clarity and gripping conviction that infant life develops in a matrix of exchanges between infants and caregivers. Infants seek more than satisfaction of bodily hunger; they hunger for the actions and responses of caregivers who give them a sense of participation in the world of others. They primarily get a sense of becoming part of the mother as a loving caregiver, and through being part of her they also experience being separate, being apart. Human infants are born with the capacity and disposition to relate to as well as withdraw from other human beings. From the moment of birth, of release from the womb, there is a search to rejoin the mother, an experience mediated through physical holding, feeding, vocalising in baby speech, and gaze interaction. These interactions begin to lay down in the infant's experience, both of mind and body, the beginnings of self in relation to other. These processes are the precursors of language and are language forms themselves, the language of gestures, 'proto-conversations' that will lead to entering culture through language (Lichtenberg 1991).

Developing boundaries

The body has boundaries that the mind does not have. Encased in envelopes of skin, we communicate over distance with other creatures through our openings, our special senses. As human beings, as persons, we are not limited by our bodies as we exist as constituents in a continuum, as members of communities. We are 'co-creatures' who communicate, converse, cooperate.

Our capacity for consciousness, for knowing others, is socially derived. We are born through coition to lead separate lives, always bound together as group animals. We grow up in families, clans, communities, nations. Our prized individuality is our personal synthesis of the formative influences of our communities. The word 'identity' means to have an identity that sets us apart from others and yet stamps us as being identical to others. We seek separateness to develop our own identity, but we also delight in merging with others through shared actions, in song and dance, games, teams, organisations. In shared activities, we experience being parts of a greater whole and for a while are released from our separateness – our skin envelopes. Sadly, the greatest force that binds groups together, a force greater than pleasure and joy, is fear of and aggression towards other groups.

Moderation

This brings us to the theme of moderation, to the management of cooperation and understanding between groups, meetings in the 'in-between'. These meetings can take place if the conditions for dialogue and mutual understanding exist. This is the credo, the raison d'être of group psychotherapy. The history of small-group and now large-group therapy as developed over the past sixty years shows us that our confidence is justified, that the group therapy approach is a recognised and important factor in psychiatry, in social services, in organisations and in helping to resolve problems in and between communities.

As strangers participate as group members, the dynamics of group processes develop. Strangers find similarities and differences and eventually experience themselves as belonging to 'their' group, an entity they have formed and been formed by, that begins to take on an identity of its own – this is 'the group'. They speak with each other of their feelings, attitudes and appraisals and they speak of the other group members; they are seen, heard, addressed, understood and misunderstood by others. These processes we call dialogue, mirroring and resonance (Brown 1994/2000). Conflicts are inevitable – fears, hostilities, rejections – and can slowly resolve into understanding of what in oneself and one's own attitude causes or helps to cause such conflicts. The mirroring, the seeing and accepting, of exploring and understanding parts of oneself as seen by others and seeing aspects of oneself in others, is a form of benign 'dialogical mirroring'. It both continues and re-enacts fundamental childhood developmental processes. We build ourselves up largely through the internalisation of the reflected appraisals of others. Inevitably, there are people who find difficulties partaking in such processes, who are not open to sharing, to mutual recognitions. They feel misperceived and misunderstood. They will see and treat others in such ways as to make others feel unaccepted and unacceptable. The more such patients function on primitive levels of projection and denial, the more such group processes will occur until the dialogue is derailed and ceases. What each sees in the other is experienced as frightening and bad. It has to be abandoned or attacked. The mirroring now is non-dialogical. Now the forces of moderation, of mediation, are needed to bring understanding and conciliation so that the work of the group can continue. This work can be done by the other group members who are not caught up in these conflicts and of course by the therapist.

We are all familiar with the interruption to the therapeutic process that occurs with borderline and paranoid patients, with impulsive and infantile characters and anti-social persons. But we also know that in many cases, through special techniques, we can overcome these barriers. A combination of group understanding and firmness and my own underlying desire to join in have helped me to discover that insight and communication are more rewarding than withdrawal.[3]

War, peace and the 'in-between': Moderation and the use of moderators

The recently signed treaty between Israel and the PLO, the Oslo Accords, heralded, it was hoped, the beginning of the ending of community hatreds, the beginning of cooperation between nations that have hated and fought each other so many times, divided yet joined by a matrix of hatred. This was a false dawn as we sadly know. The process was facilitated by patient behind-the-scenes negotiations by Norwegian diplomats and social scientists. I shall give you a small-scale example of local efforts within Israel to bring Arabs and Jews into dialogue. A situation was set up for high school youths of both sexes from Arab and Jewish schools to meet in a residential setting. The aim was to get them to know each other and, hopefully, to increase understanding and cooperation between the ethnic groups. This project was a failure. Both groups closed ranks, speaking with one voice and blaming their opposing group for all the problems. The staff tried to analyse the reasons for this failure and to devise other approaches, and they succeeded. What they did, which was simple yet brilliant, was to get each of the two ethnic groups to meet separately and beforehand in their own settings, each in their own schools. There, the process of talking about and thinking through the issues that divided them began, without the presence of the other group against whom they had to present a united front. Each group, Arabs and Jews, began to use dialogue in separate groupings within which they expressed their own differences of opinions, facing their differences, learning to understand and to cope with conflict. When they met the other group, which had been going through the same process, the grounds for discussion and understanding were already there. They could meet in the 'in-between'. This small yet encouraging example is, I am sure, one that has been repeated in many places.

Finally, to elaborate on the underlying dynamics of this Arab-Israeli experience, when the groups first met without preparation, they united to show a common face to their enemy. They could not allow for internal differences, for separate voices; the members ceased to act as responsible individuals. They gave up the most developed parts of their mentality and formed a group mentality, a process we can understand as Bion's (1968/1998) basic assumption of fight-flight, adaptive to conflict situations.

When they met beforehand to discuss the issues under trained leaders, their differences could emerge and be discussed. Thus, their higher mental capacities were exercised, retained, maintained and enhanced by the mental work of discussion over difficult issues. The group as a whole maintained a higher level of social organisation, respecting and valuing differentiation. The strength of the group lay not in its primitive unity, its cohesion, but in its capacity to discuss, understand and negotiate, to value similarities and differences among themselves and with the others of the opposing group. This strength arose from a structural differentiation within the group. Each of the members of each group contributed as individuals to its strength and to its unity. This is the strength of coherency, a much more developed and flexible strength than cohesion. Cohesive strength is not flexible or adaptive. It is strong until it breaks, when it disintegrates into fragments. Coherent strength can be adaptive and flexible; it can accommodate differences and allow for growth and change (Pines 1997). This is the essence of a group therapy that is informed by psychodynamic principles. We know that the strength and unity of an individual human personality is based on similar processes taking place in infancy between the child and its caregivers. Rigid intrapsychic formations can dissolve, resolve and reform through the shared construction and formation of new dialogues, new 'in-betweenness' of group psychotherapy.

Evolutionary considerations about the 'in-between'

The virtuoso scientist J. B. S. Haldane (1932) was a physiologist, scientific populariser, politician and population geneticist, among his many other accomplishments. One day, sitting in a pub, he announced he would willingly lay down his life if he could save two brothers or eight cousins (Smith 1975). Haldane's reasoning was about the genetic advantages in altruism and the overriding importance of kinship. In kinship, there are overlapping genetic boundaries between individuals; self includes parts of others. Thus, genetics gives biological support to the fundamental thesis of group analysis that we are inextricably embedded with others in a psychosocial matrix throughout life. As persons striving to realise our unique individual potentials, we also know consciously and unconsciously that our potentials arise from and are realised through the lives of others, primarily our kin. We are both self and other; the other is partly self; self is in them.

Evolutionary forces in the deep design of the human animal make us innately loving, nurturing and allied to the interests of others. Slavin and Kriegman (1992) call this 'the adaptive design of the human psyche', a natural adult disposition to experience interest and mutuality with offspring which leads to altruistic acts. Human beings are intrinsically divided between self-interest as individuals and self-interest in others as social beings.

Altruism is not restricted to the relationships of kin. Concern for others is a present capacity in us to varying degrees – it is a powerful cohesive force within natural and artificial groups. We see it in friendships and in organisations, with work mates and in teams dedicated to caring for others at risk to themselves like fire services, ambulances and rescue teams. Caring for others who are not kin is accounted for by geneticists as 'reciprocal altruism', which means that at some point an altruistic act may be repaid. We may help the helpless, our neighbours, even strangers, from an inner sense of the rightness of such acts. We are part Pharisee and part Samaritan. Such altruistic acts may not be repaid to the actor, but there is a possibility that they will be repaid to members of the extended network to which the actor belongs, *the chain of interdependency*, to use Norbert Elias's (2000) term. My colleague Robin Skynner (1989b) wrote eloquently about 'the myth of altruism'.

Evolutionary pressures for such interconnections also develop our capacities to discriminate between reciprocators and non-reciprocators, those we would call cheats, who use us in their own interest and do not repay our investments in them. We must know how to look into and look through people to detect cheats and deceivers, the seductive salespersons of themselves. We need also to know how to keep secrets, tell lies and deceive, for at times this is necessary for the maintenance of our own safety, integrity and self-interest. There are tricky depths to the 'in-between'.

Conflicting interests are part of the human condition; they exist between parents and offspring, between siblings, within extended families and in social life. Freud described the eternal, dynamic pull between separateness and togetherness as the eternal struggle between Eros and Thanatos (Freud 1930). It has been recently demonstrated how infant and mother struggle with each other at the placental barrier; the foetus invasively implants into the mother's body, competing for the vital nutrients needed for its survival and growth. A healthy child may be responsible for an ill mother. Siblings' competition for love and attention from the limited resources of their parents can generate illness in them.

Parents are genetically equally invested in all of their children and therefore have an interest in encouraging altruistic behaviour at the sibling level, but siblings do not have the same genetic involvement with each other as the parents. Freud noticed that children hate each other as competitors, though this hatred may lessen with maturity and the lessening dependency on parents (Mitchell 2000). Of course, on the psychological level, parents are not equally invested in all their children.

The practice of psychotherapy: Psychoanalysis and group analysis

Psychoanalysis presents us with two radically different concepts of human nature, broadly speaking: the antagonistic and the cooperative. On the one hand are Freud and Klein, on the other, Ferenczi, Fairbairn, Guntrip, Winnicott and Kohut: drive theory versus theories of object relations and self-objects.

From its origins, group analysis has this second paradigm that acknowledges the essential sociability of mankind as well as the conflicts inherent in social life – this is Foulkes's model of persons as nodes in the social matrix. When there are dysfunctions and disjunctions between members of the matrix, as within the family, these nodes become focal points of disturbance and show up as a figure against the ground of the family, organisation or therapy group. Morris Nitsun's (1996) thesis of the anti-group has focused attention on these universal components of group life, though he has not taken his argument through to the biological and genetic level.

Another tenet of group analysis is that the healthy individual is an open system, open to change and learning. When we become closed systems, we fall sick, no longer adapting to and thriving from exchange with the encompassing human environment. *Homo sapiens* learns from his own experience and from cultural inheritance. Norbert Elias (2000) tells us to think of human animals as 'homines aperti', open people, not as the single 'homo clausus', the closed person. Bachelard (1992) calls us 'half-open creatures', expressing the view that we cannot stand excessive exposure; we need solitude, sleep, day and our night dreams to balance our sanity. Openness also denotes vulnerability; we may be overwhelmed, misled and deceived. Scepticism is an essential aspect of self-preservation, safeguarding the development and integrity of the self-system. Doubt can be crippling, but we cannot do without it. Children are right to question their parents' motives and actions, for parents will act in their own self-interest and attempt to impose their own solutions on their offspring, so transmitting family pathology. The turbulence of adolescence is a time to reorganise the self, to discover the individual's own capacities and goals, to renegotiate the relations of past, present and future.

The reorganisation of the self, particularly in adolescence but throughout life, is a process of recognising, revisioning and revising aspects of the self that are both compatible and incompatible with the encompassing environment, to use Foulkes and Anthony's term (1975; 1986). The adaptive aspect of repression is that buried unconscious schemas are in storage and are capable of being revived and reviewed when conditions allow. The adaptive view has important consequences for psychotherapy. Patients use the transference to probe the capacity of therapist and group to understand what these unconscious forces represent as they surface in the interpersonal, the 'in-between'. The task of therapy here is to find mutual and reciprocal ways to arrive at new adaptive solutions. Foulkes anticipated this when he wrote that group analysis is 'analysis of the group including the conductor' (Foulkes 1975: 3). The therapist responsible for a group cannot take the patient in the group farther than the therapist himself or herself has been able to go.

The 'in-between' is the space for review and revision of the 'fit' between individual and environment. 'Goodness of fit' is a principle of Gestalt psychology, the optimal adaptation of organism to environment as was emphasised by Foulkes's mentor Goldstein (1939/2000). The subjective experience of this, the sense of a good fit within the self system, is the sense of vitality, effectiveness and resourcefulness, of living better, of being able to transform tension into attention.

In group analysis, the subject is exposed to the multiplicity of others, to many responses from and towards oneself. Becoming attuned to the variability of the group situation involves capacities to listen, reflect, discover, react and respond to the mentalities and experiences of the several others. There are wide differences between people in their capacity and willingness to engage with the mentalities of others. Such differences span the dimension from the single tenaciously held viewpoint, 'I don't understand you; I have no experience of what it is like to feel like that, to be you' to the capacity (true or false) to be in relationship and to the many different mental experiences brought by the others. There will inevitably be both meetings and missings.

Mirroring and resonance represent modes of meeting. The experiences of one may be amplified through the responses of others, responses of similar and of different self-states, differing perspectives on shared experience. Monologue can transform into dialogue when individuals shed some of their separateness, as self-boundaries become more open. The therapeutic process reopens an internal dialogue, the recognition of the multiple voices of each single self. Each can begin to recognise that there is a multiplicity of selves within the illusion of the unit self, which compete to represent the whole person, to substitute dialogue for monologue (Schlapobersky 1994/2000). Monoglossia can replace heteroglossia, as Bakhtin (1981; Holquist 1981; 1990) describes the progressive movement from one tongue to many. Within every closed political system of tyranny or control, one tongue purports to speak for many. In open societies we gradually differentiate ourselves as persons, subjects, citizens and selves.

We are all formed in the experiential and linguistic world of many. Is the presupposition of a unitary self a healthy necessity, a comforting illusion? We each possess a framework for dealing with experience. Frames are essential: they set limits, they filter the booming buzzing confusion of the world, in William James's (2013) memorable phrase. Frames filter, contain, accept and deflect internal and external perceptions.

Bakhtin (1981; Holquist 1981; 1990) calls our point of view 'a surplus of vision'. It is our own, developed in our lifespan, and we can offer it to others. Each has a way of experiencing the world, and in the course of our lifespan we may eventually come to see this from without – the Archimedean principle of 'give me a lever and I can move the world'. When the invisible frame is seen, a choice can be made as to whether it is adaptive or maladaptive. An example: A patient who led a hectic life, running from one appointment to another – I used to see him running past my window for his appointment – was hugely relieved when I suggested that he was the slave of time, not its master, as he had believed. My viewpoint was the lever that enabled him to change his pace and live within time, abandoning his futile attempt to live outside of it. Each person brings their own framework to group analysis, of which they are only partially aware, as we cannot see ourselves. What is unknown to self may quickly be known by others, to use the language of the Johari window (known to self, known to others; unknown to self, known to others; unknown to others, known to self; unknown to both self and others). Learning to see ourselves through the eyes of others can be both painful and releasing, confirming and disconfirming.

The unstructured group-analytic situation allows for the emergence of many different viewpoints. The solidity of each subject begins to melt as the group process takes hold. As in a kaleidoscope, patterns seem ever changing, but in time, a recognisable coherence emerges, a coherence of personal styles, relationship patterns, meetings and disjunctions. Conflicts emerge and resolve as persons come to recognise and understand the meanings of their oppositions and alliances. The process is not linear; it is more spiral, circling around many of the same issues – authority, sexuality, intimacy, emotional development – as the group process unfolds over time. The capacity for emotional and mental health may reside in the 'ability to stand in the spaces between realities without losing any of them – the capacity to feel like one self while being many' (Bromberg 1993: 166). This possibility to be both one and many is there in the group for those who can take it.

In conclusion: Freud, Janet, Ferenczi, Goldstein, Foulkes, Gregory

At the end of the nineteenth century, Freud and Pierre Janet were the great explorers of the mind, each with a vision of the complexity of mental processes. In the understanding of their time, Janet's account of dissociation gave way to Freud's model of repression based on scientific positivism. In his account, the hierarchical organisation of the psyche is based on the neurological model of this time drawn from Hughlings Jackson (Critchley and Critchley 1998) in which the forces of the mind are understood to work on linear terms. Today there is a new interest in Janet's contrasting, originating theories of dissociation for their relevance especially in the understanding and treatment of trauma (Craparo 2019; LeBlanc 2001). In Freud's repression model, there is a barrier between conscious and unconscious. The structures of the psyche (id, ego and superego), though interconnected, are separate psychic entities. But Janet, more than Freud, was able to entertain the concept of multiple selves, of constantly changing levels of consciousness and unconsciousness. He did not postulate 'the' unconscious. He was much like Ferenczi who – more than Freud – could see the subtle, differentiated landscapes of the psyche. Foulkes was closer to this way of understanding. Influenced by Goldstein, he conceived of mind as social, as multiple, as the emergence of self from a social matrix, always intertwined and sustained through this matrix. His own account of this is most accessible in a short section of the book written with Anthony where, in 'Model of different levels of communication', they explore 'the frontier between what is normally conscious and normally unconscious'. They describe twelve different layers of human experience, stratified by their levels of conscious or unconscious awareness (Foulkes and Anthony 1965/1983: 160). Foulkes returns to these ideas about differentiated levels of conscious and unconscious experience in groups when, writing on his own in his 1964 text, he simplifies and reduces the earlier account to four levels – current, transference, projective and primordial (Foulkes 1964/1984: 114–116).

His ideas give access to a more relational than a unitary self, and we see the same ideas emerging in self psychology and intersubjectivity. The concept of a 'relational unconscious' in which conscious, preconscious and unconscious emerge in response to and in relationship with the minds of others is current. This is the conscious and unconscious of the 'in-between', emerging through the gaps opening within the group, when understandings appear as background to the foreground of misunderstandings. Misunderstandings, recognised and explored, can lead persons back to the origin of their incompatibilities within their own primary groups (Lyons-Ruth 1999).

The group-analytic experience opens up the possibility of moving fluidly between different experiences of self and other. The idiosyncratic, the I, emerges as foreground against the experience of self with and interrelated with others as background. Gregory, the great explorer of vision and of mirrors, writes that the beliefs and hypotheses of the sciences are 'gap filling'. Perception and scientific hypotheses bridge gaps in data to predict unsensed properties of things and act in the service of prediction. He declares that the mind abhors gaps and, making the presumption that this is because they block action, he points to a major difference between science and myth. Science draws its strength, he says, from admitting and examining sometimes frightening gaps in perception and understanding. Myths do the same but fill the gaps in very different ways. Mirroring reality remains difficult and controversial, depending on how the eye and brain are focussed (Gregory 1997).

Notes

1 This presentation was given as a keynote lecture to the 1993 regional meeting of the International Association of Group Psychotherapy held in Taipei, Taiwan. It has not been published previously. (Ed.)

2 Freud kept a statue of a bronze porcupine amongst the artefacts in his consulting room. It is on display in the Freud Museum in London. (Ed.)

3 The clinical material with which Pines illustrated this part of his lecture has been removed because it was not possible to identify those described nor to seek their consent to its inclusion. (Ed.)

14 Problems with Freud's constitutional aggression and the virtues of group analysis[1]

My talk tonight is addressed to the problems I find in Freud's theory of innate, constitutional aggression – it underlies much of his thinking and is extended in the theory of Melanie Klein and the Kleinian school. I shall begin with the well-known exchange of letters between Freud and Albert Einstein in 1932, published one year later as 'Why War?' (Freud SE XXII:1964: 199–201).[2] Reading Freud's reply to Einstein and thinking about my response to it, I am, as always, impressed by the broad sweep of Freud's vision and by his exposition of the complexity of human life, followed by his reduction of this complexity to the two great principles of Eros and Thanatos. Let us return to the complexity. Here is the gist of his position as set out to Einstein (and the world at the time). He declares it to be a general principle that:

> Conflicts of interest between men are settled by the use of violence. This is true of the whole animal kingdom, from which men have no business to exclude themselves. . . . In a small human horde, it was superior muscular strength which decided who owned things or whose will should prevail. . . . From the moment at which weapons were introduced the winner was the one who had the better weapons . . . but the final purpose of the fight remained the same, to subdue the other, to eliminate the opponent permanently and/or to kill him. Killing an enemy also satisfied an instinctual function. . . . There was a path which led from violence to right or law. . . . Violence could be broken by union, and the power of those who were united now represented law in contrast to the violence of the single individual. Thus, we see that right is the might of a community. It is still violence, ready to be directed against any individual who resists it. . . . The union of the majority must now be a stable and lasting one. The recognition of a community of interest leads to the growth of emotional ties between the members of a united group of people—communal feelings . . . the true source of its strength. If the security of communal life is to be guaranteed each individual must surrender his personal liberty to turn his strength to violent uses. . . . From its very beginning the community comprises elements of unequal strength—men and women, parents and children and soon, as a result of

DOI: 10.4324/9781003494713-18

> war and conquest, it also comes to include victors and vanquished, who turn into masters and slaves. The justice of the community then becomes an expression of the unequal degrees of power obtaining within it; the laws are made by and for the ruling members and find little room for the rights of those in subjection. (Freud SE XXII:1964: 199–201).

We can summarise the complex sweep of his account thus:

1 Men have no business to exclude themselves from the animal kingdom.
2 Conflicts of interest in the animal kingdom are settled by the use of violence.
3 The path from violence to law is by the union of the weak against the strong. Right is the might of the community, a form of violence ready to be directed at any who resist it.
4 To guarantee the security of communal life each must give over his personal liberty to turn strength to violent use and surrender it to the community at large – the state.

The last two of these statements will surely remind us of Norbert Elias (2000), who traced the evolution of the modern psyche with its strong ego and the capacities of the superego to exercise restraint and foresight to inhibit immediate outbursts of violence. According to Freud, violence was formerly adaptive for man – a means of defence to protect his safety and that of his family. The evolving development of society saw emerging superior powers in groups that began to monopolise the use of force, affording protection to individuals and families that lay within their circle. In Freud's letter to Einstein we see him attribute the emerging rule of law in societies to the definition of these circles of protection and to the codification of the relationship between individuals and their society. The internalisation of these social forces leads to the presence of a power that is both protective and punishing: the protective and punishing superego.

There is a developmental thrust in Freud's story of the evolution of law, but in the final account the weight is on the elemental, eternal force of aggression: the death instinct. The death instinct at work in every living creature makes it useless to try to get rid of mass aggression. Before turning to Foulkes and the group-analytic attitude to man's unquestioned capacity for destructiveness, I would like to fill out Freud's true statement that humankind has no business to exclude itself from the animal kingdom. There is a growing body of knowledge of the complex social relationships in the animal kingdom, best studied and analysed in the primates. What is being learned in this newer literature should excite the interest of all students of human behaviour, particularly those of us who accept the primacy of the social for the evolution of the individual. A great deal in these advances can be found in one form or another in the following seven books:

1 De Waal (1996): *Good Natured: The Origins of Right and Wrong in Humans and Other Animals*
2 Wrangham and Peterson (1977/1996): *Demonic Males: Apes and the Origin of Human Violence*
3 Donald (1991): *Origins of the Human Mind: Three Stages in the Evolution of Culture and Cognition*
4 Oliner et al. (1992): *Embracing the Other: Philosophical, Psychological, and Historical Perspectives on Altruism*
5 Slavin and Kriegman (1992): *The Adaptive Design of the Human Psyche: Psychoanalysis, Evolutionary Biology, and the Therapeutic Process*
6 Ridley (1996): *The Origins of Virtue: Human Instincts and the Evolution of Cooperation*
7 Margalit (1996): *The Decent Society*

These books are rich sources of information and speculation about the evolution of social capacities in primates, which both genetically and culturally are so much more evident in humankind. I will discuss Freud's primary argument in the light of this literature and begin with Adam Smith, whose *Wealth of Nations*, written during the eighteenth-century Scottish Enlightenment, provided a founding text in political economy that explained prosperity as a product of free enterprise.

> In almost every other race of animal, each individual when it has grown up to maturity is entirely independent, and in its natural state has occasion for the assistance of no other living creature. But man has almost constant occasion for the help of his brethren, and it is vain for him to expect it from their benevolence only. He will be more likely to prevail if he can interest their self-love in his favor and show them that it is for their own advantage to do for him what he requires of them. It is not from the benevolence of the butcher, the brewer, or the baker, we expect our dinner: it is from their regard to their own interest. We address ourselves not to their humanity but to their self-love and never talk to them of our own necessities but of their advantages. Nobody but a beggar chooses to depend chiefly on the benevolence of his fellow citizens.
>
> (Smith 1776/2003: 19)

We have to go further than Adam Smith. In the complexity of human society and the complete interdependence we have on each other for survival and development, a community is a web of interdependences. Hence, we recognise that we are parts of the invisible chains that make our life forms possible. So let us now ask: what is the biological foundation of our capacity to live and flourish in complex societies? Is there a biological foundation for benevolence? We need the neurological hardware that enables us to recognise, appreciate and cope with complex and multiple social relationships. Human children grow up in societies that present them with rules of conduct, obedience and conformity, to recognise rank and hierarchy and the social obligation and rewards of work. Nowadays, it is evident that most of these issues are already present in monkey and ape societies and that the necessary hardware is provided by the growth of the brain. There is a tight correlation between brain size and social group. The bigger the society in which the individual lives, the bigger its neocortex relative to the rest of the brain: 'To thrive in a complex society you need a big brain. To acquire a big brain you need to live in a complex society' (Ridley 1996: 69). Interdependent relationships involve the development of the capacities for reciprocity, for exchange, for recognising trustworthy fellows and distinguishing them from the untrustworthy. For these, we need good memories and a social intelligence, social awareness that informs us of the boundaries of the possible and the acceptable and what lies without these boundaries.

These facts are missing in Freud's overview of the evolution of society, accounted for by the state of the evolutionary biology of his time and by his personal conviction of the strength of human destructiveness. Freud was a staunch Darwinian and did not attend to or appreciate what Peter Kropotkin (1902/2008) had foreshadowed in his famous book *Mutual Aid*. Kropotkin pointed out that cooperation is an ancient animal tradition with which man, like other animals, was endowed. Animals who demonstrate mutual aid are the fittest to survive. So what do modern sociobiology and genetics now tell us about the genetic basis of sociability? Frans de Waal, recognised as one of the world's leading primatologists, writes:

> It is hard to imagine human morality without the following tendencies and capacities found also in other species. Sympathy-related traits include attachment, succorance and emotional contagion; learned adjustment to and special treatment of the disabled and injured; and an ability to trade places mentally with others (cognitive empathy).
>
> (De Waal 1996: 211)

Sympathy is shown when animals give care or provide relief to distressed or endangered individuals other than their progeny. De Waal calls this 'succourance behaviour'. If we, or animals, are vicariously affected by someone else's feelings and situation, we are being sympathetic, and this behaviour is shown through the individualised bonding, affection and fellowship of many mammals and birds. De Waal and others have observed that injured and handicapped monkeys are not as a rule abandoned or maltreated; they receive extra tolerance, vigilance and care. Monkeys respond to the distress of others of their group, especially amongst friends and relatives, which seems to indicate that there is an awareness of 'social mirrors', that others and self are in some ways alike. We can conclude that such animals are attached by emotional bonds, that they exhibit emotional contagion – they are affected by the emotions of others – and that this leads to caring behaviour and, possibly, to what De Waal terms 'cognitive altruism': behaviour in the interests of the other. He says: 'Despite its fragility and selectivity, the capacity to care for others is the bedrock of our moral system which functions to protect and nurture the caring capacity' (De Waal 1996: 88). In Freud's language, this is the function of Eros, the principle that serves to bind entities together and mitigates destructiveness.

The next feature De Waal emphasises is 'norm-related characteristics': presumptive social rules that organise group behaviour which are internalised and obeyed. They derive from a hierarchical organisation in which the subordinate pays close attention to the dominant: 'Without agreement on rank and a certain respect for authority there can be no great sensitivity to social rules, as anyone who has tried to teach simple house rules to cats will agree!' (De Waal 1996: 92). But it is not only fear of punishment that provides respect for rules and norms; the desire to belong to, to fit into the group, is involved. As the social structure becomes more elaborate, as in chimpanzees, there is a shift from the despotic towards a social arrangement; there is room for sharing, tolerance and acceptance from those above and below one another in the power structure. 'The dismantling of despotic hierarchies in the course of hominid evolution brought an emphasis on leadership rather than on dominance and made the privilege of high status contingent upon services to the community, such as conflict management' (De Waal 1996: 142).

Reciprocity is a factor that is essential to moral behaviour: do unto others as you wish them to do unto you. This capacity seems to begin with food sharing. To give some of one's food to others establishes the system where one can expect to receive from others. Reciprocity leads to alliances. We do things together and our interests benefit each other. For these systems to work, there must also be ways of detecting cheating – and of punishing cheats – which is another step in social sophistication!

The last capacity found in primates that lays the foundation for human society and morality is that of 'getting along'. This involves peacemaking, conflict avoidance, negotiation to accommodate conflicting interests, and concern for the community as a whole through the maintenance of good relationships. Returning to Freud's answer to Einstein, he states that it is a general principle that conflicts of interest are settled by violence. We now know that this is not so: there are elaborate social procedures for settling conflicts without violence and which serve the interest of the community as a whole. We know that negotiators of conflict resolution receive social prestige, that communities are regulated by norms that benefit the community and that norms are acquired by learning, so that animals are not simply creatures of instinct.

What, I wonder, would Foulkes have thought about these sociobiological ideas? He admired Julian Huxley's concept that man is a new and unique kind of organism whose evolution is no longer purely biological but primarily cultural (Foulkes 1964/1984). He thought the time was ripe for the study of psychosocial evolution. In his far-reaching review paper, 'Psychotherapy in the 1960's', he writes that Freud could not find the biology to link with his psychoanalytic findings. The id, the mental reservoir of unconscious drive, was a no-man's-land of the earlier developmental phases of the human individual. Foulkes, ever respectful to Freud and psychoanalysis, tactfully mentions modern zoology, anthropology and ethology as fields of study for the psychotherapist, all contributing to the study of 'living beings, most of all man . . . born with incomplete adaptive structures. These are completed in a transactional reality, the nature of which is transmitted from generation to generation' (Foulkes and Stewart Prince 1972: 148).

Two psychoanalysts who have studied evolutionary biology have offered a psychoanalytic schema that incorporates this knowledge. Slavin and Kriegman's (1992) central thesis is that the entity we call the self cannot be strictly individual, nor a thoroughly social entity. The self is a 'semi-social' entity, social through genetic adaptation over countless generations. Crucial adaptive challenges faced by countless ancestral generations, through differential survival and reproduction, have powerfully shaped aspects of the psyche's deep structure before the individual child encounters the world for the first time. This semi-social psyche concept is a way of describing the tension between individual and society that characterises the human being. Through our genetic kinship with others, the locus of self is both within the skin-bounded individual and with related others. With this, there is also the tension between the essential affects that drive the person to particularise the self versus the affects that promote and maintain deep connections with the interests and subjective experiences of related others. We semi-social creatures are inherently divided between eternally conflicting aims and that is what we are – both intrinsically individualistic and innately social, inherently selfish and self-promoting, also inherently primarily altruistically disposed towards those whose interests we share. The family of generation and of nurture is an arena of conflicting interests. Infants, children and parents have conflicting as well as mutual aims, and it is through the recognition and negotiation of these conflicts that the process of psychic growth and individuation takes shape.

On returning to the second part of this chapter's title, 'The virtues of group analysis', I mean to say that the framework of group analysis fully recognises the semi-social nature of the human being. We can now go beyond Foulkes's starting position, where he grasped the importance of cultural change in shaping the psyche – a theme so productively developed by Norbert Elias. We now also have the modern biology of which he saw the necessity. Ridley (1996) offered us the striking recognition that we define virtue almost exclusively as pro-social behaviour and vice as antisocial behaviour. This formulation does not take into account the inborn tension between the individual and the social, but it serves the useful function of bringing virtue back to our attention.

Margalit develops a theme that connects with that of virtue. He asks: What is a 'decent society'? His answer is that a decent society is one whose institutions do not humiliate people (Margalit 1996). He differentiates this from a civilised society, which is one whose members do not humiliate each other. Thus, the decent society is a 'macro-ethical' concept, a setup of society as a whole in contrast to the 'micro-ethical' concept of the way that individuals treat each other. Influenced, I should imagine, by the conflicts within the Israeli society in which this author lives, and by its relationship to the encompassing Arab world, Margalit looks at the way in which societies provide the possibility of the primary good for human beings – of self-esteem. He bases this on a theory of justice advanced by Rawls (2005), who speaks of the distributed good, the social conditions that enable people to have self-respect. Margalit is well aware that in his own society this good is only distributed to people who are seen as belonging to the community through religion or ethnicity.

Margalit, looking at humiliation, evokes the distinction introduced by the philosopher Bernard Williams between 'red and white' responses to humiliation. The red response is that of blushing, of shame experienced as if one were in the eyes of others. The white response is more that of guilt, where the eyes are those of the inner world (Williams 1969: 159). Humiliation can appear in our ways of treating other people not as fellow humans but as things, as machines, when we impose on them feelings of helplessness and defencelessness. The humiliating agent is he or she who can create a situation that puts the other into this degrading position.

On the social level, Margalit introduces the useful concept of the 'encompassing group'. What is an encompassing group? It is not the intermediate group that we know about in sociology, those smaller groups that mediate between individual and society. The encompassing group has more powerful emotional connotations:

1 There is a common character and culture that encompasses many important and varied aspects of life and that shapes peoples' lifestyles.
2 Growing up in an encompassing group, people acquire the group culture and possess its special traits.
3 There is a mutual recognition between the members of an encompassing group, which is informal and does not require formal procedures. Conditions such as birth, or belonging to the culture, are generally considered reasons for such identification. It is not a formal setting with clear explicit rules for membership.
4 Thus, membership of the group is important for self-identification of those belonging to it. Membership in such a group goes hand in hand with the identification of the members as belonging to the group, and therefore it is an accepted way for people to present themselves to others.
5 Membership in the group is a matter of belonging rather than achievement. One need not prove oneself or excel in anything to be accepted

> as a full member in the group. Being a prominent member of the group may be a matter of achievement, but just belonging is not. To be a good Irishman is a matter of achievement; being Irish is solely a matter of belonging.

People do not decide to belong to an encompassing group; they belong because of who and what they are. This makes it a focus for self-identification because one's very membership in the group cannot be threatened in the same way it can be threatened in groups based on achievement.

Lastly, these are not small face-to-face groups; they are anonymous groups that may be stretched out throughout the world, as are the Jews in the diaspora or the Irish in emigration. This makes it necessary to have a whole range of symbols – ceremonies, rituals and other events and accessories – that enable the members to identify friends and foes.

The significance of the encompassing group is that ejection or rejection from or by such a group is a very powerful and painful source of humiliation. This can apply to the individual who is ejected from such a group or to the group itself if it is rejected by society as a whole. These are forms of cultural violence which can, of course, lead to outbreaks of physical violence. The most powerful violence can be between the group as a whole that is rejected by society, as is shown in ethnic conflicts that, for instance, have followed the breakup of the Soviet empire or the former Yugoslavia.

A decent society is also one that respects personal privacy. Margalit describes the private realm as the minimal sphere for individuals' control over their interest. Violation of privacy is restricting individuals' control, against their will, over what is supposed to be within their control. A society that closely surveys the activity of individuals, as in totalitarian states, invades personal privacy, showing a lack of consideration for the vital interests of the person. The overthrowing of totalitarian communities is one manifestation of the enormous pressure that builds up inside people as a result of such invasions. Thus, we have here another source of violence based on 'despotic societies' that have not learnt the lessons of our primate cousins: authority should be based on acceptance from those below in the power structure.

> The dismantling of despotic hierarchies in the course of hominoid evolution brought an emphasis on leadership rather than dominance, and made the privileges of high status contingent upon services to the community (such as effective conflict management).
>
> (De Waal 1996: 132)

We can see the evolution of this form of leadership in our large-group events, when informal forms of leadership seem to develop from the chaotic conditions that prevail in the early stages of such groups. The chaotic conditions eventually give way to an informal structure, with distributed leadership being acknowledged in those persons who have the capacities to understand and guide the group in its social evolution.

In conclusion I will offer two important distinctions provided by Mikhael Bakhtin (1981; Holquist 1981; 1990). The first is between monoglossia and heteroglossia. The normal state of human society is one of different voices in dialogue and debate – heteroglossia. When one individual voice, a dialect, attempts to legislate itself as the sole voice of a society, this becomes a totalitarian feature, the state of monoglossia. To this, we can add that humans have the capacity to assess fairness and outcomes of both government and private performances critically, which provides a constant selective pressure for change in both rules and performance. By this means, governed populations ultimately select morally significant reforms through pressure and choice. This process is dependent on the degree to which such talk is allowed: critical assessments, from pulpits, arts, press, social science and intermediate organisations, constantly attempt to voice individual unfairnesses and to aggregate them in order to initiate reforms.

Bakhtin's second distinction is between the voice of authority and the voice of persuasion. The voice of authority has to be taken as a whole, in one piece without loose edges; no part can be critically evaluated separately from the whole; there is no place for critical assessment. A persuasive voice can be taken piecemeal, taken apart and responded to with questions. This voice is an 'utterance', not an edict. The natural fundamental human speech form is that of the utterance – a voice that seeks its completion through the response of the other. The group analytic situation favours the persuasive voice, though the group may seek the voice of authority.

These voices, the voices of heteroglossia and the persuasive voice, represent the move from tribalism to universality, the extension of moral boundaries to encompass those marginal to the dominant core social group. These are the 'others' within the group, in contrast to those without. Within the group will be the sick, the criminal, the refugee, the other ethnic and religious groups, the sub-dominants. Can we move towards what is being called 'civil society', one in which altruism can be incorporated into cultural regulations? Is there an emergent quality that selects for the rapid expansion of commonly held moral constraints? These significant questions lead us into a whole area of the nature and development of altruism, of the pro-social in conflict with the antisocial. There are enough questions here to keep us occupied for a lifetime, let alone an evening!

Notes

1 This paper was first delivered as a lecture to an unknown audience in the late 1990s. It has not been published previously. (Ed.)

2 The context for the correspondence between Freud and Einstein was set by a proposal by the League of Nations and its International Institute of Intellectual Cooperation to have people of note – in this case Einstein – 'invite a person, to be chosen by myself, to a frank exchange of views on any problem that I might select

(which) affords me a very welcome opportunity of conferring with you (Professor Freud) upon a question which, as things now are, seems the most insistent of all problems which civilization has to face . . . is there any way of delivering mankind from the menace of war?' He poses a series of questions for Freud's attention based on Einstein's own premise that 'man has within him a lust for hatred and aggression' . . . 'and so we come to our last question. Is it possible to control man's mental evolution so as to make him proof against the psychoses of hate and destructiveness? . . . Here lies, perhaps, the crux of all the complex of factors we are considering, an enigma that only the expert in the lore of instincts can resolve.' (Freud SE XXII:1964: 199–201) (Ed.)

15 From social mind to social brain[1]

Introduction: Human sociability

What is the social brain? We are social animals embedded in networks of relationships without which we cannot survive. Human beings have the greatest capacity of all animals to create and control their environment, their portion of nature. Humans are cultured animals who have the brain capacity to develop cultural communities.

Merlin Donald (2007: 215) states:

> Human beings are cultural entities. We share mind. We construct cognitive collectivities called symbolic cultures. Raised in isolation from such collectivities, we have quite limited, non-symbolic minds. Culturally isolated human beings are not much different from their large-brained anthropoid relatives. However, embedded in a cultural network from birth, human beings become something unique in the biological world: symbolizing intellects bonded to a community of minds.

This understanding of our sociability is rooted in many strands in the history of ideas since the Enlightenment. Emma Rothschild (2001: 3) writes in the introduction to her magisterial work, *Economic Sentiments: Adam Smith, Condorcet and the Enlightenment*, that in the years 1770 to 1820,

> economic life was intertwined . . . with the life of politics and the life of the mind. Economic thought was intertwined with political, philosophical, and religious reflection. The life of cold and rational calculation was intertwined with the life of sentiment and imagination.

The most exciting of her discoveries was finding in the writings of Adam Smith, author of *The Wealth of Nations*, a beautiful, clear exposition of society as a *mirror* for the person (the *mirror* is Smith's own word). Without this mirror, the person will never come to know himself or herself. In 1759, Smith, then holding a chair at Glasgow University, published *The Theory of Moral Sentiments*, in which he asserts that man is a social animal and that

DOI: 10.4324/9781003494713-19

without the society of his fellows, the individual has no mirror for his own actions. If a human being were to grow up in solitude, he writes, he could no more think of his own character – of the beauty or deformity of his own mind – than of the beauty or deformity of his own face, being without a *mirror*. But, he writes, bringing him into society places a mirror in the countenance and behaviour of those he lives with through which he can view the propriety and impropriety of his own passions and the beauty and deformity of his own mind. Because mankind approves or is disgusted by his passions, life in society can moderate extremes of feeling. He demonstrates how the individual is drawn towards social norms, desiring not only praise, but *praiseworthiness*. Admiring the excellence of others, we wish ourselves to become admirable, desiring not only their respect but – through them – our own self-respect. Introducing the famous – or infamous – term, 'the invisible hand', he anticipates spontaneous self-determining social order in concepts leading to the idea of cybernetics and negative feedback.

Contributions from group analysis and neuroscience

S. H. Foulkes (1964/1984: 81) defines mirroring thus:

> Mirror reactions are characteristically brought out when a number of persons meet and interact. The person sees himself, or part of himself – often a repressed part of himself – reflected in the interactions of other group members. He sees them reacting in the way he does himself. . . . He also gets to know himself – and this is a fundamental process in ego development – by the effect he has on others and the picture they form of him.

The emphasis that Adam Smith and Foulkes both give to the role of social mirroring, separated by over 200 years, has been confirmed and amplified in child development research. The research points to such crucial factors as empathy and sensitive responsiveness, contingency and agency, and protoconversations that can lead to dialogue. Infants have been found to be visually active from birth, to seek visual intercourse; they are able to imitate others' facial expressions within a few minutes of birth, such as tongue protrusion and sucking movements. Adults are programmed to respond by providing 'biological mirroring'. These are essential steps in the birth of intersubjectivity, the dawning awareness that there is someone who understands and responds knowingly to the process through which the infant begins to know himself – steps towards the theory of mind. I will refer here to the groundbreaking work of neurophysiologist Giacomo Rizzolatti (Rizzolatti and Craighero 2004; Rizzolatti and Sinigaglia 2008), described by neuroscientist V. S. Ramachandran as the single most important 'unreported' (or at least unpublicised) story of the decade (Ramachandran and Blakeslea 1999). I shall also be referring to the work of another neuroscientist, Walter

Freeman (1995), to whom I was first attracted by the title of his book *Societies of Brains: A Study in the Neuroscience of Love and Hate*. He has followed this up with *How Brains Make Up Their Minds* (Freeman 2001).

Culture is of fundamental importance in forming the mind. Fiumara (1990), writing as both a group analyst and neuroscientist, described the brain in an evolutionary context as a 'Darwinian Machine'. As a result of natural selection, humans are subject to fixed evolutionary laws that guarantee survival and genetic success, along with strategies through which these laws are fulfilled. The mind can be defined as a functional apparatus of the brain (Panksepp 1998). It is considered as natural a function of brain circuit dynamics as digestion is of gastrointestinal actions, although the former is vastly more complex. The functions of the brain begin in the babies' intrauterine experience as an awareness of a 'bodily self' contained and limited by the amniotic fluid and uterine walls. At birth, the mental function has to cope with a sudden transition from its intrauterine state to the totally new experience of being no longer contained in the maternal space; what begins then is the relationship to the maternal facilitating environment, to the environmental culture.

The contributions from group analysis, particularly Foulkes's exploration of the social unconscious, play a significant role in understanding the social mind. The concept of the social mind is implicit in Foulkes's writings. Powell (1991) has extracted passages from his writings that clearly show Foulkes's approach in his 1948 and 1957 books (the latter cowritten with E. J. Anthony). Unfortunately, these writings are not included in the definitive study *The Social Mind* by the historians of psychology Jaan Valsiner and René van der Veer. They ask, 'How can the mind be social, and why do we need to mention it?' (Valsiner and Van Der Veer 2000: 1). The word 'brain' does not appear in their index. In the writing of Norbert Elias, the word 'brain' only appears once with a reference in *The Society of Individuals* (Elias 1991/2001) in more of an aside.

The Social Mind explores the history of the socially constructed mind, focusing on key theorists: Lev Vygotsky from Russia, G. H. Mead and James Mark Baldwin from the United States and Pierre Janet from France. Leslie Brothers (1997), a clinician and neuroscientist, introduced the term 'social brain' in her book *Friday's Footprint*. Neurosurgeon Michael Gazzaniga (1985), known for his research on the corpus callosum's removal, authored *The Social Brain: Discovering the Networks of the Mind*. His later work, *Human: The Science Behind What Makes Us Unique* (Gazzaniga 2009), delves into contemporary neuroscience, highlighting the distinctions between the human brain and those of other animals, especially higher primates.

In the past three decades, the social brain concept has gained significant traction in ethnoprimatology, developmental psychology and neuroscience. Advancements in neuroimaging techniques like PET scans and small fMRI have allowed researchers to explore the functions of the normal brain beyond clinical studies of disorders of the central nervous system. Notably,

Foulkesian group analysis, although not acknowledged in discussions of the social mind or brain, exhibits important parallels with the study of social networks and concepts like matrix, mirroring and resonance.

Foulkes (1937), in his psychoanalytic paper 'On Introjection', challenged the traditional separation of the developing psyche from its environment, culture and various dichotomies like inside and outside world, individual and society. His assertion that these aspects are inseparable has gained acceptance over time, reflecting a shift from the old to the new perspectives. Foulkes's insights marked a departure from the dominance of projection and projective identification mechanisms promoted by the Melanie Klein school in the psychoanalytic world.

Foulkes wrote on the permeability of the developing psyche to its human environment and its culture. He argues that the 'old juxtaposition of an inside and outside world, constitution and environment, individual and society, phantasy and reality, body and mind and so on, are untenable. They can at no stage be separated from each other, except by artificial isolation' (Foulkes 1948: 10). On prescient terms, the old has given place to the new, and these issues are now far better understood and accepted than when Foulkes wrote his 1937 paper.

The personal as social

The American sociologist Charles Horton Cooley enumerated the terms that relate the person to the social. Among them are the social self, the looking-glass self, the social mind, the elite as the social brain, making up the group mind, and the social process (Cooley 1902). In *The Social Mind* we find that 'in contemporary sociocultural theorizing, disputes about internalization/externalization, appropriation, mastery, guided participation, etc. abound. All these indicate efforts to overcome the limits of the either-or thought model that is firmly entrenched in human everyday language' (Valsiner and Van der Veer 2000: 6–7). The dialogical principles of 'now me, now you; in and out' escape from the polarities of projection or introjection and fit well with current developmental studies such as those of Alan Schore (1994), Peter Fonagy and others (Fonagy and Target 1996–2000).

In much of his writing Foulkes does not refer to the four major theorists of the personal (Vygotsky, Mead, Baldwin and Janet) as social. He acknowledges Trigant Burrow but not in detail. His reference figures are, from psychoanalysis, Paul Schilder, Erik Erikson and Ives Hendrick; from sociology, Norbert Elias; from anthropology, Bronisław Malinowski and Jacob Moreno. But Kurt Goldstein is absent from his references until *Therapeutic Group Analysis* when Foulkes (1964/1984) asserts that man's social nature is basic to him. Goldstein takes his proper place from then on. Foulkes also acknowledges Helen Jennings (1947), a sociologist, for introducing the term 'psyche group' in the 1950s, when he also references Ruesch and Bateson (1951) for their introduction of communication theory. In Foulkes's developmental perspective, he turns to Erikson's schema of (1) autocosmos, where the world is experienced and reacted to exclusively in terms of the child's body; (2) microsphere, when object relations are formed but the child's psyche is central, which Foulkes relates to Melanie Klein's findings in child play analysis; and (3) macrosphere, where object relations are experienced in a world genuinely shared with others (Holman 1999).

As Foulkes's library was distributed after his death, we have little to go by on factors that have been influential in forming his theories. We know that through his thorough German classical education he was well versed in the writings of Goethe, Schiller and other authors of the German Enlightenment. We also know that through the teachings of Goldstein, Foulkes was well versed in neurobiology and continued to maintain an interest in evolutionary biology as presented by Julian Huxley (1992; Huxley et al. 2010).

Major contributions to social brain theory

Merlin Donald's (1991) *Origins of the Modern Mind* was and remains a great stimulus to our thinking about how our human social brain emerges from primates. He insists that culture is fundamentally important in forming the social brain and mind. Our human mind, he writes, evolved through a series of three major adaptations, at each of which new representational systems emerged, leading to our symbolic capacities. The progression he describes is:

1 From primates by developing gestural, linguistic and thought structures. In this first stage of 'mimes', gestural communication, cooperation and social coordination of actions were central to species' survival strategies. Mimetic cultures allowed individuals to create group structures with social roles and group norms. Knowledge can be transmitted, acknowledged and shared: 'Social brain, distributed knowledge'.
2 The second transmission is from mimetic to mythic cultures. Collective knowledge about survival is passed on through a vast heritage including oral lore, totemic art, mimetic song, dance and ritual. Language gives rise to narrative, and storytelling and symbolic art appear.
3 The third transition involves the synthesis of symbolic art and symbolic language. Writing emerges and memory can now be held in 'external storage systems'. Knowledge can be retrieved and critically examined, leading to theoretic culture. As humans evolve through these stages, brain structures and capacities appear, not an increase in brain mass but in brain capacities, encephalisation and network capacities. Biology and technology now are a single evolutionary continuum (Gazzaniga 2009).
4 In the fourth transition Donald describes how we become 'cultural entities', with cognitive collectivities bonded through symbolic consciousness. At this stage we become something unique in the biological world – symbolising intellects are bonded through a community of minds. Knowledge is distributed and, using coded communication like

> alphabets and systems of enumeration and technologies, networks engage other minds. Today's World Wide Web is the latest of these stages (Donald 2007). He does not refer to Elias's (1991/2001) studies of networks of dependency but expresses similar ideas, saying it is difficult for us to accept the degree of our dependency; our 'grand illusion of individuality' is defined by our fixed places in a particular community network. We gain intellectual status when we are wedded to a community of mind.

Robin Dunbar's (2009) work links brain size and complexity to the ability to live in complex large groups. He uses the volume of the neocortex as the measure of brain size because this accounts for most of the brain expansion in primates: measures of social complexity correlate with relative neocortical volume. The volume of the brain's neocortex imposes a limit on the number of relationships that individual primates can sustain in their mental model of their social world. Dunbar asserts that the human social group and clique size are determined by the neocortical volume of the brain. We are limited to a number of 150 individuals for a proximal social group size and 12 for a more intimate clique size. Dunbar cites as evidence for the 150 group size the average village size in the Domesday Book and the common size of self-sustainable military groups such as a company. Within these groups of 150, there are hierarchical structures of friendship: 5 intimates for support and 15 for close friendships and sympathy. Fifty is the next larger group size and then 150 as the outer limit of proximal relationships.

Frans de Waal's (2009) observations of chimpanzee groups revealed constant power struggles, drawing parallels with Machiavelli's political descriptions. The 'Machiavellian mind' observed in primates involves tactical deception and power manipulations, reflecting the complexity of primate social systems. The term 'social brain' signifies a brain with structures suited for living in complex large groups. In primates, social complexity correlates with the volume of the neocortex, impacting social interaction time, skills and tactical deception. Differences between male and female sociality, with affiliative tendencies in females and competitive behaviour in males, suggest varied responses to social pressures. As male competition increases, cortical control decreases (Dunbar 2009).

The evolution of the social brain, explored through diverse lenses, uncovers its intricate nature and profound implications for human cognition. Whiten and Byrne's (1997) Machiavellian intelligence hypothesis, later termed the social brain hypothesis, delves into primate social complexity, emphasising tactical deception and coalition formations. Dunbar expands on this, connecting storytelling and religion to social cognition capacities. These phenomena demand the ability to imagine virtual worlds, a unique cognitive feature of species with large neocortices like great apes and humans. Cooperative breeding, as proposed by Sarah Blaffer Hrdy (2009), emerges as a key contributor to the evolution of the social brain, facilitating extended lifespans, prolonged childhoods and larger brains.

Pro-social impulses, driven by cooperative living, maintain the survival web of social relations. Blaffer Hrdy's (2009: 11) notion that 'to care and share is to survive' underlines the importance of cooperation. The mirror neuron system, facilitating the detection of similarities, is described by Meltzoff (1997: 149) as 'seeing others like me is our birthright'. This system evolves into *tangible* modernities like art and language, along with *intangible* modernities such as emotional understanding.

Blaffer Hrdy (2009: 285) characterises infants as 'little connoisseurs of commitment', highlighting their innate capacity for empathy, mind-reading and collaboration, shaped by both genetic and environmental factors. Cooperative breeding, according to her, was crucial for the evolution of extended lifespans, prolonged childhood and larger brains in humans. This cooperative living allowed for slower maturation, resulting in individuals with bigger brains, bigger bodies and robust immune systems. The distinctive features of the human story include larger brains with higher metabolic costs, extended female lifespans beyond menopause, and unique pro-social tendencies, particularly in the context of food sharing, setting humans apart from other primates.

Social brain pathology

Exploring social brain pathologies, Brüne et al. (2003) highlight disorders stemming from severe brain disorders, often rooted in social isolation. Loneliness, recognised as social pain, activates brain areas associated with both physical and emotional pain. The UCLA Loneliness Scale measures interconnectedness, revealing the impact of social isolation on health.

Cozolino (2002: 5) introduces the concept of the 'social synapse', emphasising the interconnectedness vital for physical and psychological well-being. Social communication regulates physiological and emotional equilibrium, impacting the neural and hormonal processes of the social brain. Chronic loneliness contributes to physiological damage, evident in heightened cortisol levels.

Neural plasticity

Neural plasticity, vital for understanding how the brain registers external and internal stimuli, involves the permanent alteration of synapses according to lived experiences. Ansermet and Magistretti (2007) explain that synaptic plasticity, dynamic and subject to modifications, shapes neuronal networks throughout one's life, forming an internal reality grounded in both conscious and unconscious inscriptions. The ever-changing synaptic network prompts the question of how identity is maintained amid such ongoing transformation.

Experience continually modifies the connections among neurons, rendering the brain a highly dynamic organ in constant interaction with the environment and the subject's psychic experiences or actions. Rejecting the notion of a fixed and determined organ, plasticity reveals the brain's openness to change and contingency, subject to modification by events and evolving experiences. Plasticity underscores the brain's transformation throughout life stages and, crucially, highlights how psychotherapy effects neuronal changes, offering an avenue to break free from repetition and fixed patterns – a biology of freedom. Ansermet and Magistretti (2007: 241) make a bold claim:

> The trace, which is at the center of the phenomenon of plasticity, lies at the intersection of the neurosciences and psychoanalysis. What we have to do is show how the synaptic trace is related to the psychic trace and the signifier.

Foulkes's concept of 'ego training in action', further advanced by Dennis Brown, aligns with the circular and spiral nature of self-development in group analysis, emphasising the role of empathy and subjective interaction. This process involves discovering inner worlds, discerning old and new internal object relationships, and attuning to others' experiences. The group composition, the balancing of diversity and similarity, aims to uncover connectedness, moving from cohesion to coherence and fostering individuality within the group matrix (Brown 1994/2000).

Clinical experience underscores the importance of active adaptation in ego training, where individuals' sense of self is confirmed through networked self-discovery. Individuality emerges in the dynamic interplay with the surrounding world.

Mirror neurones

The discovery of mirror neurons by Rizzolatti in the 1990s sheds light on the neurological basis of shared experiences (Rizzolatti and Craighero 2004). Mirror neurons enable the brain to match observed movements with those the observer can perform, forming the foundation for individual and societal actions. The mirror neuron system proves essential for imitation, learning and communication, highlighting the deep bond that connects individuals to others. The shared activation of brain areas during the perception of emotions further underscores the profound interconnectedness that underlies human sociality.

While initially identified in monkeys, mirror neurons have also been found in humans, affirming their critical role in shaping human behaviour and social interactions. The presence of this brain mechanism and capacity provides us with the data to support the theories of George Herbert Mead. He described what he saw as 'the language of gestures' in animals, who seemed to understand and respond to the intentions of another, and he extended this to humans (Mead 1934/2015; 1964).

Mirror neurons play a crucial role in our ability to understand and interpret the actions and gestures of others. Research, initially conducted with monkeys, revealed that when a monkey either grasped an object or observed another performing the same action, neuronal stimulation occurred. This mirrors our human capacity for understanding and grasping meanings.

To understand, etymologically meaning 'to stand under', involves placing oneself physically and mentally in the position of the other. Grasping refers to the mental act of comprehending meaning. Mirror neurons allow us to comprehend the meaning of motor events and actions performed by others, recognising specific types of actions and differentiating them. We utilise this information to respond appropriately to the movements of others, perceiving the intentional aspects of actions.

From an evolutionary perspective, mirror neurons are integral to our brain-activated motor system, providing knowledge on how to defend ourselves by parrying the movements of others. This concept is illustrated in Japanese martial arts like aikido, where practitioners learn to anticipate and parry the actions of their opponents. Cozolino's experience learning aikido exemplifies how, without physical contact, the master could quickly and effectively throw him to the ground by leveraging the anticipatory and parrying aspects ingrained in the brain's motor system:

> My teacher was a master at activating and manipulating balance, reflexes, mirror systems, and resonance behaviors. He was playing my body like a familiar instrument. It was a humbling lesson on my lack of skill as an aikidoist and on the power of our automatic and unconscious resonance reactions.
>
> (Cozolino 2006: 227)

Resonance

The concept of resonance as first described by Foulkes (1937; 1977; 1990a), and further developed by Brown and others, aligns with neural networks and the way situations trigger unique responses in individuals. In a group, neural networks are activated by emotions, themes and verbal acts, leading to automatic, reflexive and implicit responses known as resonance behaviours. These behaviours contribute to social cohesion, group identification, safety and learning through imitative processes.

Resonance behaviours are rooted in mirror systems and can be seen positively as supporting gestural communication, language development and social relating. However, they also have negative aspects, including the potential for groups to exhibit characteristics described by Freud (1921), such as emotional contagion, mob behaviour, gangs, and rigid autocracies.

The capacity for resonance is crucial in attuning to the emotional states of others, allowing, for instance, a mother to understand and respond to an infant's affective internal state. This form of attunement forms the foundation of a healthy infant-caregiver relationship.

Identifying a patient's neural network involves therapeutic principles like giving attention, exploring unknown aspects of the self and paying attention to language patterns that provide pathways for exploration. The concept of neural networks adds a layer to traditional psychoanalytic and group-analytic concepts, emphasising the search for latent patterns that can emerge when unblocked.

Edelman's (1987) theory of neural group selection describes how synapses actively form neural circuits to communicate and shows how the brain's basic operating unit is composed of groups of neurons. These groups fire together, creating structures and maps that coordinate sensory inputs and other neuronal activities through re-entrant connections. Neuronal group selection, akin to neural Darwinism, involves the reinforcement and elimination of patterns, providing a mechanism for the brain to recognise objects and form coherent experiences. Edelman's mention of values aligns with Foulkes's concept of 'norms' – shared values that guide groups toward mature patterns.

Individuality is not to be found in isolation from the world in which it moves. As a being, the individual is forever forming and transforming himself through interactions between himself and his sustaining natural ground and social world. Individuality can only be known in the world *with* which, *in* which and *by* which it is coming to be. The individual, furthermore, constantly re-enters this world through activity of its own. A self is a self only in its fruitful interplay with its world. The value of individuality lies less in its separate uniqueness than in its unique way of making itself part of the world (Pines 1978a). At the time of writing this, I was unaware of Edelman's neural network theory and the significance of re-entry, through which the brain communicates with itself, generating new patterns.

Cozolino (2006) highlights our interdependence, emphasising communication across space through gestures, expressions and language – he describes this as the 'social synapse'. Though Foulkes never used this term, its implicit connection to his approach in group therapy and our interdependent existence is evident in the way he put to work in his own writing the conception of interdependencies as 'figurations', as coined by Elias (1991/2001).

Freeman's (1995; 2001) work emphasises the interdependence of individuals and the importance of communication in shaping neural patterns and social bonds. His exploration of brain structures in animals, particularly the olfactory cortex in rabbit brains, points to the biological and evolutionary basis of brains working in pairs, families, tribes and larger social structures. The involvement of the social hormone oxytocin is highlighted in the progression from pairs to larger social groups, indicating the significance of social cooperation and the dissolution and reformation of language, music, rhythm and dancing in creating and sustaining group bonds.

The notion of unlearning, proposed by Freeman, underscores the dynamic nature of biological and cultural evolution in mammals. The release of neuro-modulators during sleep is suggested as a mechanism for this unlearning process. Freeman also distinguishes between private meaning and meaning learned through interaction with others, emphasising the importance of shared gestures and cooperation in confirming similarity to others. The permeability of individual boundaries, facilitated by gestures and language, is crucial for building trust and forming cohesive social groups.

Freeman's observation that reading others' expressions allows us to see only the surface of the deep ocean of meaning within each individual highlights the complexity of human interactions. Trust, seen as the unquestioning acceptance of others and the basis for predicting the behaviour of people we know well, is at the foundation of forming cohesive social groups. This trust is built through the unlearning and relearning that occurs in various social activities, training programmes and team-building exercises.

Overall, Freeman's (1995; 2001) work underscores the intricate relationship between neural processes, social behaviours and the formation of cohesive social groups, providing valuable insights into the deep interconnectedness of individuals in social contexts. His conclusion in *How Brains Make Up Their Minds* describes how

> each brain, and the mind that is its function, is a unity that is isolated within a solipsistic barrier. This is a barrier only in the sense of a horizon, which endlessly recedes as it is approached. We cannot directly experience the qualia and meanings that exist in another brain, nor can any other outsider enter your own private world. You have to learn to understand and unlearn to empathize.
>
> (Freeman 2001: 154)

Bridging the solipsistic gulf

Humans employ chemical mechanisms (oxytocin, vasopressin, endorphins) to influence behaviour, bridging the 'solipsistic gulf' in societal formation. Music, dancing and sports serve as archetypal techniques. Neurons, which emerge through biological evolution, collaborate in pairs, families, tribes and, through cultural evolution, in larger societies. Freeman's thesis centres on intentionality – the brain's active process marked by unity, wholeness and intent. Unity distinguishes the self from non-self in various entities, while wholeness involves a bounded process leading to maturity. Intent signifies a relationship that allows the self to conform to non-self aspects.

Freeman underscores the importance of intentionality, evident in the brain's neuropil – nerve cells, axons, dendrites and surrounding glia. The concept is manifested in the 'stretching forth' between brains. Piaget's work reveals children's exploration through body movements, while Merleau-Ponty's (1968) intentional arc highlights bodily adaptations to achieve maximum grip. Paul Schilder's (1938/1999) concept of body image emphasises the body's continuous change through multiple different experiences, particularly emotional and physical contact with other bodies. It is a puzzle his work does not enter Freeman's account.

In *Baboon Metaphysics*, Cheney and Seyfarth (2007) delve into the intricacies of baboon behaviour, drawing inspiration from Darwin's musings on the connection between understanding baboons and metaphysics. In his notebook M, Darwin (1838) contemplated the nature of the mind, challenging John Locke's associationist view. Darwin's theory of evolution became a pivotal framework, suggesting that animals, like baboons, act on instinct shaped by hereditary tendencies. *Baboon Metaphysics* explores the social lives of baboons, revealing that their minds, shaped by natural selection, excel in observing social dynamics, computing relations and predicting behaviour. Unlike humans, baboons lack a strong ability to recognise others' mental states, emphasising computational and representational processes without language or a theory of mind. This raises intriguing questions about thought and cognition in the absence of language. Despite the stark contrast in brain size between humans and baboons, the book prompts a re-evaluation of cognitive processes in the absence of language and therefore without a theory of mind.

We suspect that as our uniquely human traits began to appear, the continuing evolution of a theory of mind played a crucial role as catalyst and prime mover. It facilitated and led to the evolution of all of the traits that are uniquely human, including speech, teaching, elaborate tool use and culture (Cheney and Seyfarth 2007: 279).

Leslie Brothers pioneers the concept of the social brain. In *Friday's Footprint* (Brothers 1997) she describes Robinson Crusoe as a metaphor for the conception, prevalent in eighteenth-century biology. Brothers stresses that culture emerges from the interactivity of human brains, which form the communal essence of the mind. The 'social order' is inherently moral, comprising 'oughts and shoulds'. An emerging understanding of autism sees the condition characterised by a lack of attention to social cues, which reveals the intertwining links between the understanding of utterances and the attribution of them to other persons. Hobson, writing with others (Hobson and Lee 1999; Hobson et al. 2000), gives emphasis to the experience of having an emotion elicited by another human being and associated in turn with the known capacity to elicit emotional responses in others. These authors identify these dynamics as the material out of which people fashion their sense of self, other, object and symbol.

Neurons in emotion-associated brain areas form a 'social module' responsive to significant gestures and expressions, creating an innate 'social alphabet'. The primate brain's specialised system for mutually regulated behaviour in complex social settings involves linking others' gestures to appropriate responses. This evolutionary process extends to humans, who add a conceptual level to perceiving others' minds and connecting this to the social order. This development correlates with Foulkes's emphasis on social norms. Brothers (1997) criticises animal experimentation on socially isolated animals, citing Klüver and Bucy's early findings on amygdala damage. This underscores the importance of considering the social network's role, echoing lessons from Goldstein, Schilder and Foulkes, though Brothers omits these references. She concludes *Friday's Footprint* thus:

> In contrast to contemporary cognitive neuroscience, which views the mind as a kind of closet with entities like emotion, linguistic rules, and memory arranged inside, I take mine to be irreducibly transactional. Rather than something packed inside a solitary skull, it is a dynamic entity defined by its transactions with the rest of the world. . . . Minds are best characterized by reference to the larger forms of life in which they play a part. Just as gold's value derives not from its chemical composition but from public agreement, the essence of thought is not its isolated neural basis but its social use.
>
> (Brothers 1997: 146)

Psychogenesis and sociogenesis

Elias (1991/2001) posits that society moulds individuals from birth, influencing attitudes towards various aspects of life. He illustrates the evolution of manners, tracking societal expectations and behaviours through time. The concept of neuroplasticity reveals that brains undergo dynamic processes, and Norman Doidge (2007) notes the reciprocal relationship between culture and the brain. Elias's work aligns with the idea of a culturally modified brain, where changes in culture induce corresponding changes in the brain. Cultural evolution relies on the transmission of knowledge, represented by memes. Experiments highlight how cultural backgrounds shape perception, with individuals from Western and Eastern cultures demonstrating distinct approaches to interpreting scenes. Cultural beliefs modulate visual experiences, influencing neural activity in the frontoparietal regions associated with attentional modulation. Studies using the framed-line test show that cultural context impacts cognitive processes, emphasising the bidirectional relationship between culture and the brain (Whitehead 2008).

Wexler writes that:

> Human beings alter the environment that shapes their brains to a degree without precedent among animals. These human alterations in the shared social environment include physical structures, laws and other codes of behavior, food and clothes, spoken and written language, and music and other arts. . . . This ability to shape the environment that in turn shapes our brains has allowed human adaptability and capability to develop at a much faster rate than is possible through alteration of the genetic code itself. Transgenerational shaping of brain function through culture also means that processes that govern the evolution of societies and cultures have a great influence on how our individual brains and minds work.
>
> Wexler (2008: 3–4)

He concludes that our brains (and minds) develop concrete perceptual structures, capabilities and sensitivities based on common reaches of the environment in which we are reared and then are more able and more likely to see those features in a sensory mix of new environments we encounter. Conversely, we have a limited ability to see even common features of new environments if those features were absent from our rearing environment. Through instrumental parenting, adults shape the child's physical world and actively engage in their object-related activities. These interventions provide frontal lobe functions, such as memory and planning, which a child's underdeveloped brain lacks. This supports the maturation of sensory, motor and association areas into more sophisticated functional systems. Human frontal lobes, significantly larger than those of other primates, develop through external structure and ongoing social interactions. Language, a cultural and social brain development, further enhances adults' influence on children's brain development.

Loewald (1989) has made the same point in psychoanalytic terms. Adults and children live in a shared psychosocial field in which the adult is at the more developed and more structured pole and the child at the less structured pole. In the course of development, and also in the course of psychotherapy, these positions alter as the child, or the patient, acquires capacities that previously were found only in the adult. This is a move towards autonomy for the child and a greater capacity for self-analysis in the patient.

Note

1 This study was later summarized in a paper, Pines, M. (2003), 'Social brain and social group: How mirroring connects people', published in *Group Analysis* 36 (4): 507–513. Acknowledgements are made to the editor of the journal for consent to its original and extended publication here. (Ed.)

16 Building on Bion, following on Foulkes[1]

I begin this paper with quotations that express better than I can the spirit of my enterprise. The developmental psychologist Alan Fogel (1993: 4) wrote: 'The life of the mind is a dialogue, most typically a verbal dialogue between imagined points of view'. And Shweder (2003: 300), a 'postmodern humanist', wrote: 'the whole world is incomplete if seen from any one point of view, incoherent if seen from all points of view at once and empty if seen from nowhere in particular'.

A paper that attempts to establish a dialogue between Bion and Foulkes, one that never actually took place, cannot possibly be empty! The facts of their cultural backgrounds are inescapably significant. Foulkes was a child from a large, prosperous, assimilated German Jewish family and was educated in the advanced school system of his time. Deeply literate, he had to choose between a career as a theatre director and a career in medicine. In his writings he refers frequently to Maxim Gorky and Luigi Pirandello.

This is from Pirandello's *Six Characters in Search of an Author*:

> My drama lies entirely in this one thing. In my being conscious that each of us believes himself to be a single person. But each of us is many people – according to all the possibilities of being that are within us. We are one person with some and with others we're someone entirely different. We have the illusion of being one and the same person with everyone we meet but it is not true. We discover this when we are, by some terrible chance, caught in the middle of doing something we should not be doing and are left dangling, suspended in mid-air. Then we see that every part of us was not involved in what we were doing, and it would be a dreadful injustice for people to judge us by this one act, as we are held there, as if we were suspended in eternity, with one's personality summed up in a single, uninterrupted action.
>
> (Pirandello 1922/1995: 14)

Possibly Pirandello's exploration of the complexity of character stimulated Foulkes's ideas. The latter's original name was Siegmund Heinrich Fuchs. During World War I he served as a communications officer on the western

DOI: 10.4324/9781003494713-20

front in the German army and then studied medicine in Heidelberg and Frankfurt, psychoanalysis in Vienna in the late 1920s and sociology in Frankfurt, where he went on to become the director of the Frankfurt Psychoanalytic Clinic's outpatient service. Displaced by Nazism to the United Kingdom in 1933, he made a successful readaptation involving a change of name – anglicised to Michael Foulkes – and retraining in British medicine, psychiatry and psychoanalysis. He did not write an autobiography, so we have problems in reconstructing his personal development and penetrating beneath his urbane appearance.

Wilfred Ruprecht Bion was of Anglo-Indian parentage. He was displaced at the age of eight from the warmth of India and the care of his ayah to a bleak British public school. He openly describes severe mental conflicts and confusion in his early childhood, in particular his fears of a fantasised, persecutory father (Bion 1990). His experiences in World War I and II, his education in history and philosophy at Oxford after World War I, and his deep interest in mathematics are all crucial to his later development. He spent many years of unproductive psychotherapy with Hatfield before meeting with John Rickman in a brief analysis that released him from isolation and enabled him to marry. Tragically, however, his wife died soon after giving birth. His postwar psychoanalytic training with Melanie Klein, who discouraged his involvement with groups, fostered his exploration of the early development of mind and psychotic disorder.

There are some commonalities in these apparently very different intellectual developments. Both acknowledge their debts to their mentors in neurobiology. Foulkes spent two years as a neurological assistant in a hospital for the brain-injured under the influence of his mentor, Kurt Goldstein (1939/2000), whose impact on him is well known. Out of the crucible of these formative influences come his ideas of network, matrix, concepts of figure, ground and figuration, the dynamic equilibrium of the organism and environment and the basic biological principle of adaptation. Running through all this is the underpinning premise of holism, of the group as a whole. Even the therapeutic community concept derives from the therapeutic atmosphere of Goldstein's hospital, where patients were encouraged to overcome their disabilities and mobilise creative and reparative forces within themselves and in their environments.

Although Bion did not have Foulkes's firsthand experiences in neurology, he was greatly influenced by the great British neurologist and brain surgeon Wilfred Trotter, to whom he was house surgeon during his own medical training in the years after World War II. Both Goldstein and Trotter were in line of descent from John Hughlings Jackson and his dynamic concept of the hierarchy of central nervous system functions, the 'doctrine of levels' discussed in Chapter 4. Trotter's influence on Bion has been amply substantiated by Nuno Torres (2003) in his illuminating piece 'Gregariousness and the mind: Wilfred Trotter and Wilfred Bion'.

Torres demonstrates Trotter's sociological influence on Bion's mental models. Trotter's (1916/2005) influential monograph *Instincts of the Herd in Peace and War* was well known in the 1920s and was even referred to by Freud. Although Trotter is little read nowadays, he has brought out the significance of his ideas and shown how they anticipated Bion's, though the latter scarcely refers to him. Trotter was brother-in-law to Ernest Jones; in fact, he had led Jones to read Freud. Together, Jones and Trotter went to the 1908 Salzburg Congress of Psychoanalysis, but Trotter, bored by the discussion, reinvigorated himself with the thought that among all the participants, he was the only one who would know how to amputate a leg!

Before explicating more of Trotter's influence on Bion, I will point out another similarity between Bion and Foulkes. Foulkes's contact with the sociological-historical approach of Norbert Elias and the Frankfurt sociological school is well known (Elias 1968/2000). Less well known and appreciated are the sociological ideas of Trotter and Bion's later mentor and analyst, John Rickman, whose work I have also discussed in Chapter 4. Of all the British psychoanalysts of the 1920s and 1930s, Rickman was the most advanced in his understanding of social dynamics. This arose from his Quaker background and upbringing and his service in Russia with a Quaker relief unit in World War I, during which he observed the social dynamics of a Russian village. Rickman also acknowledged the importance of Kurt Lewin (1977) and field theory. Letters exchanged between Bion and Rickman show clearly how much Bion learnt from Rickman in forming his ideas about leaderless groups which Trotter had already written about thirty years previously. Another pioneer who benefitted profoundly from his relationship with Rickman was E. James Anthony.[2]

What are Trotter's contributions that inspired Bion? Man as a gregarious animal; group mentality; social valence; the drive to search for truth, for certainty; intolerance of uncertainty; learning by experience; the conflict of new and established ideas; mental turbulence; the mind digesting food for thought; mind as muscle.

During World War I, Trotter (1916/2005) was viewing the powerful primitive forces dominating mentalities. He saw the great struggle in how to reconcile the rational mind with the enormous forces of the herd mind. To survive, groups have to establish and maintain high morale and good group spirit. The herd will blindly follow the leader who presents them with simplified ideas, and the more complex the mind, the less inclined it will be to adopt the simplified viewpoint of those who want to establish leadership.

Trotter wrote that the British had developed their powers of cooperation and did not follow aggressive leadership in the way the Germans had done. For him, the British were more like bees, the Germans like wolves! He stressed the need to see through idealisations and to develop mature cooperation. The voice of the herd, he thought, would produce mindlessness. Clearly Bion's (1962) concept of basic assumptions leads us in the same direction as Trotter had already outlined. The concept leads on to Bion's ideas about genius and establishment in opposition to each other, the struggle that new ideas have to survive in the conflict between innovation and stability. Trotter had already written how the herd will choose stability and the maintenance of old ideas rather than face the uncertainties of new ideas.

There is some connection between Trotter's ideas and those of Trigant Burrow, the radical American psychoanalyst discussed in Chapter 4. Burrow had tried to get the psychoanalytic community to see that unless they studied their own dynamics, they were simply replicating the dynamics of neurosis. Bion wrote that if we equate psychoanalysis with 'treatment' and improvement with 'cure', this restricts psychoanalysis and places limitations on the analysand's growth. The interest served by these limitations is simply to keep the group undisturbed. If psychoanalysts are unaware of the expanding nature of their universe, difficulties will arise between analysand and analyst: the container restricts the growth of the contained.

Expanding worlds

Now, fifty years on, I can review what has been done with the legacies of Foulkes and Bion. In the first edition of his book *The Theory and Practice of Group Psychotherapy* (1975), Irvin Yalom was dismissive of Foulkes, Bion and the Tavistock approach. It was one of the most widely read and influential texts in the field and remains so in its successive editions, but Foulkes's and Bion's contributions find no place in his writing.

Bion's (1968/1998) *Experiences in Groups* has remained a seminal, even inspirational, text, though it is often misunderstood and misapplied. Robert Lipgar (2003) has illuminated Bion's intentions and style in 'Re-discovering Bion's Experiences in Groups'. He writes that Bion's interventions are aimed towards promoting 'learning from experience' in the context of the group experience. Here, Bion's work is fundamentally psychotherapeutic, taking psychotherapy as an enterprise that is directed towards individual self-definition, interdependency and capacity for intimacy. His commitment is in searching for insight and truth. Bion's writings on binocular vision (1961), container and contained, and narcissism and sociability (2000) show that he remained deeply aware of our need to retain the vision of mankind and society as discrete but inseparable, with constant tensions arising between narcissism and sociability. The legacy of his work has been most productive in the study of institutions, in ideas that social scientists have used in studying the dynamics of societies. Basic assumption theory has shed light on ethnic and national conflicts, though he had not explored the dynamics of power in groups, a notion which was central to Norbert Elias's views on the dynamics of group relations.

It can be argued that in small-group therapy and the part that group therapy can play in mental health services, Bion's ideas have had somewhat negative effects. Novices attempting to take their first groups, who use *Experiences in Groups* as their compass, have been discomforted, finding that it is not a guide to effective therapy. The original enthusiasm for group therapy at the Tavistock and other such centres post–World War II quickly waned and David Malan's (1999) follow-up study, which showed how unpopular group therapy was for the patients, gave no encouragement. However, the Tavistock 'approach' with Bion's work at its centre has grown into a different, primary model for group psychotherapy in the United States.

Contrasting the legacy of Bion and Foulkes, we can use the story of the hare and the tortoise. Bion's early work makes a tremendous start, but Foulkes goes slowly and steadily. His experience in running a successful outpatient department at the Maudsley Hospital set the model for many later developments in the application of small-group and large-group therapies in outpatient units, day hospitals and community psychiatry. There are also particularly impressive examples in the Scandinavian mental health services. I note especially the network of Norwegian day units for the successful treatment of borderline patients. This regime makes extensive use of group-analytic small and large groups. Another impressive example is that of the University Department of Psychiatry in Geneva, where Professor José Guimón (2007) is using a group-analytic model as his basic framework. Two hundred mental health professionals from Geneva and other cantons have taken part in a training programme that covers a one-, two- or three-year period, taking the form of seminars that last four days each.

The conceptual basis of group-analytic psychotherapy includes free-floating discussion; facilitating communication; the holding in mind of the concepts of group matrix and network; processes of universalisation and socialisation; the group-specific features of mirroring and resonance; and the belief in the fundamental rule that a group will gradually move towards a healthier set of norms than each participant brought with them to the circle.

Stacey (2003: 145) writes about group process and complexity:

> Healthy minds and healthy social relating are characterized by the paradox of continuity and transformation at the same time, where health is a paradoxical dynamic of stability and instability at the same time and illness is the repetition of thematic patterning with very little potential for transformation.

Health and illness are always reflected simultaneously in individual minds and in social relations. The move from illness to health progresses from emotional stability to more complex, variable patterns of relating of a body to itself and of bodies to each other. Therapeutic change can never be either individual or social; it is always both individual and social *at the same time*. The medium of therapy is the group, understood through the processes by which individuals relate to and communicate with one another. This relating and communicating is individual and social at the same time. What Stacey adds to Foulkes's original account, drawing on Elias, is that we focus attention on emerging narrative themes and power relations in the group and on the inevitable dynamics of inclusion and exclusion as an aspect of power-relating. He suggests that we focus attention on the vicissitudes of attachment and separation rather than on the vicissitudes of the drives.

Foulkes drew attention to the importance of mirroring and resonance as group-specific factors (Foulkes and Anthony 1957/1983). Developments in neuroscience are bringing out the significance of these factors in a way that could not possibly have been envisaged previously. In Chapter 15, I refer firstly to the writings of Adam Smith (1776/2003), who in 1759 wrote of society as a mirror for the person. Without this mirror the person would never come to know himself or herself. Mankind is a social animal, and without the society of fellows, the individual would have no mirror of his or her own actions. Growing up in solitude, people cannot know themselves, but if you bring them into society they will discover that they know themselves differently from the way society views them; this discrepancy gives birth to self-reflection. Jumping to the twenty-first century, neuroscientists led by Rizzolatti (Rizzolatti and Craighero 2004) at the University of Parma identified what they call 'mirror neurons', multimodal cells located in Broca's area of the brain activated both by the subject – animal or person – in their own actions, and also by viewing similar actions performed by another organism. The chapters in section III of this collection – Chapters 5 to 12 – track the progressive development in our relational understanding that rests on foundations in the work of both Foulkes and Mead. Mead (1934/2015) showed that the development and the emergence of self is inseparable from the recognition of the existence of the other. Foulkes's account of resonance has become a feature of current neuroscientific interest also (Foulkes and Anthony 1957/1983), and taking this into neuroscience, Damasio (1994) states that our experience of ourselves arises from the brain activity that is registering the internal state of the body. These body states constitute the background to the sense of self which is repeatedly reconstructed by activities: mind arises when bodies interact with each other; changes in body rhythms constantly affect mental states and the sense of self. It seems likely that knowledge of our own self states also gives us knowledge of the body state of the other. Here, both mirroring and resonance contribute to our sense of being in the world and being in the world with others.

Bion's (1962) model of container and contained assumes and relies on the processes of projection and introjection. The emergence of greater knowledge of attunement and empathy in early infant-caregiver relations moves our understanding in a different direction. Within psychoanalysis, the model to which I am closest is the one Hans Loewald (1989) gave us many years ago – that infant and caregiver together create needs and satisfactions. Building on Winnicott's (1951) ideas, Loewald posited an original psychic field or matrix, the mother-infant unit, within which individuation processes start. Instinctual drives, as psychic forces, are processes taking place within a field; the mother-infant psychic matrix and their characters' instincts, as well as the character of the emerging individual psyche, are determined by the changing characteristics of that matrix field and their evolution into differentiated but related separate psychic fields.

Motivational psychic forces are relational phenomena that do not presuppose life and death instincts or destructive envy per se: drives are fashioned through the matrix of early relationships. When these processes go well enough, the separating and separate persons have a sense of being in oneself and being with another; a sense of basic trust and value in oneself, in the relationship to the other and in the representation of the other. Being 'good enough', to use Winnicott's term, to have an internal sense of value, becomes part of the core self. There is an inner conversation between the asking and responding parts of self, which maintains a sense of a good enough fit with the world. Meares (2000) describes how the pleasure that generates a sense of value comes from a harmony or resonance between inner states and the outer world. This kind of relatedness, which is more than mere congruence, is essential to development.

When there has not been a good enough fit, when there has been a failure of matching between inner feelings and outer responses, the sense of inner value is absent. Meares describes this as a state of 'non-resonance' that can show itself in a group as the inability to take part in exchange and dialogue. The slow transformational potential of a group-analytic group enables the non-resonating person to find that these resonances can begin in part through the sense of universality of feelings between persons but much more specifically through dynamic interchange.

The psychoanalyst Betty Joseph has written that there are certain patients in whom there appears to be no resonance to interpretations, nor to any emotional understanding (Feldman and Spillius 1999). Unconsciously there is no expectation of being emotionally understood and no expectation that the object, in analysis the analyst, can stand up, tolerate and contain the patient's anxieties and impulses. To maintain their equilibrium, these patients erect a kind of pseudo-container of a rigid type, which prevents real resonance in the analysis between patient and analyst, and within the personality in their inner world. This is well put, as regards individual practice, but the possibilities of developing resonance to others are much greater in the dynamic field of the group matrix.

Bion: The hare

Bion had been in analysis with Rickman for a year before World War II, but quickly the former analyst and analysand formed a creative working couple. Both realised the great psychological problems that faced an army and a nation at war. To this, Rickman would apply his experiences in Russia during World War I, when he observed the dynamics of decision-making in a community. His contribution was shaped by his deep immersion in psychoanalysis as an administrator of the British Psychoanalytical Society and its publications, as an analysand and analyst, and as a pioneer of the psychoanalytic exploration of the psychoses. He died suddenly in 1951, when he had a coronary thrombosis sitting under a tree in Regent's Park, to which overwork and conflicts within the Psychoanalytical Society must have contributed. Following his death, his work was quickly forgotten, but it has been brought back to our attention by Pearl King (Rickman 2003), his former analysand and a great admirer of his work. Nor was it forgotten by Bion, his other analysand and collaborator.

At the beginning of World War II, Rickman had helped to draft the *Wharncliffe Memorandum*, assisted by Eliot Slater and described more fully in Chapter 4. The document is sadly lost. It outlined an active rehabilitation program for traumatised soldiers. Bion, with his own traumatic experiences of World War I, knew how important these ideas could be, and we can see how they developed from the letters Bion and Rickman exchanged during the war.

In 1942, Bion wrote to Rickman about the officers' selection programme he was working on:

> The first point about selection . . . has been the emergence of the psychiatrists as the leg on which the whole organisation hangs. . . . The presence of the psychiatrist in the unit has exerted a quite unmistakable influence in inducing a sane and fairly balanced approach to the problem of the unit as a whole. We first taught our lay colleague, by refusing to be certain when we were not certain, that in the selection of potential officers there really was a problem. . . . We paved the way for an absence of dogmatism in our approach to the selection. . . . Our influence in this direction has I think been as invaluable as it is difficult to measure. But some hundreds of officers strange to this work here have seen it and have been unmistakably struck by its importance.
>
> (Vonofakos and Hinshelwood 2012: 75)

Bion goes on to write:

> I felt myself to have played a big part; because when I first met the adjutant general, he was saying that officer material was bound to deteriorate, and this indeed had been published in an official document circulated through all boards and elsewhere. I tackled this point at once and pointed out that it was quite fallacious. . . . By all precedents, officers should not deteriorate in an army at war. On the contrary, if all were well, an army should sprout officers. . . . If it was not doing so, it was because the climate was wrong and as soon as a new atmosphere was abroad, one could expect the new shoots to come on instead of being frozen off.
>
> (op. cit. 75)

Later he writes:

> No candidate should be allowed to come forward unless he has been voted for by his platoon or company. . . . Every officer I have mentioned this to, including many hard baked regulars, have been thrilled by the idea. . . . I pointed out to the A.G. [adjutant general] that if this privilege of election was granted as a sort of regimental privilege to the best regiments, a great increase of keenness was to be expected. . . . Officers and men would be compelled to think seriously about the problem of leadership [which] would lead to a growth of leadership.
>
> (op. cit. 76–77)

Still later on he says: 'There have been many difficulties in pushing this to the present point and I have learned the power of the mediocre mind as a really obstructive force' (op. cit. 77). At the end of this letter, he urges Rickman to come and join him in the spearhead of an advance.

In 1946, he wrote to Rickman:

> I suspect that group therapy may one day have a good deal to say about the factors making for health, or continued dependence, in a hospital for physical ailments. I think I am still learning a good deal and to this extent there must be a lot in the [group therapy] technique. I am certain we must have a study group. This business needs studying. I find that one important thing with patients—dreadfully important and I kick myself for not having seen it before—is the need to let them make their own experiments and approaches however hard and sterile they may appear to be. This time they need to feel in a family in which their sprouting curiosity and intelligence is not frosted off.
>
> (op. cit. 91)

Foulkes: The tortoise

Tom Harrison's (2000) research into the records of Northfield shows that after the departure of Bion and Rickman, Foulkes became the acknowledged teacher of group therapy. However, his ideas would be vigorously contested by Tom Main, Harold Bridger and others. For them, this approach to group therapy was too tame, too conventional. In 1945, Main complained to Rickman that the present state of development, which he saw as insufficiently dynamic, came about because of a cult of 'Foulkes worshippers', an assertion Harrison feels was quite unfair. This issue of dealing solely with the here and now in the Bion/Rickman model continues to pervade our approaches to dealing with large groups. Gerhard Wilke (2003: 102–103) offers a Foulkesian perspective:

> It is clear that Foulkes's lessons are mostly heeded in the small-group world and that his ideas have been under-utilised for the large group.

> Foulkes claimed that the group conductor has to develop three roles in the service of the group . . . the analyst, dynamic administrator and translator. Through training, supervision and learning from experience, the conductor eventually integrates these roles and develops a clearly identifiable group analytic self which the members of any group can use, abuse, cathect and de-cathect as an object. What holds the conductor's personality together is his humanity, and more important than his technical tools are his integrity, honesty, directness and care. The boundary between the analytical role, the responsible citizen and the human being has to be transparent in the large group.

Harrison (2000: 241) shows that in his last year at Northfield, Foulkes's approach to the ward was very similar to Bion's, concentrating on the here and now and encouraging men to face up to the realities of their situation: 'Perhaps this was the time when the two men's practices came closest to each other' (2000: 241).

In his first book, *Introduction to Group-analytic psychotherapy*, Foulkes (1948/1983) clearly states that group analysis is not simply applied psychoanalysis, that it stands alongside it, draws its strength from the study of social processes, from dynamic network theory, from the practical experience of Northfield and from clinical, small-group therapy.

Rickman wrote some very influential, short papers on number and the human sciences (e.g., 1957b), trying to schematise the different names of one-body, two-body, three-body and four-body psychologies. From the table of psychosocial relations discovered in his archives by Pearl King, we can see how deeply Rickman continued to think about the significance of the human as always immersed in group experiences, from the one body to a multi-body, to mankind as a single united group.

For my focus on divergences and convergences between the theories of Bion and Foulkes, I draw from Ralph Stacey's (2003) *Complexity and Group Processes*. He looks at the foundations of Western intellectual traditions and draws out the differences intrinsic in following either Kant or Hegel. Bion is avowedly Kantian, influenced by his Oxford tutor, Herbert James Paton, a distinguished Kantian. Bion searches for a model of the mind for his basis in the search for 'the thing in itself', an unseen, non-sensory reality, an ultimately ineffable '0'. Schermer (in Pines 1985b) writes that Bion was well-read in, and utilised, the ideas of logical positivism, mirroring his interest in mathematics and logic, eventually manifested in the grid and the concept of transformation. Later, Bion moved to the other end of the spectrum of thought, to the great Eastern and Western mystics. Driven by the search for Truth, he moved from the philosophico-scientific logic, finally to the mystics and art as ways to get to the truth. In a personal communication, Torres described to me how many flaws the human mind is troubled by that prevent encounters with the truth, including negation, projection and hallucination. Bion opted for an intuitional path for growth at the end of his life, instead of the intellectual one he had been following. But the tension between these two extremes is always there and can be mind-shattering.

And what now of Foulkes? Stacey (2003) places him firmly in the Hegelian path: individuals, groups and society are all interwoven; society is both inside and outside us. Indeed, the dividing line is itself a false construction governed only by our need for categorisation. Elias (1968/2000) drew to our attention the notion of 'homo clausus', the gradual withdrawal of the person into the recesses of the self in response to the increasing complexity of modern society. The aim of therapy is to move us towards 'homo apertus', the open person, which is achievable through our immersion in the dynamics of small and large groups. In contrast to Kantian thinking, where there is a duality of the individual and the social, Hegel presents a perspective in which they cannot be separated. Indeed, individuals arise in the social, which they are simultaneously constructing. This is clearly a paradoxical or dialectical perspective, in which individuals are simultaneously forming and being formed by the social.

Foulkes is not drawn to the 'formless infinite', the ultimate truth, which Bion strove to reach. His interest is in trying to find out why and how individuals and groups go about trying not to understand. In his last book, Foulkes (1975/1986) offers a number of maxims:

- Try to find out why and how the group goes about not understanding. (Also, how each patient goes about not changing.)
- Always follow the group. Listen before you intervene. When you think you understand, listen again and see whether it is confirmed.
- You should not have to communicate to the group to satisfy your own need – like relieving your own anxiety – speak only for what the group needs.

I think that I can see here a similarity of spirit for exploration and a search for the truth that is common to both pioneers.

Here is Foulkes again:

> Honesty towards oneself and others is fundamental. There must be a love of truth, even if it is disagreeable and contrary to personal advantage. Nothing has impressed me more than the degree to which people bend their minds, their emotions, their convictions, their opinions, even the very structure of their minds, according to their personal advantages or disadvantages, and [according to] changes of all sorts in their fortunes.
>
> (Foulkes 1975/1986: 157–158)

Of the spiritual, so central to Bion's search, I heard him quote Goethe: 'He who possesses science and art also has religion; but he who possesses neither of those two, let him have religion!'

I have written about 'Bion and Foulkes on empathy' (Pines 2003b). Foulkes says: 'We need to have the capacity for empathy with our fellow humans. . . . [It] comes from a certain philosophical attitude, by seeing things in proportion, as part of the human problem in which we are all continuously involved'. He goes on to write about a therapist's receptiveness, the 'creative function – in a way like an artist, in a way like a scientist, in a way like an educator. . . . I have sometimes compared this function with that of a poet' (Foulkes and Anthony 1957/1983: 254).

Bion never uses the word 'empathy': 'truth' and 'compassion' are his words. In *Cogitations* (Bion 1992), he writes that these are centres of man, compassion as a feeling he needs to express, an impulse he must experience in his feelings for others; likewise, compassion is something he needs to feel in the attitude of others towards him. Here, he evokes the essential qualities in human relations of reciprocity and intersubjectivity.

Both Bion and Foulkes created vectors that have points of convergence that help us uncover the deeper truths which groups so often try to hide from themselves. The place of empathy, sympathy, compassion and pity continues to call for our attention. When we annihilate those feelings, we become inhuman, arrogant and capable of horrific actions towards others whom we cease to regard as in any way being of the same common stuff as ourselves. Bion's experience in World War I immersed him in the horrors of fundamental warfare, and he never ceased to draw on those experiences in his exploration of primitive psychic processes. In the case of Foulkes, neither the full extent of his combat experience on the western front nor the losses he suffered as a result of the Holocaust was ever told – he remained at a distance from primitive psychic processes.

Notes

1 This paper was prepared as a lecture for an unknown audience and delivered in about 2003. (Ed.)

2 E. James Anthony (1978) gives an account of John Rickman's influence on him during World War II in his Foulkes Lecture, 'The Group-Analytic Circle and Its Ambient Network'. He returns to this in his historical preview in Schlapobersky (1996), pp. xxvii–xxxiii. (Ed.)

Section V

Final papers

17 Training in group analysis

Where we have come from[1]

Where we have come from

I am pleased to join you here at the EGATIN [European Group Analytic Training Institutions Network] meeting in Copenhagen to deliver this keynote lecture on where we have come from in group-analytic training. Group analysis has emerged from the mind and experience of S. H. Foulkes – experience that he brought with him from a formative background in Austria and Germany, then from his teaching at the Northfield Military Hospital during the war, and then from his subsequent teaching and development at the Maudsley Hospital. I first met him at the Maudsley in the early 1950s. Coincidentally, he became my training analyst for the Anna Freud group at the British Psychoanalytical Society; indeed, we began analysis in his consulting room at the Maudsley. It felt peculiar, lying on his couch, hearing passing footsteps of colleagues, nurses and patients, anticipating disruption, the room guarded only by the 'engaged' notice on the door. Now I can see that anxiety as the externalisation of my fears of unconscious disruption from within. Foulkes did not seem to find the situation at all peculiar, but I was relieved when we transferred to his rooms at 22 Upper Wimpole Street. This personal memoir serves to introduce Foulkes as teacher and trainer of a generation of psychiatrists at the Maudsley for some twenty years. It was there that he collaborated with James Anthony – then Reader in Child Psychiatry – on their famous book, *Group Psychotherapy: The Psychoanalytic Approach*, first issued by Penguin in 1957 and now published by Karnac. It has been continuously in print since it first came out. He also took part in the fierce ordeal of Professor Aubrey Lewis's Monday morning conferences, which was the baptism by fire of all of us junior doctors. Foulkes was not inclined actively to participate in the discussions unless directly called on. The psychodynamic flag was carried by Clifford Scott and by us juniors.

Now I am setting the scene: a large room in the outpatient department, where all the junior staff running groups came once a week for supervision. Foulkes describes his teaching and his observations on that situation in *Therapeutic Group Analysis* where, in section III, he says that teaching and psychotherapy have much in common, insofar as a change of attitude is essential in both, but therapy is not enough for training:

DOI: 10.4324/9781003494713-22

> Experience as a patient is not all that the future therapist requires. Not only does he himself have to make the experience of being a therapist in the therapeutic situation, but the fullest acquaintance with the experience of other colleagues from personal observation as well as from perusal of the literature is indispensable. . . . My experience points to a procedure in which such teaching takes place in a number of situations, graduated according to the degree in which the psychotherapeutic element, in a frankly personal application, enters into the admixture.
>
> (249)

Foulkes describes the supervisory group seminar, where all therapeutic groups in progress were reported and discussed by therapists, observers and visitors. The advantage of learning from each other, under the consultant's guidance, was generally recognised as every participant experienced himself and others in a variety of roles, such as that of conductor, observer and third person. The keynote of the supervision seminar was the desire to change attitudes in both therapist and patient, seen as interdependent. Problems of countertransference played a considerable part in our meeting and were more impressive as they in turn were brought to light and analysed by all those present. Foulkes emphasises that the boundaries regarding personal and interpersonal aspects were carefully chosen and respected.

He goes on to describe some of the supervisory experiences at the Maudsley. He notes that in the course of time, most supervisory groups split into two factions: radical and conservative – an interesting anticipation of Farhad Dalal's radical and conservative Foulkes! He also notes the same happening in therapy groups which can split again into radicals and conservatives. Later participants could recognise that this split was also an internal one and thus a phenomenon that recurs in every group.

You can get an idea of *'Le style c'est l'homme'* from this description. Supervision is done by the group and for the group: communication is the key and the learning process is shared by all participants. I witnessed how even naive and resistant therapists, new to and often hostile to analytic psychotherapy, could see how their patients benefitted from therapy. And I had the pleasure of working with Eduardo Cortesão and Juan Campos, who went on to pioneer group analysis in Portugal and Spain, respectively. One of the visitors was Ebbe Linnemann from Copenhagen, and it was through this contact that I later received an invitation to meetings in Copenhagen that led on to our successful training there. This resulted in the Institute of Group Analysis (IGA) Copenhagen and later to the Institute in Aarhus. Norway followed soon after. The Oslo IGA became a source of valuable research in outpatient and inpatient group analysis and in a diversified range of applications spread across their vast country.

Foulkes always favoured the seminar method. He applied it at Northfield and after the war with a group of interested colleagues, including Norbert Elias, when he established the Group Analytic Society, some of whose early members had trained as analysts. But we can now carry the story back to Northfield. Tom Harrison's (2000) important book *Bion, Rickman, Foulkes and the Northfield Experiments* has given us vignettes of the seminars at Northfield in which Foulkes, Tom Main and Harold Bridger were the leaders. Some of the tensions can already be seen between the position Foulkes adopted towards the management of group tensions and dynamics, and those who represented a different position, the kind of approach favoured by Bion and Rickman who had already left the hospital by then. Foulkes was the only psychoanalyst and was regarded as the leader, but his authority was challenged and was always under scrutiny. These supervision seminars were attended by psychiatrists who had no previous experience of group therapy. They came from a conventional psychiatric background and therefore, in a discussion about therapy, were insecure about their roles and technique.

According to Harrison (2000), Foulkes encouraged doctors to abandon a directive and organised role. He encouraged them to avoid rules of behaviour, techniques and attempts to tackle symptoms rather than causes. This led inevitably to the question of what skills a psychiatrist needed to be a group therapist. As clinicians admitted their lack of confidence, Foulkes elaborated further, pointing out that he (the experienced psychiatrist) would consider taking this issue to the group members themselves. He would encourage clinicians to discuss these issues with group members at their own level, suggesting that for many patients, confidence may be a concrete thing they feel they have lost, and seeing the therapist inviting comment could help restore it.

Most of the group discussed technique in as dispassionate a manner as possible. Foulkes was looked on as the fount of information about this, and for much of the time, attempts within the group to examine the state of mind of the doctor presenting a case were ignored. However, as many of them became more confident, there were sporadic attempts to reflect on the impact the therapy had on themselves and how their own emotions influenced their patients. Foulkes underlined how responsive the group was to its therapists and stressed that the patients had the same emotional difficulties as the doctors in facing the group idea.

Harrison shows how Foulkes himself developed confidence. He began by being cautious, conciliatory, supportive and caring for the individual members of the group and later progressed to caring for the group, which in turn cared for its members.

The same split between radicals and conservatives can be seen at Northfield: Main was the leader of the radicals and constantly challenged Foulkes. Those of us who knew Main knew how he was driven by his own need to be leader. Perhaps he projected this aspect of himself onto Foulkes, for in a letter to Rickman he wrote that Foulkes was a leader of a cult of Foulkes worshippers. Harrison writes:

> Foulkes . . . had to fight for every insight. His own understanding of the purpose of group therapy evolved as he gained experience. He moved from conducting individual therapy in a group setting to a position that was not far removed from that of his predecessors at Northfield (Bion and Rickman). However, he had to contend continually with his tendency to avoid confrontation and his reparative, protective nature. This led to misunderstandings, particularly with Tom Main, who was himself struggling to understand the full implications of Bion's approach.
>
> (Harrison 2000: 62)

Foulkes had evolved his own style of teaching that he developed in the Group Analytic Society which he founded with a group of colleagues and former patients in 1953, described in my own introduction above. His teaching style also continued in the private seminars he conducted with groups of interested colleagues. Systematic teaching was not his forte, and he was disinclined to discuss his own ideas in relation to those of other group therapists or analysts who were exploring the group field, whether in Britain or in America. The demand for systematic teaching came from a group of social workers who wanted to apply group work to their clients and felt they had not received sufficient training in their core profession. By then we had founded the Group Analytic Practice with Foulkes and others, and from its premises in Montagu Mansions near Baker Street, Robin Skynner and Pat de Maré took up the challenge. In 1964 they offered a year of weekly seminars on group analysis which unleashed a flood. The next year the numbers doubled, and after that the increase was almost exponential until the Introductory Course, or General Course, would number perhaps up to 150 persons. Here began the intimate link between the Group Analytic Practice and teaching of group analysis that led – in due course – to the Institute of Group Analysis, the training centre we established on the practice premises in 1973. Most of the teachers on this course were from the Group Analytic Practice, and we continued on these premises until the IGA – as we became known – moved into premises of its own in Daleham Gardens, Belsize Park.

I had the responsibility of organising and chairing this Introductory course for a number of years (it is now known as the Foundation Course) and it represented our first steps towards a more systematic outlining of group analysis and establishing the group-analytic method. The well-known formula of lectures, seminars, personal group experience and large groups came into being between 1964 and 1973. Large groups were pioneered by Pat de Maré and Lionel Kreeger at Halliwick Hospital and then brought into the training. The responsibility for teaching drove us to clarify our own ideas and to adapt our methods to the needs of the participants.

The training needs we were presented with went further than we had anticipated. The participants wanted more after the first year, so we initiated an advanced course. A second and a third year were asked for, and this led us to the radical step: to form the IGA. Foulkes himself was not too keen on this for reasons that we can only speculate on. Perhaps he preferred his own way of working in his own seminars and in the Group Analytic Society. Perhaps he felt his influence would be diminished. I can only briefly sketch our procedures: careful selection of candidates for training towards membership of the Institute (not very carefully upheld to begin with), and no 'grandfather clause': however senior and experienced members of the Society were, they could not become members of the Institute without undergoing the Institute training. This led to many protests and disappointments, but the position clearly established the boundary of this new Institute. Candidates seeking qualified membership were required to have group therapy twice a week and a more systematic set of seminars was created which included a more general introduction to psychotherapy as well as to the group analytic model we favoured.

After some years, I insisted that we establish a Curriculum Committee to systematise our teaching and to look at its strengths and weaknesses. This committee remained at the heart of our teaching for many years, and eventually a core group headed by John Schlapobersky undertook a complete revision. This resulted in a handbook which outlined to candidates and teachers the scope of group-analytic training as it stood and remained for several years more. For some years we worked to find an academic link with a university department that could offer us a university accreditation for the training. Our curriculum and its handbook were a key to opening the door to university programmes. Sometime after I left the training programme, Birkbeck College at the University of London became our academic partner. Our jointly administered master's programme in group analysis continued for some twenty years under the helpful guidance of Stephen Frosh, then head of their Department of Psychosocial Studies.

Where are we now?

I will continue with the history of the London institute, which is what I know best. For several years I took the opening seminars under the rubric of 'Mind, Self and Society' (you will recognise the derivation from G. H. Mead). We had a dual track set of seminars in which the development of the individual and the development of the group were looked at in parallel. I used my seminar to stimulate the candidates to think socially. There was a strong emphasis on the impact of culture, so we began with the ancient Greeks and progressed through European culture looking at the birth of individuality, until we reached the processes outlined by Norbert Elias. These seminars stimulated active debates among the members about the nature of self. I was considerably influenced by the development of self psychology at that time, so I introduced those ideas. Later, training candidates would be exposed to a very considerable tranche of seminars on object-relations theory in which Winnicott was key. I cannot outline here the details of the training, which are obtainable by looking at the handbook, but now we have again come to a point of major revision. This is because the candidates have experienced a very heavy burden in having to combine their therapy, supervision of their own groups, reading for their seminars and taking an active part in conferences.

The major revision at present consists of introducing a modular system: students are able to make choices as to which modules they wish to take part in after the first year. This modular system allows people who have had sufficient training and experience in one area to eschew that and choose another they are particularly interested in or feel they have inadequate knowledge of. One such module is 'Victims and Perpetrators'; another is 'Groups for Children and Adolescents'; another is 'Organisations and Psychiatric Services'. This is a new experiment, and there are clear snags as well as advantages. The expenses are high as more staff is needed; the returns can be low, as some modules are chosen by relatively few persons; and the organisation is complex and demanding. However, the modular system might make possible a shortened form of training for experienced therapists who want to train as group analysts but do not want to go through the whole lengthy and elaborate training.

Continuous and block trainings

There is a well-known debate amongst members of EGATIN, the European Group Analytic Training Institutions Network, about the merits of these different approaches to training. I will not elaborate on it here. You will know that strong support and strong criticism have followed the development of the block trainings, which were devised to meet the inevitable problems of teaching group analysis away from capital cities. Thus, in the British Isles and Ireland, as well as training in London, we developed training to Qualifying Course level in Manchester, Glasgow and Dublin, and there is a further training associated with the IGA based in the South West – in Exeter and Bristol. You will know of the successful training schemes in Denmark and Norway, the less successful ones in the former Yugoslavia, and the sadly unsuccessful but now renewed training in Israel. There are many lessons to be learned from the less successful enterprises. These include the importance of contracts that have to be carefully drawn up and defined; organisers and teachers that have to be appointed by the responsible local institute that takes charge of the enterprise; and the content and structure of the programme that has to be carefully monitored.

Many of you here have participated in training programmes in Germany, Greece, Poland, Lithuania or Russia. Each of these has its own character, its 'genius loci', and EGATIN, originally sponsored by Ioannis Tsegos and a team of others from Croatia, Germany, Greece, Norway, Switzerland and the UK, has been an essential link between the different institutes.

I was recently privileged to participate in the first meeting of the Czech Institute of Group Analysis in Prague. These graduates have been trained by staff from the Institutes of Group Analysis in Denmark, where their trainers developed through the work in Copenhagen and Aarhus where earlier teams of trainers from the London Institute and elsewhere had worked over years. Norwegian group analysts, trained in Oslo by a team from the London Institute, have worked in Lithuania, and now Lithuanian group analysts may work in Russia. The network develops through these chain reactions of endeavour.

The Prague group analysts have worked fruitfully with the concept of the social unconscious in exploring and undoing the deep permeation and perversion of personality by totalitarian ideology, as our German colleagues have done following the collapse of Nazism. The democratic message of group analysis will hopefully reach to many other lands, disempowering doctrinaire practices and re-empowering people and organisations.

Where are we going?

This is an idiosyncratic section. I will reflect on my own view of the development of psychoanalytic psychotherapy and the inputs from our surrounding fields, which powerfully impact our training. In some ways, I will be outlining an 'ideal model'. What do we have to take account of that is not at present part of our training, at least in London?

Genetics and neuropsychology

Vast progress has been made in these fields. The nature/nurture debate has been rekindled, and new integrations are taking place. The impact of the early infantile environment on the developing brain and mind are beginning to be clearly established. Concepts such as neural networks, social networks and internal working models seem to share in their fundamental aspects. To my mind, this indicates and celebrates the genius of Foulkes in so far anticipating these findings and in his ability to transcend the accepted psychoanalytic view of the mind as located within the individual. The dynamic neuropsychology Foulkes had learned from Goldstein allowed him to look beyond the confines of the individual, long before others across the range of depth psychologies. This is more fully discussed in Chapter 15.

The most interesting contribution to psychoanalysis of modern genetics for me has been a monograph by Malcolm Slavin and Daniel Kriegman (1992), *The Adaptive Design of the Human Psyche*. There is fascinating work on the sociality of primates, most clearly and accessibly presented by Frans de Waal (1996; 1982) in *Good Natured* and in his earlier book *Chimpanzee Politics*. Two books that bring together psychobiological and social theory that I think are important to us are *Connexity* by Geoff Mulgan (1997) and *The Origins of Virtue* by Matt Ridley (1996).

We must continue to develop group analysis as a comprehensive theory of human relationships and development. We can both borrow from and add to those trends within psychoanalysis that are steadily moving towards what is nowadays called 'the two-person unconscious' (Lyons-Ruth 1999), the relational unconscious, the newer interest in differentiating preconscious and unconscious levels of mentation, the basis of human personality in the intersubjective processes (Stolorow et al. 1988), with advances in the theory of mind (Fonagy and Target 1996–2000), and newer aspects of self-psychology (Ornstein 1978).

Developmental Psychology

There is a significant shift within psychoanalysis, led by developments in attachment theory, from drive to relationship, from drive to affect regulation. The well-known work of Daniel Stern (1998) is being filled in with research from others such as Robert Emde (1980: 1981; 1983; 1988; 1990; 1992a; 1992b) and Alan Sroufe (Sroufe and Waters 1977). A very interesting development within psychoanalysis is the recognition that there are 'non-interpretative' therapeutic processes, which involve nonverbal mechanisms; the distinction between implicit procedural memory and semantic memory is increasingly emphasised, as is the difference between knowing how and knowing what. In group analysis, we have known for a very long time 'how' things happen when therapy progresses well; we are less clear in being able to establish 'what' it is that makes things happen. Foulkes's framework of therapeutic factors, such as mirroring, resonance, activation, location and condenser phenomena, are still our guidelines, but they stand in need of elaboration. Much recent work relates to mirroring: the discovery of 'mirror neurons' in the primates; mirroring as a social bio-feedback phenomenon; a deeper understanding of resonance and its failure; empathy, altruism and reciprocity. Dialogue, as the basis of human personality, means that we have to increase our knowledge of language genres. Personally, I find the work of Vygotsky (1962/2012; Rieber 1987–1999) and Bakhtin (Holquist 1990) to be most constructive in these areas.

Research

Vital to our future, to obtain recognition and financial support from funders of health services, is the search to validate the effectiveness and cost benefit of group-analytic therapy. The appreciation of this need has begun to produce results. Effectiveness of group psychotherapy is well proven (Bergin and Garfield 1994; Burlingame et al. 2003). Our own research is beginning and must progress. We number some good researchers in our network, and we must encourage and support their work and not be afraid to examine our own record.

This is a very incomplete sketch of the future of the developing field of group analysis as I see it. Seeing things in a round will hopefully bring together all the ideas that those of you from your own backgrounds can contribute to our shared field. That there is a future for organisational group analysis is shown by the Copenhagen group-analytic training in organisations, and this is also developing through our colleagues in Aarhus, Oslo and Stockholm. A final glimpse of the future: computer modelling of complex biological systems will be applied to large groups; medium and large groups will reconnect people in small communities as Pat de Maré has shown us (Lenn and Stefano 2012). The iron cage will loosen its grip on the isolated mind and group analysis will go on evolving.

Twenty-five years ago, after the death of Foulkes, I edited *The Evolution of Group Analysis* (Pines 1983a); after the death of Bion, I edited *Bion and Group Psychotherapy* (Pines 1985b). I am now finishing work on a second volume, *Building on Bion* (Lipgar and Pines 2003a; 2003b). After *The Evolution of Group Analysis*, I thought that it might be the first in a series; when will it be time for the second volume in this series, and then the next? This year there will be a millennium issue of our journal *Group Analysis* with a look back to our past and a glimpse towards the future. Modern science shows that complexity arises from simplicity, that design flows upwards. Dyadic therapy led through Burrow to Foulkes and Bion; de Maré leads to median and large groups and now there is an internet large group. What will come next? The answer lies in the minds of the next generation of group analysts.

What I have not looked at are the political, cultural and economic issues that face group analysis. Economics reminds me of how we are trying to develop a group-analytic view of economic theory, which will be the subject of our next European symposium in Bologna. A final word about median and large groups: how much of our future lies in developing our understanding and expertise in these fields? How much in organisational theory and practice? How many more questions?

I end with a rediscovery. This translation of a poem by Goethe was read to us in Prague by Thor Friis, the Danish group analyst who was one of the trainers of the Prague group:

> In exploring nature, always look at each thing and the whole;
> Nothing is inside and nothing is outside,
> For what is within is without.
> Hurry then, to grasp this wholly open secret,
> Rejoice in the true illusion, in the earnest gain,
> No living being is a single thing, it is always a many.
>
> (Goethe, 2005)

Note

1 This paper was given as a keynote lecture to the Study Day of the European Group Analytic Training Institutions Network held in Copenhagen, Denmark, in 2006. It has not been published previously. (Ed.)

18 Group analysis and the affective disorders[1]

In 1988, a Special Section on Group Therapy with Affective Disorders was published in the March issue of *Group Analysis*. An authoritative review supported the optimism of group therapies for depression. In general, group treatments compare favourably to individual psychotherapy, though the conclusion was that no one model or form of group therapy has great advantage over others. In this article, published nearly twenty years later, I shall discuss the nature of depression and the therapeutic aims of the group-analytic approach and will attempt a group-analytic typology of depression. I shall then present some observations based on patients with bipolar affective disorders with whom I have worked in group-analytic and couples therapy.

The fundamental features of depression – pessimism, hopelessness, withdrawal and lack of motivation – can logically be linked to the therapeutic aims of participation, interaction, responsiveness, acceptance and mutual support. Powles (1989) profiles the two main features of depression. First, giving up: the experience of helplessness, loss and defeat leading to a state in which a person's powers of resolution give way to a state of despair. The second feature is severe self-blame, where the self is experienced as helpless and despicable. Self-blame is very largely a defence against rage towards significant others. Powles usefully distinguishes between therapeutic aims for the patient who is in a state of depression and what needs to be done once the patient is out of depression. When the patient is in depression the group must act as an ally, a friendly critic, urging activity at learning or in recovering the capacity for active coping. Once out of depression, the person must learn how to maintain the non-depressed state. This involves reviewing one's developmental history, one's lifestyle, and the nature of relationships both towards oneself and one's inner world and towards the significant others of the present social life. Powles believes that group therapy may hasten the remissions which are part of the natural history of affective disorders and that the therapeutic factors are those of empathy, group solidarity, installing and maintaining hope, sharing distress, encouragement to keep trying to recover and peer pressure to become more active. Many depressed patients have a low and precarious level of self-esteem. They have negative

DOI: 10.4324/9781003494713-23

attitudes towards themselves and are ambivalently and strongly dependent on significant others; their locus of control is external rather than internal.

The main group-therapeutic approaches to the affective disorders can be classified as: (a) cognitive – short-term homogeneous groups with a considerable educational component; (b) interactional heterogeneous groups which are longer term and have a strong here-and-now emphasis, again with a considerable psycho-educational component; and (c) group-analytic, long-term heterogeneous groups, with the therapeutic measures aimed at reaching to many levels. Homogeneous groups focus on such emotional issues as coping with loss, dealing with anger, and the initiation and maintenance of satisfying relationships. Such issues will naturally emerge in group-analytic groups as part of the natural history of joining a group, developing and maintaining relationships, and coping with loss. The loss element comes to the fore when other group members leave the group or when the person themselves has to face parting from the group. And, of course, throughout the group-analytic work the person is having to recognise their relationships with others as transference figures (Pines 1990; 2007).

Yalom (Yalom and Leszcz 2005) singled out four therapeutic factors as the most important in the affective disorders. They are universality, altruism, the installation and maintenance of hope, and interpersonal learning. The importance of universality is to bring the person out of self-blame and isolation into a universe that includes the suffering of others. Altruism enables the person to become a helper of others rather than someone who might do them harm. The hopelessness of the patient is comforted by the hopefulness of others. The term 'interpersonal learning' is a very wide one, but the most important lessons the depressed patient learns include the recognition of their own ambivalence; tolerating their own dependency; the defensive idealisation of others; the working through of depressive anxieties and of the defences mobilised against this painful anxiety.

When dealing with depressed people – including our patients – the theoretical concepts we need to keep in mind include seeing their loss of self-esteem as a fundamental ego state and not solely as a pathological condition. It is a state to which we are all vulnerable through 'the slings and arrows of outrageous fortune'. In our patient population depressions may be precipitated by different kinds of losses and perpetuated through a patient's inability to recover. Deep ambivalences towards lost objects have long been recognised as a fundamental characteristic of the depressed patient, as has been the precarious maintenance of self-esteem through narcissistic object relations and defences. Thus, many patients have repeated disappointments in love which can be traced back to early childhood relationships. The unrealistic goals of many patients in the search for glory – a form of neurotic pride – inevitably leads to disappointments in the self. Uncovering with the patient what their goals are in life and how their relationships may be controlled by the need to maintain an idealised relationship with a dominant other are also important therapeutic steps.

Here is a brief clinical example:

> **Vignette 1:** A single woman in her fifties was seen some months after leaving a twice-weekly group she had attended for some three years. She said she missed the group, which had become her family, but now she was more able to make use of the ordinary opportunities for relationships, some with neighbours and some with people at work. She is more aware of and more able to express her feelings towards herself and others. She recognises how for most of her life she has only allowed herself to have painful feelings and has therefore engaged in self-defeating and masochistic relationships. Her predominant relationship for many years has been with a very abusive and alcoholic man whom she has maintained financially and sexually. An early memory with her mother was of sitting on her mother's lap when her mother, it seems, accidentally burnt her with a cigarette and she had to conceal that she felt pain. Later when her partner abused and abandoned her, she burnt herself on her hand with cigarettes. Painful feelings stood between her and the sense of abandonment and emptiness.
>
> Looking back on her experience in the group she saw how negative her own self-concept had been; how unattractive, unworthy and unfeminine she had felt. She had taken very little care of herself, of her living conditions and of her appearance. It had helped her that in the group others had been concerned with her, angry with her and angry for her. They had pressed her to recognise the masochistic attitude she had towards herself, to recognise what she gained from this and to become more self-caring, and this she now does. She is left with a good deal of shame about her life, for the mess she has made of things, and does not know what she will be able to make of the rest of her life. She is still in a stage of appropriate sadness and mourning for having left the group.
>
> During her time in the group she had been seriously suicidal but had been able to reach out both to the group conductor and to other group members to sustain her. She had also become a very important person for other members of the group. She cared about them, expressed her feelings towards them, remembered their dreams, carried much of their histories in her mind and became a sensitive and empathic significant other for her fellow group members. She has experienced appropriate sadness at the loss of fellow group members who had left the group before, and as much sadness at her own leaving.
>
> She had been a companion to, and support for, a severely depressed man in the group who had a long history of depressive illness with strong genetic factors. For the first three years of his group participation, he went through several months of a retarded depression, which was very painful both for him and for the other group members. He, in his turn, became the one who, as he recovered, was able to support and work with the woman I have described.

Fiumara and Zanasi (1989) make an important distinction between depression in the group and depression of the group. Depression in the group refers to the work that has to be done with the depressed individual members of the group; depression of the group refers to the stage in the group development when the group as a whole goes through periods of depression. They link this to a developmental process, the point at which the group members attempt to reject and expel the group conductor in order to deny their dependency and exert a collective narcissistic grandiose form of strength. This stage of illusionary self-sufficiency inevitably gives way to a sense of depletion and loss and to an acceptance of the dependency and the ambivalence intrinsic to it. In some ways this is the equivalent to recognition of the depressive position and depressive anxieties that have been elucidated by Melanie Klein and her school.

The phase of magical omnipotence when the group member joins in an omnipotent illusion of self-sufficiency and grandiosity is a manifestation of a manic defence. The term 'manic defence' covers the features of omnipotence with denial of psychic reality, of the importance of object relations, the significance of object loss and the experience of guilt towards objects. As part of the omnipotence, there is a need to obtain control and mastery of objects which do not exist in their own right as persons with whom one has full reciprocal relationships. There is an idealisation of the self, a splitting of objects into the idealised and denigrated, and an absence of true reparative feelings and concerns. In their place comes the omnipotent manic fantasy of reparation, that of being able to repair damage and restore relationships through magical gestures. These manic defences may be seen at times in the group as a whole, particularly in denying the significance of separation, loss or absence, but they can be more clearly seen in individual members of the group.

Before I turn to deal with manic patients, I will summarise some of our group-analytic experience in dealing with the depressive disorders:

1 Treatment needs to be sustained over long periods and with the more depressed patients should take place in a twice-weekly group.
2 Severely depressed patients will test the capacity of the group for containing and holding their despair, often by inducing despair in others.
3 The capacities depressed patients are unable to maintain for themselves have to be carried for them by other group members. These include a sense of 'aliveness', of the reality of time and memory, of hopefulness, and a knowledge that empathy and understanding will eventually bring the person out of their solitude and despair and into the movement and progression of the group as a whole.
4 The group context can provide a sustaining holding and responding attitude, enabling very basic levels of trust and a sense of safety to be internalised.

Two clinical vignettes of manic patients I have worked with

Vignette 2: I worked with a physician in his mid-fifties who had a twenty-year history of manic depression with several hospitalisations. He has a family history of this disorder. In his teens he had homosexual fantasies and used to exhibit himself, about which he has great shame. He is now married with children and has a successful professional career. In his initial interview with me he made a powerful response to my comments that he had had a heavy burden of shame and guilt to carry throughout his life. He felt very understood and released by this. He hated his father, who represented himself as a saintly and perfect man who had achieved an international reputation in his own profession. After seeing the patient three times on his own I introduced him into a once-a-week group, having advised him not to force the pace in making premature self-disclosures. His exhibitionism took the form of forcing other members to listen to his sexual history.

He was quickly attached and involved in the group and maintained a predominantly positive transference relationship both to me and to the group. This enabled him to cope with a very difficult relationship with a woman member. She was very dominant and used narcissistic defences of omnipotence, intellectual arrogance and contempt. For over a year she was unable to accept her own dependency needs and to be open about her vulnerability. Her own mother had had repeated hospitalisation for a paranoid illness, and as a child she was often homeless when her mother was in hospital, having been abandoned by her father. A bitter paranoid relationship developed between these two after she had declared that in her opinion, he had not been a good father to his children. On one occasion he walked out in a rage and threatened to leave the group. This position was finally resolved through interpretation and reconstruction. The man had experienced the woman as the bad father, 'the devil himself, my phantom father', as he later wrote. In her he had condensed both the devil father, the adored mother and a dominating older sister. It emerged in the group that he had a lifelong delusional belief that he was Jesus Christ and that his father was Herod; that he was a Jew and that his father was Hitler. Therefore, he lived in mortal fear for his life. During his manic episodes he believed himself to be the Omnipotent Christ and crashed a car because he did not need to keep control of the steering. He has given me the book that he read during his journeys to the group, a study of two omnipotent persecutors, Hitler and Stalin, and he has inscribed in it a dedication to me as his good grandfather.

Vignette 3: Another patient with a history of affective disorder is a young woman from another country who has lived through short-lived delusional psychotic episodes with religious and grandiose features, for which she has been briefly hospitalised. She had been in psychoanalysis for some years before coming to England and joining a once-weekly group. She is the youngest member of a large family and was frightened of her father, who could be paranoid and violent. She maintained her self-boundaries through silent withdrawal and paranoid attacks which she repeated in the group. She was devastatingly accurate in pointing out to others all my faults and errors. She accused me of neglect of herself and of others, of having favourites who in the transference were her older siblings. She tried to stir up rebellion against me, seeing me as becoming old and incompetent. Now she feels a good deal stronger and more integrated and able to return to her native country without the fear of being overwhelmed by a powerful family. She experienced a 'mini-psychosis' whilst in the group during which she began to feel grandiose, but with the aid of the group she was able to master this within a week or two.

The background of the mini-psychosis was that it occurred after a session when the theme of the group had been that of anality and penetration. She had told how she treated her baby's constipation by inserting a thermometer into its anus. She disclosed a few days later that after that session she had gone away with her mind feeling very expanded and felt that she was becoming psychotic. This was because they had talked about holes. She began to get peculiar ideas, a feeling of having discovered the secrets of the world, but now she knows how to check these experiences and get everything back under control. She disclosed that when her father had had a psychotic episode, he had himself been deluded about holes in walls. Because of other material in the group that had to do with violent sexuality, with memories of standing outside parental bedrooms frightened that the parents are going to kill each other, it seemed that the conflict was between good, obedient, clean and controlled, an anal level of control; and the release from that control, which leads to fears and excitement. I linked this with the way in which, in childhood, we learn to close our ears to the sounds that are going on around us, which are bodily sounds that express many different forms of activities.

Conclusion: Group-analytic typology of depression

Depressed patients may present themselves as inducing feelings in others of emptiness, hurt, anger and paranoia. Seeking out a pathological response from others can thus perpetuate cycles of maladaptive interpersonal relationships. A paranoid depressive seeks rejection, the angry depressive is trying to gain attention, the hurt depressive is seeking soothing and the empty depressive courts abandonment. As these patterns of self-other relationships become evident, so they become clearer both to the patient and to the other group members, who then begin to question and reject these transference patterns. The paranoid person is questioned as to why they seek rejection, why they reject the understanding and identification that others can offer them; the angry person can gain attention through vulnerability rather than through anger; the hurt person can receive understanding and care not solely for being hurt and will have to begin to see how being hurt oneself is a disguised way of hurting others; the empty depression that seeks abandonment can eventually be understood as a flight from dangerous and painful relationships. There are different group processes that can be observed with these patients. The paranoid person induces splitting, which is a challenge to others to remain integrated. The angry person receives understanding; the hurt person learns about reparation and the empty person learns that they can be found. And all the time these experiences are taking place in a group that makes demands for each member to be honest in their attitudes towards others and to be caring.

Note

1 This is an edited form of a paper first published with this title in *Group Analysis* 24 (2): 99–109, 1991. Acknowledgements are made to the editor of the journal for consent to its publication here. (Ed.)

19 Myths and mirroring[1]

I shall explore what we can learn from two Greek myths whose stories incorporate vision and hearing – the story of Narcissus and Echo and that of Perseus, Athena and Medusa. Myths are primordial: woven webs of meaning, cultural texts of attitudes and behaviours that both bind us to and enable us to speak out about their hidden meanings. Myths are stories that renew themselves and always have something new to tell us.

Narcissus and Echo

I will begin with the dyadic myth of Narcissus and Echo. Narcissus is the child by a demigod's rape of the water nymph Liriope. The blind prophet Tiresias tells Liriope that her son will live 'so long as he does not know himself'. Though attracted to his companions, both male and female, Narcissus does not reciprocate their feelings and remains solitary. For this he is to be punished – he will experience the pain of unrequited love.

The nymph Echo had earlier fled from the god Pan, who had fallen in love with her. She feared him because Pan, the bringer of panic, represents frightening totalities that obliterate individuality. When Echo appears in the Narcissus story, she too carries a punishment. It came from the goddess Hera, wife of Zeus, as by her chatter Echo had so distracted her that she created space in which Zeus could have sex with her sister nymphs. Hera's punishment deprives her of independent speech and now she can only repeat the last part of another's words.

What meaning can we find in this Hera/Echo story? Hera constantly tries to control her partner Zeus. Her attitudes are rigid; she is a stickler for facts, form and order and she is trapped in The Real. Zeus escapes from her to procreate the world because, had she retained control over him, there would be neither genesis nor development and nothing would be left to chance. Echo opened to Zeus the way to fertilise the nymphs and allow new forms to be born.

Through Hera's curse, Echo is condemned to be repetitive and can herself no longer create new forms. In search of a new form for herself she develops a passion for Narcissus, hoping that by winning his love she can break out

DOI: 10.4324/9781003494713-24

from Hera's curse. Though Narcissus is trapped by a self-mirroring beauty, he also attempts to go beyond this, to direct his longing downwards, seeking depth. This depth is what Echo longs to find for herself by attracting his love.

In their verbal interplay, words circle within themselves, auto-generatively. The words are not direct, object-related – they are not dialogue and they lack depth. When Narcissus calls out for the company of others, all he finds is Echo. Thus, every occurrence between them is a reoccurrence, a duplication. Narcissus flees from Echo because he is seeking his own identity, based on separateness and sameness, whereas Echo is totally dependent on her surroundings. Her painful passion, her longing for the unrealisable, represents painful intrapsychic and interpersonal distance. When Narcissus repudiates Echo, who symbolises dependency on one's surroundings, he returns to his own self-entrapped world.

Patricia Berry (1992: 429–433), a Jungian analyst who has looked in depth at this myth, writes: 'To develop the echo in one's narcissism, one must achieve a certain painful distance in and by which this echo can sound'. This 'echoing distance' creates an aesthetic space that can lead to transformation. In psychoanalysis and group analysis there is a developmental 'distant nearness'. We hear echoes and transform them into resonance.

We use the term 'echolalia' when a person's speech simply echoes the speech of others and seems to lack any sense of inner significance for the speaker. Working with mentally handicapped patients, Sinason (2010), a British child analyst, found echolalia in the speech of sexually abused girls. She considers that this is because the mother has not been able to enter into or sustain a sexual dialogue with the father and therefore colludes with the father's sexual attention to the daughter, who experiences this sexual abuse as punishment by an angry internal mother. The girl's echolalia mirrors the parental couple who cannot sustain their own sexual dialogue. According to Sinason, echolalic speech changes when the therapist helps her patient actually talk about the abuse she has experienced. Psychotherapy mirrors and reflects back a commentary on the false echoing in the family dynamics and thereby gives Echo an opportunity to find her own speech.

Echoing and resonance

I will now explore the differences between echoing and resonance. The *Oxford Dictionary*'s (2018) definition of resonance is, 'The reinforcement or prolongation of sound by reflection'. In all four of his books, Foulkes (1964/1984) described mirroring and resonance as group-specific therapeutic factors. They involve seeing oneself in and through others, as well as responding in one's own particular way to the events of the group and to the emotions of another. We are all familiar with patients in psychotherapy who relate on only concrete terms, who have no reflective resources and whose emotional reactions to others are flat, unempathic and sometimes entirely absent. Contrary to all expectations, these are the very people who, seemingly intractable and unreachable through individual psychotherapy, can make progress in our groups. As they witness fruitful exchanges amongst others, they can begin to model and replicate a participating role. Self-understanding can develop out of this, and they can become more sensitive of and sensitive to the situation of the group and of other members' needs. As their range of responses widens, they can begin to resonate, as well as to echo. In Chapter 16 I have written about the British analyst Betty Joseph's account of 'non-resonance' as a factor militating against psychic change (Feldman and Spillius 1999). She describes patients who seem impermeable, unable to resonate to the analyst's attempts to reach their emotions. They do not seem to have a notion of what it is to be emotionally understood by another, one who can tolerate, understand, feel for and contain another person's experiences. They seem to have a rigid, narcissistic, defensive structure, providing a pseudo-container that seems to protect the person against unconscious psychic catastrophe. Preoccupied with themselves, they seem unaware that they have a particular way of being that is different to others. They often respond to the analyst's attempts to gain access to their mental life as if these were forceful, cruel attacks, a penetration of the container. Without a notion of what it is to be understood by another person and without a concept of mind, they have no way of being with another person that could lead to understanding between two separate individuals.

Non-resonance stands out in a group as an inability to take part in exchange and dialogue. We see this in borderline patients, psychosomatic patients and people who seem emotionally illiterate and for whom the language of emotions is utterly alien. Over a lengthy period, non-resonance can progress to resonance in a way that may well not be possible in dyadic therapy. The patient eventually manages to become part of and contribute to the emotional life of others, thereby entering into an intersubjective world.

Meares (2000) writes about resonance. Those of his patients who do not resonate provide the therapist with 'chronicles', boring recitals without complexity. They cannot use metaphor and they bring a sense of deadness to the therapist. Meares makes the point that such patients can slowly acquire the capacity for resonance, helped by a very patient therapist who can gradually introduce metaphor and imagery, who can move from the dead 'linear' account of mental and emotional life into one that becomes complex and kaleidoscopic. This is what we provide small children with by play, where adult and child play with the same object, yet endow it with multiple meanings.

Perseus, Athena and Medusa

I now go on to explore the other myth, Perseus and the mirror. This is a more complex story; it introduces a family drama with clear Oedipal themes. Perseus is the great redeeming hero of Greek mythology: a son of Zeus, who symbolises the spirit, and of Danaë, a mortal woman, the symbol of mother earth. Although Danaë's father, Acrisius, imprisons her in a tower, Zeus fertilises her with a shower of gold. We take the tower to represent a symbol of phallic narcissism, for Acrisius imprisons Danaë in his attempt to escape his predicted fate: that he will be killed by his grandson. When he finds out about her pregnancy, Acrisius decides to kill her and her son by exposure, but they are saved from his filicidal rage. The same conflict between father, mother and son re-emerges when Perseus reaches manhood, for their rescuer and protector, King Polydectes, tries to force marriage on Danaë. He tricks Perseus into promising that to save his mother from having to marry him, he has to secure the head of the Gorgon Medusa.

What does Perseus's struggle against the Medusa, queen of the Gorgons, symbolise? It is the universal human struggle against the enemy within. She is one of three sisters, monsters who symbolise different aspects of the enemy within. She has the dreadful power to petrify all who look upon her, to stop all psychic development; she symbolises guilty vanity, the narcissism that blocks development. Medusa has been a beautiful maiden, serving Athena in her temple. Athena, goddess of civilisation, is the daughter of Zeus, born asexually from the head of her father. Medusa is so proud of her beauty that she allows herself to be seduced by her uncle, the sea god Poseidon, brother of Zeus, the dark side of the spiritual god. Horrified by the sexual desecration of her temple's purity, Athena punishes Medusa by turning her hair into serpents and by destroying her facial beauty, though her bodily beauty is left intact. Now she has the face of fear and rage with power in its staring eyes to turn anyone who sees her into stone. She is a split-off part of Athena, the embodiment of Athena's envious rage, of the violent emotions that can play no part in 'civilised' behaviour – emotions that are not integrated into a self who can take part in undamaging exchange.

Medusa lives out a life of punishment for her guilty vanity and can only be released by the hero Perseus, who can only approach her with the aid of the gods. Athena teaches him the power of self-reflection and gives him part of her armour to act as a mirror. He also needs the helmet of invisibility, magic winged sandals and a magic wallet that has the capacity to contain the powers that remain vested in Medusa's head, even after her death.

The symbolic meaning of these figures and their accoutrements – the reflective mirror and the shield – gives us a reflective perspective on ourselves. The myth helps us see Medusa as part of ourselves: through her we can see our own destructive narcissism, our own guilty vanity, our own envious rage, our own fear of and hatred for our own incestuous fantasies. Until these things are faced, we cannot integrate the lower with the higher parts of our psyches.

Diel's analysis of Medusa's powerful symbolism suggests she stands for the shock and despair that can seize the very soul when, during flashes of lucidity, it finds a mirror to its own unacceptable face (Diel 1980). These words capture the power with which shame can paralyse. He goes on to describe how she symbolises the deformed image of the self that can be glimpsed during those moments in which vanity collapses. This is the face we must not see or we will suffer the consequences of horror. Instead, we must find this image reflected in the mirror of truth – Athena's shield. This is the mirror in which man sees himself as he is, not as he imagines himself to be. Thus, Perseus can bear the sight of Medusa's lucid image, which is the sight of his own guilty vanity. His sword, symbol of the lucid force of the spirit, can cut through to the heart of the problem, to the blindness that comes from the encapsulated, narcissistic structures.

The beauty of this myth is extended by what follows. After Perseus has decapitated the monster, two new entities are born from the blood which spurts from Medusa's neck: one is Chrysaor, the golden sword, a symbol of spiritualisation; the other is Pegasus, the winged horse, symbol of a capacity to rise into the heights of the imagination, to sublimate. Pegasus is the horse of the muses and represents art and beauty. When he struck the ground on Mount Helicon with his hoof, poetic inspiration gushed forth. Art plays imaginatively with the most deformed and destructive parts of ourselves. Art is the mirror of life in which we can see the most destructive aspects of ourselves contained and elevated.

Now, Perseus is able to use the head of Medusa, contained in the magic bag, to destroy his enemies, those parts of his own self that cling to perverse vanity – destructive jealousy and rage. The legend of Perseus and Medusa is concluded when the dying Perseus bequeaths Medusa's head to the goddess Athena, who places it in effigy on her own shield; thus Medusa and Athena are made one. The goddess of Truth, who had condemned Medusa, shows us the possibility that Truth will liberate us from guilty vanity. The shield of Athena is the mirror in which we can see our self-reflections, through which we can recognise the Medusa in ourselves and continue the eternal struggle against the essential Lie, the subconsciously deliberate lie, that comes about through fear of the truth.

We begin to see those many-faced truths about ourselves in psychotherapy, reflected in the mirroring responses, which give back to us some of the truths we can never see, amplified in the mirroring and resonance of the group situation.

Narcissus and Echo today: Eva Hoffman's novel

In the novel *The Secret* by Eva Hoffman (2001), this myth renews itself and is projected into the near future. The story is about Iris, a little girl who grows up in a Midwestern American town where her mother, Elizabeth, goes to live, thinking it will be a good place to bring up a child. Mother has left her financially successful career in New York and devotes herself entirely to her child. They keep themselves away from other people; Iris has no friendships amongst other children and mother keeps her out of school as long as possible.

Inevitably, Iris begins to ask what has happened to her daddy, particularly when she discovers that other children have both a mother and a father. She is told it will be explained to her when she reaches eighteen, so she avoids speculating or fantasising about her father. The daddy space is left mostly blank. Mummy is an enfolding comfy place; she folds her child into her body and absorbs her unhappiness. Mother and daughter look very much like each other; when they look into each other's eyes, Iris feels she enters into her mother, into a looking glass, in which she dissolves, becoming her mother and feeling full and safe.

Yet she knows something is wrong. At seven, she starts to look into mirrors, wanting to discover a secret, yet what looks back at her is an It, not her. To her, mummy is not quite a mummy; she is more than one. She is a sibling: as much her as her limbs and her bloodstream. They seem to move in tandem, as if joined by a connecting passage or cord.

When Iris is twelve, her mother meets Stephen, an anthropology lecturer at the local college. Mother soon takes him into her home. Iris adores him and they become a threesome. She wants to sleep with them, as she used to with her mother, and cannot understand why Stephen always takes her back to her own bed. He talks to her about her not having had a father, telling her she has to accept that he now comes first in mother's affection.

Gradually, she becomes aware that for others there is a strangeness about them. Stephen leaves home after having confronted Elizabeth over her refusal to disclose the secret of her daughter's early life. That is when Iris becomes desperate to uncover the secret. At seventeen, she finds where her mother keeps her personal documents and at last finds her birth certificate. It says she has been cloned from her mother and has no father. Confronted with the birth certificate, mother avows that it changes nothing: Iris is still her daughter and Elizabeth is still Iris's mother. Enraged, Iris calls her mother her identical twin and demands to know how 'a copy' can have desires of its own.

A few days later, Iris leaves home and looks for her grandparents, now in their nineties, who may explain her secret to her. They are mystified and confused by her appearance. Grandmother sees her as her daughter, as Elizabeth, who had completely severed ties with them. The shock is too great for grandmother, who has a massive heart attack and dies.

Iris traces the scientist who cloned her and asks how she was made. The scientist is pleased that his experiment has turned out so well; he has no understanding of her torment. Iris then has an affair with a fierce Eastern European who tries to bring depth to their relationship but fails. When she is nearly knocked down by a bus, she is shocked to find that she has a self-preservative impulse. She begins to think about the existence of both her and her mother, considering that there are two objects occupying the same space that cancel each other out. She begins planning how to murder her mother. Returning home, she tells her that grandmother on her deathbed had not called for Elizabeth – that she, Iris, had been what grandmother had wanted. Hate mounts between them. Iris feels her mother is still the mirror and she the reflection. But the 'Echo' has said something of its own and can no longer be contained. She strikes her mother, more than half strangles her but does not kill her. When mother sits up, she finally sees she gave life to a copy of herself, which metamorphosed into this strange, alien creature.

Later, Iris meets Stephen, her mother's former lover, the man she had wanted to think of as father. Inevitably, they are drawn together and have one sexual encounter which both know they have to stop. Staying in her aunt's flat, she begins to try on her clothes. As she looks at herself in the mirror, she feels transformed into a three-dimensional solid that can be inferred to have real, internal existence.

There is a good ending to the story. Iris has a relationship with a scientist she meets on the internet who is working on origins. Through their online exchanges, he solves the secret, discovering that she is a clone. When they meet, she feels he is looking at *her*, to find her 'me'. She begins to feel pleasure in developing a relationship and eventually in their lovemaking.

As their relationship develops, she enjoys their quarrels, the intensity of feelings, the pleasure in forgiveness and reparation. When they are on holiday in France, she walks into a little village where people look at her with curiosity. She realises why when, as she later walks home, she meets her mother. Mother turns away without speaking. Over the next few years, she gets occasional gifts, letters and videos from her mother. Feeling sympathy for other human beings, she begins to feel herself a human being and to feel the pain of the other. As she mourns her own future ending, she feels her humanity. She is mortal and she knows it. This myth is played out in the future. Iris is born in 2005 and lives out later experiences in 2025. The mirror and the echo are subtext: in her, the Echo finds a voice and enters into separate experience.

Note

1 This paper was prepared for publication in 2007 but has not been published previously. It is a preparatory study for Chapter 20. (Ed.)

20 Narcissus and Echo: Vision and hearing in early development

Applications to individual and group psychotherapy[1]

'Desire is a desire for inconsolability'

(Verhaeghe 1999)

Narcissus and Echo represent a pair who cannot create life-giving dialogue and who suffer psychic death. Ovid's myth is a story of desires that lead to death. The story fascinates the Western mind and is constantly renewed through new interpretations. It is a primordial story that is not only ancient but woven. A primordial myth is a woven text of meaning that both binds us and permits us to speak. We can speak of the inability of one to acknowledge the Other, of entrapment in the self, of absence of intimacy, and of the vital importance of human mirroring and resonance. I will consider the emergence of dialogue in early development through the interplay of mirroring and resonance. Clinical vignettes that illustrate both the presence and absence of mirroring and resonance are given.

Introduction: The goal of desire – to go on desiring

When we look up at the stars, we are de-sidering. The word 'desire' has its Latin origin in the heavens: *de sidere*, from the stars, to look *vainly* at a star. Desire, a mixture of wanting, lusting, yearning, hoping, is the motion, which drives us to reach out, makes us aware of the needs and wishes of the self. Desire is psychic motion. Our fascination with art is because the artist is perpetually driven to reach for the unobtainable, for the stars. I shall evoke the powers of the artist to illustrate my theme. Some years ago, in a commentary by Edward Lucie-Smith to an exhibition of photographs entitled *Desire*, I found these words:

> Desire is an energy that brings about change and it always means a leap into the frightening unknown. It is an unpredictable force that defines the limits of life and death.
>
> (Lucie-Smith et al. 1995: 1)

Life without desire can be a release from vain cravings, but it can also be a form of psychic death. The myth of Narcissus and Echo is a story of desires

DOI: 10.4324/9781003494713-25

leading to death: they represent a pair who cannot enter life-giving dialogue and who both suffer psychic death. Why retell this story that descends from Ovid? Because it is a story that has fascinated the Western mind and has been repeated and renewed over the centuries. A myth is a story that renews itself through interpretation. The myth of Narcissus who refuses the cries of Echo and longs to seize the image of himself in the water and is – in the end – changed into a flower is woven into our culture. It is *primordial*, which means not only ancient but basic; it means being woven. Through this myth we encounter the inability to acknowledge the other, entrapment in the self, the mystery of self-reflection and the absence of intimacy (Ovid 1993).

These two are a non-dialogical pair whose speech has not reached the level of the social. The philosophers George Herbert Mead (1934/2015) and later Mikhail Bakhtin (1981; Holquist 1981; 1990) asserted that speech is irreducibly social, intrinsically dialogical; that mind is the product of language. Speaker and listener can only converse if each can assume the role of the other: we speak to ourselves when we speak to others. This is how we come to know that we can be understood, for I am both listener and speaker, and we are a community of interlocutors.

Through emotional communication with others and with others to the self, intimacy evolves in a context of interpersonal equality. It lies between autonomous persons who are open to discussion and to the force of better argument; accountability stands in tandem with trust. Love's lust is trust, and love without selfishness can lead to friendship; love for the other is as her-/himself. Michel de Montaigne, when asked why he had such a deep friendship for Étienne de La Boétie, replied: 'Because he was he: because I was I.' Aristotle says a friend is another self.

In sexual love, even between persons who have achieved sexual maturity and who are defined and differentiated sexually, there is always the possibility – indeed, the inevitability – of suffering. For, while union with the other elevates the self, paradoxically love also threatens to infantilise, debase and deplete the self. This is because in sexual love, a self has been rendered no longer whole in itself; the other always remains essentially unknowable, and we are also made aware of the essentially unknowable part of ourselves. There are paradoxical aims to possess, to destroy and to preserve the existence of the other.

In the wake of infatuation, passion, ambivalence and then forgiveness, compassion and gratitude are entertained, and the intimacy of lovers becomes invested with feelings of empathy and mutuality. Through love, others than ourselves are perceived as having their own contours and life: we celebrate otherness. Ortega y Gasset (1963) defined the self as 'myself and the circumference of others'. Narcissus fled from otherness and sought for the immediacy of love without experiencing the exploration of difference. His fragile existence could not bear the pain of entering into differentiated reflections with non-identical others through whom he might have become less fragile and more tolerant and self-aware. New people with their distinct personal histories teach us new knowledge and expand experience in unexpected ways. Narcissus did not know that through love with, for and from others, he could – in a roundabout way – restore some of his lost infantile narcissism. He could have affirmed himself as a separate but equal centre of the universe. He died alone without having experienced the warmth, connectedness, reciprocity, intimacy and mutual identification that are the rewards of taking the risk of plunging into the deep waters of sexual love. He fled from Echo's offer of sexual love into the trap of self-love.

Analytic groups offer a special form of intimate life available to almost anyone who acknowledges needs they cannot meet from their own resources. They enable an intimacy of minds, of partnership in a search for truth that enables each to see the world twice over. Through the group experience we can enter into each other's minds, becoming partners in listening while remaining separate persons. The diversity of the group makes possible an exploration, separately and together, which each cannot attempt alone. The diversity helps to guard the intimacy that otherwise could become stiflingly close. People forgo the power of defensive isolation, take the risks of hurt, rejection and misunderstanding, and discover in the appreciation of others the rewards of self-disclosure. In playful tolerance and the suspension of judgment, people hand control over to others briefly in the sharing of mutual dependency. Rewards arise out of reciprocity, mutuality, turn-taking within a common time frame, where productive and receptive roles alternate. Understandings are shared and skills can be acquired that fortunate children learn at the knees of their mothers and fathers, or with their siblings in the family and with peer groups as they grow up.

It was Ovid who first linked Narcissus and Echo in legend. Though the better known of his two protagonists is Narcissus, we shall begin with Echo, for we are born into sound, which surrounds us, a sound bath into which we emit sounds of our own. Didier Anzieu's (1989) concept of the psychic envelope, the sense of the body enveloped first by a skin boundary, was later extended to that of the sound envelope. This notion of the psychic envelope, the experience of containment within a psychic boundary that delineates each of us, functions for the psyche as does the skin for the body. The skin is the site of contact between the individual and the world, the boundary that holds and contains the newborn and the nursling. The physical skin becomes the site for the elaboration of mental and emotional experience. Anzieu does not deal with gender. The newcomer to the world exchanges the maternal sea for the territory provided by its parents, with the provision they have made for the 'baby bunting whose father went a-hunting', to find a rabbit skin to wrap the baby bunting in. Something must be provided, and what is offered represents the summation of psychological, social and cultural factors. The infant is born into an experience of touch, temperature, sound and sight. Though now it is known how very soon infants respond visually, undoubtedly the most immediate and continuous sensory experience is that of sound. Sound surrounds us, goes in and out of us, is continuous, comes simultaneously from many sources and directions and cannot be stopped or grasped. We have to learn how to locate the sources of sound, beginning with whether the sound belongs to and is emitted by ourselves or by another and then to differentiate the language of sounds. This is the beginning of the lifelong search for meaningful communication and interaction. What we produce are utterances, the term Bakhtin preferred to speech. To utter is to speak out into the world in search of a response from another, a need for the other to respond to and thereby complete the act, which is incomplete without that response (Wertsch 1991).

The earliest sound languages are the proto-conversations, the language of sound gestures that seek and produce responses. Mead spoke about language as the conversation of significant gestures. I return now to the ideas of Anzieu, which were further elaborated by Edith Lecourt (1990). Because of these characteristics of sound that have been outlined – continuity, simultaneity, ungraspability – sound cannot itself form a psychic envelope, for an envelope has to be clearly delineated; it has an outer and inner face, it is a container, with an internal capacity and potential volume. The envelope is more a product of tactile and visual experiences that are localisable, for the sense of touch discriminates inner and outer, the eyes can focus and grasp objects in space in a way not available through sound. Psychic elaboration, the mentalisation of the body skin, is the basis of the body ego. It is the ego skin which Anzieu suggests is the psychic surface that interconnects diverse sensations as figure upon the ground of the psychic envelope. This envelope forms the basic substrate of mind. Where the ego skin, the psychic envelope, is intact, there is a sense of safety and containment. Where it is weak, leaky or broken, there is profound unease, a continuing sense of being unheld and unsafe, and there are fears including the fear of dismemberment.

In Lacan's theory of the mirror stage, the infant is entranced and entrapped by the visual illusion of a whole body and self in the mirror, as Narcissus was trapped in the pond's mirroring surface (Kernberg 2006). Lacan assumes that the infant is still in a state of psychic dismemberment when it sees itself as a whole in the mirror and is entranced and entrapped by the visual illusion, the fateful alienation of the ego from the self. Lacan does not properly consider the mirroring provided by responding others who give infants their sense of completeness by gaze interaction, smiles, vocalisations with their rhythms of engagement and disengagement. Sight is separated from sound in his thesis, as Narcissus was from Echo. However, we can apply the idea of the mirror stage to the concept of a sound mirror and a sound bath. We interact sonorously with infants, tuning in to their auditory range and styles, mentalising their sounds. We listen for and respond to the intentions of the infant, and not only that: we attribute intentionality to the sound gestures, thereby teaching the infant how to communicate. By understanding and responding to the baby's needs, it feels carried, cared for, immersed in a sound bath. Its own surface and volume are contained within a greater volume, the psychic equivalent of the baby held in the water for bathing.

Though the primary voice is that of the mother as principal caregiver, the baby is immersed in the sounds of the family group, its acoustic womb. The sound bath introduces the baby to the human environment where it begins to experience containment, continuity and hopefully harmony, though sadly we know how often the sound bath is cold, unreliable, discordant or intrusive. In the sonorous experience, we begin self-to-other exchanges that lay down the pathways for relationship experiences that are remembered and sought for in patterns of neural and emotional experiences.

We return to Echo, whose power to communicate verbally has been taken from her. Why was this so? The jealous goddess Juno, wife of Zeus, had discovered him in sexual intercourse with Echo's sister nymphs. Echo, detaining Juno with the chatter, enabled the nymphs to escape Juno's wrath. As punishment for this, Juno condemned her to lose the power of speech and only echo the sounds of others.

Echo is punished for her intrusion into the parental primal scene. She is banished from the responsive dialogue of mother/infant and therefore is fixated in a non-dialogical state. She longs to overcome her expulsion by reaching out to Narcissus, but he is also developmentally fixated in his non-responsiveness – a non-resonant state. Juno, the jealous pre-Oedipal figure, had earlier transformed her beautiful priestess into the horrifying Medusa for having attracted Zeus. Her task had been to mirror exactly Juno's beauty, but Zeus was attracted to her difference. The Oedipal theme appears. Exact mirroring cannot open a dialogical process; it is a narcissistic preoccupation by the mother of her infant's own inborn developmental need for differentiation and growth into openness. Echo sees Narcissus hunting in the woods with his companions at first, but when he loses them, she follows him into the cold, lonely glade where he is to meet his fate.

The story of Narcissus and the fateful encounter with Echo

Narcissus comes from a single-parent family and knows only his mother. He was fathered when his mother, Liriope, was raped by the river god, Cephissus. His mother brings the newborn to the blind prophet Tiresias, who lost his power to see as a punishment by the same jealous goddess Juno. Tiresias had betrayed her jealously guarded secret, that a woman's sexual pleasure is much greater than a man's, and was cursed with blindness, though compensated with the capacity for inner prophetic sight. He tells Liriope that Narcissus will live a long time if he does not know himself, and we can hear this as a prohibition of masturbation.

Narcissus was described as a loveable child, companionable but, though liked by others, he did not reciprocate and resonate. He was indifferent to the love of others. Consequently, a rejected male suitor asked the god Nemesis to punish Narcissus so that he too should know the pain of rejection by others – the pain he had caused them. He had not acquired the developmental capacity to recognise the mind of the other; he was without mentalisation.

As well as the English words, I shall use Ovid's Latin, for there are subtle nuances in the words that are difficult to reproduce in English. Separated from his friends and finding himself in this lonely glade, Narcissus calls out: 'Ecquis adest?' (Is anyone present?). Echo replies: 'Adest' (Present). Intrigued, Narcissus pursues the conversation with Echo, saying: 'Huc coeamus' (Here let us meet). Hearing what she wants to hear, Echo understand this as 'Let us mate' since *coīre* means 'to come together' but also 'to have a sexual union'. She comes forth and throws her arms around Narcissus, who flees, crying out: 'I'll die before you have your will of me'. Echo replies: 'Have your will of me,' but rejected, she flees and hides in the woods and caves.

Echo is described as being *prudens*, one who looks ahead, one who is shrewd. She sees what she wants to see; she hears what she wants to hear; she sexualises the words of Narcissus, who himself hovers between boyhood and young manhood and has had no sexual experience. Her responses, her echoing, are self-gratifying; they are not empathic responses that create the possibility of dialogue; there is not a conversation of people who get to know each other through understanding each other's subjective feelings. Her responses are pseudo-empathic, pseudo-responses, pseudo-intimacy. But bound to Narcissus by a fatal bond – the bond of rejection – she returns to stay with him until he dies.

The desire that leads to death

Narcissus does not have the capacity to develop and enjoy the reciprocity and resonance either. Entrapped by his own gaze in the fateful pool, intrigued by the beautiful other whom he sees in his own reflection, he tries to reach through the surface of the water and finds that the image always retreats from him. It appears to come to meet him and the desire that leads to death is born in him. What is he reaching for? In one version of the myth, he is reaching for his lost, dead twin sister, but another earlier reading remains constant to the theme that in an unrecognising way, he is seeing himself. His gaze is indeed his punishment – that in this way he may not possess his beloved; he will know desire but never achieve possession or consummation. His thirst and need for water is replaced by the insatiable desire for the elusive other with whom he has fallen in love, for the very first time. Lying transfixed by his own gaze, his body becomes as still as marble. He is mesmerised but then begins to feel the pain of longing. Both need and desire are born in him; as he bewails his fate, gradually he comes to recognise himself in the image: 'Iste ego sum' (That is me). Now in accordance with Tiresias's prophecy, he knows himself. His cries are echoed by the nymph Echo, who loves him but cannot come to help him. At death, his body is transformed into the flower narcissus, a flower whose extract is toxic, causing stiffness and numbness, and Echo is transformed into the rocks that surround the pool. Thus, the coldness, stillness and hardness that surrounds him may be seen to represent the failure of empathic mirroring. Echo herself is transformed into the cold Juno, whose face never warmed lovingly to arouse the infant's desire to love and be loved.

There are many lessons to be learnt from the Narcissus myth. They include the dangers of illusion and captivation by a deceptive image; of a lack of knowledge of the self and of one's origins; the dangers of vanity and pride; of turning away from reciprocal relationships with others; of self-absorption and illusion; the developmental cul-de-sac that can lead to psychic death; and a sadomasochistic bond. Echo's masochistic fidelity to her rejecting beloved is also instructive. What I want to emphasise here is that there is no recognition, no re-cognition. Narcissus does not see Echo – there is no gaze interaction between them; he only sees the image with whom there is no alive responsiveness. Echo cannot converse; she cannot create dialogue and acts solely according to her own possessive wishes. Echo and Narcissus can both relate only to themselves or to an imagined Other, who cannot respond with a difference. Where there should be difference, there is only similarity, identity.

Inherent in this myth is an incapacity to develop psychologically and emotionally to the stage where it is possible to reflect upon oneself as an entity, a self, a person, not only one's visual or auditory image. The achievement of such perspectives, where the person becomes aware that he or she is both subject and object, a perceiving and an experiencing self, a self to oneself, but also a self to others, comes about through the relationship with others who reflect both sameness and differences within a given relationship (Dowrick 1992).

Both Narcissus and Echo in vision and in sound receive responses that exactly match the emitting source. In the discovery of difference, what I give out to the other, the other gives back to me, provides a response similar enough to be recognisable to me as a return but a return with a difference. That difference tells me there is an Other out there whom I have reached, who has responded and who, in good circumstances, enjoys the interchange and gives back to me more than I gave out. Bakhtin points out that each one of us has what he calls a surplus of vision. Each of us has a unique point of view and can see things that are similar to what others see but always with a significant difference. He adds this is how the human personality is constructed – through alterity (Wertsch 1991). It is through this responsive and reciprocal exchange of sight and sound, especially verbal, that the human personality is built up in a process he calls the architectonics of personality. The female child and mother find themselves deeply in the Other. Eventually, the growing child, both male and female, will have to dis-identify to proceed along the developmental path of achieving separateness, yet remaining connected. Separateness and connectedness are the double helix of psychological growth. The male child has to tread the path of dis-identification from mother much earlier than the girl, taking father as his model for maleness. For both male and female, children have to recognise the triangulation inherent in being the product of the two parents (Tyson and Tyson 1990).

The sense of the unheimlich, the uncanny, can come from the experience that there is a double out there that haunts us. The doppelganger, who shadows us, creates the sense of fear. Many interesting phenomena occur in relationship to physical mirrors, but here the point is that what we call mirroring and echoing are both inborn biological human capacities. The busy interaction between infants and caregivers from birth onwards is being intensively studied (Stern 1998). Some of these studies are relevant to the understanding of the Narcissus and Echo dyad. Beebe and Lachmann (2012) point out that mothers and infants match the direction of affective change in their interactions but never exactly: they are closely together but never exactly at the same level of intensity. There is a basic rhythm of turn-taking, I to you, pause, you to me, pause, you to me, and so on. (The pause was given prominence by Winnicott 1960; 1967/1971). This turn-taking gives time and opportunity for both intrapsychic and interpersonal processes to occur within the same time frame and within the same relationship (Wright 2009). Through such processes of turn-taking and matching but not matching exactly, infant and caregiver, usually the mother, can begin to enter into each other's perceptual and temporal worlds and feeling states. When we discover that we are similar but not the same, that we take turns in this dialectic, this dialogue, the Other becomes familiar and with this familiarity comes the security of being able to predict the other's feeling state.

Feelings of familiarity allow for internalisation of the relationship with the Other as one which is pleasurable, satisfying and safe. There is a great deal of unconscious mirroring and matching of facial expressions and sounds. The mirroring by oneself of the expression of the other seems to generate autonomic sensations, which produce similar feeling states in both partners. This can be repeated experimentally with adults, in whom facial muscular actions and patterns generate more autonomic changes than actually attempting to experience emotion through ideation and recall. In these ways, infants and caregivers can create similar psycho-physiological states, participate in the subjective state of the other and thereby have access to the feeling state of the other. This is the beginning of intersubjectivity. Through shared experiences of matching come further expectations of matching and being matched. In the course of these anticipations there are inevitable mismatchings. It is through an understanding of the nature of these mismatches and learning what they are about that infants and caregivers learn to get along with each other (Wright 2009).

Clinical illustrations

Vignette 1: A patient I saw over a decade ago came back recently. She had been a silent entrapped person, who felt more a machine than a human being. She felt sufficiently understood by me to accept referral to an older woman therapist with whom she stayed for many years. She became alive in that relationship with this sensitive woman who treated her, as she put it, developmentally. This means that the therapist as well as being a reliable presence, an engaged therapist, also taught her how to look up words in a dictionary if she did not know their meanings; she taught her to withstand gentle teasing. Sadly, the therapist became old and somewhat incapable, and though the patient remained loyal to her and continued to visit her until her death, the therapeutic relationship was over. The patient undertook a course in child development and therefore was referred to another therapist, a woman, this time much younger, probably not much older than the patient herself. She found this therapy intensely intrusive and disturbing. Not only did the therapist have a theoretical orientation which led her to be a much more active interpreter, but what the patient felt most acutely was that she felt her new therapist to be a chatterer, meaning that there was constant verbal interaction between them. There were few silences, no pauses, mostly an immediate and what was felt to be intrusive response, and on top of that there were noises and interruptions to the therapy sessions. There also seemed to have been some contempt on the part of the new therapist for the work of the former one. The patient fled from this new encounter and wandered through the rooms of several other therapists, trying to find a place to settle and finally came back to me. Though I only intended to see her once, she asked for a second interview, now feeling safe enough to recount something of her painful experiences, and remained in once-weekly therapy. The emphasis here is on the differences in rhythm, pace, sound and empathic interaction. There was a good match between her and her first therapist and a poor match, a mismatch with the second.

Vignette 2: A young man who was in individual therapy with me for a couple of years said that when he thought about his mother, he realised that he always had to draw in his horns; he always had to match her mood. Her mood was one without much liveliness and joyfulness, or pleasure in his own liveliness, noisiness and naughtiness. He always knew that she would approve of his working hard, especially when he went away to boarding school. He could always get an echo from her by being a good boy, but he couldn't be a naughty boy with her. He was always afraid she might treat him as if he were being like his lively, noisy father. His father could go away and ignore his mother's moods. It was exciting to be with him and do sporty things, though he always had a fear of whether he was going to be able to keep up with his father. Mood-matching is a feature of the transference with me. He is often occupied by trying to sense whether I have approved or accepted what he has to say and whether he is reading my mood appropriately. Indeed, he felt that before he could leave me he had to get the Good Housekeeping seal of approval, which he could get by working hard and bringing problems which had to be solved, boxes to be ticked. When it became clear that this was what he was doing with me, we could both laugh and he felt released by that. Getting his mother to laugh was always hard work.

Sonorous experience in therapy groups

In the group the therapist offers a privileged and protected space where – for a limited time – the members speak with and listen to one another. The therapist himself/herself listens to the themes, counterpoints, rhythms. Gradually he or she weaves the sounds and silences together into themes, stories and significant dialogues, offering the participants a view of themselves as interconnected parts of a whole, figures against the ground of the group matrix. We do not create the interconnections, the patterns of responses, articulations and disarticulations, for they are already there in the life of the group, in its comings together and partings, in the time intervals between sessions when, as individuals, each one faces out to their own worlds. When we reassemble, we face inwards towards each other and in what is brought to the group. What is disclosed and what is enquired about or inferred provide a linking of the in- and out-of-group experiences, revealing two aspects of the same person. As I write, I begin to think of inspiration and expiration, systole and diastole, turning in and turning out, of each session as a breath or as an immersion in the sonorous and visual group experience.

Speaking, listening, pausing, responding: looking, being looked at: looking towards, looking away: engaging, disengaging: mirroring, resonating, articulating responses: enquiring, answering, tuning in to oneself and to others: the slow difficult process of deepening our understanding of one another and ourselves – these are the ground-base experiences of being in the group. They underlie all other processes.

Isaiah Berlin (1976) describes how the eighteenth-century German philosopher Herder asserted that the principal link between humans is language because we think symbolically: to think is to use symbols. Words connect passion with things and the present with the past, making possible memory and imagination and creating family, society, literature and history. Shaped by our association with others, swimming in an inherited stream of images and words, we must accept these media on trust; we cannot create them. Herder wrote about empathy, sympathetic insight that conceived and cast light on the crucially important social function of belonging – what it is to belong to a group, to a culture. Man lives in and belongs to a cultural network, and without this he dehumanises and destroys. Narcissus and Echo, our mythological duo, are separated from their own natural groups: Narcissus from his group of adolescent companions and Echo from her sister nymphs. Because of this separation, neither can develop their own mature humanity. Going beyond the individual to the group and nation, we must mark Herder's observation that those societies are truly human which may follow a leader but have no master, for the man who needs a master is an animal and as soon as he becomes human, he needs no master at all (Berlin 1976).

Herder states that without society there can be no self-criticism, for self-criticism is social criticism. Both Narcissus and Echo are without society and furthermore have no society within as a basis for their self-awareness, no sources for inner reflection. They cannot sustain human existence and are transformed into non-human forms, he into the flower narcissus and she into bare rocks that only reflect sound. Neither has developed into those recognisable human entities who can sustain themselves as centres of their own initiative and continuity. Neither has acquired what the anthropologist Clifford Geertz (1973: 59) defines as a self: a bounded entity, a more or less integrated centre of awareness, emotion, judgement and action, organised into a distinctive whole and set contrastingly, both against other such wholes and against its social and natural background. What Geertz emphasises is the integration of cognition, conation and affect. Herder's passion is connected to things by thought, and language, and this integrated entity is connected with culture and society. The self is a bounded entity inseparable from its context as figure is to ground.

Echo and resonance

> **Vignette 3:** Jane, a woman in her early fifties, spent many years in psychoanalytic treatment since adolescence. Three lengthy analyses have ended unsatisfactorily, the most recent one experienced as a vindictive persecution by her analyst. In the analytic group she will sometimes caricature like Echo, her previous analyst's interpretations, making them sound like moralistic injunctions. She comes to a group that meets twice a week where she has attended for some five years. Often, she slumps into sleep when having to listen to others; when waking she often asks factual questions as if the concrete details of what a person had said were of the greatest importance: details as to time, place, event. Paranoid rages, temper tantrums when she rocked and banged her feet were frequent in the earlier years, particularly when she heard herself addressed moralistically – for instance, unrealistically hearing that she had been told to put up with her lot and give up hope for a sexual relationship. Here I am reminded how Narcissus fled from Echo's sexual approaches. Jane had to release herself from pathological narcissism before she could be approached sexually. Much has changed over the years, and now she often takes part sensitively in verbal interactions and has shown a good capacity to penetrate to fellow members' underlying problems.

Through this patient I want to bring out some of the qualities and differences between echoing and resonance. The *Oxford Dictionary*'s (2018) definition of resonance is: 'The reinforcement or prolongation of sound by reflection'. Foulkes stated that mirroring and resonance were group-specific therapeutic factors, the seeing of oneself in and through others, responding in one's own particular way to the events of the group and to the emotions of another. Jane has displayed echo-like qualities; she only hears and listens to what directly and concretely seems to echo her own conflicts, ideas or emotions. She often misheard and misinterpreted what others were saying to each other, to make their words fit with her own preoccupations. Much of her life is lived in the realm of what she regards as the factual: deprived, exploited, jealous and envious of others. Despite this unpromising, difficult and frustrating way of being in the group, she has received much good attention as well as confrontation. She has been fought with furiously and is sometimes responded to with sustained and patient understanding and sometimes with great impatience. Gradually other group members have come to recognise and articulate what it is they find themselves experiencing in the relationship with her. There are two concurrent and intermingled processes. Jane functions at the level of Echo, calling out into what she experiences as a hard, uncaring world both within and without the group. She hears herself in the words and responses of others and transforms their words into her own, as did Echo with the words of Narcissus. The other level is based on the individual responses of the other members, who find in their dealings with her a variety of attitudes and affects that deepen their own self-understanding. Sometimes she is the mad mother or the mother who does not hear and respond to her child; sometimes she is the greedy child who wants to monopolise all attention. Gradually, she has begun to understand and accept these responses and become more sensible of and sensitive to the situation of the group and to other members' needs. As her range of responses widens, she begins to resonate as well as to echo.

The British psychoanalyst Betty Joseph (Feldman and Spillius 1999) has written about non-resonance as a factor militating against psychic change. She describes patients who seem impermeable, who do not resonate to the analyst's attempts to reach to their emotions. Such patients seem to have no notion of being emotionally understood by another who can tolerate, understand, feel for and contain another person. A rigid, narcissistic defensive structure provides a pseudo-container that seems to protect the person against unconscious psychic catastrophe. Such patients, preoccupied with themselves, seem unaware of their way of being. The analyst's attempt to gain access is responded to as if it were a forceful, cruel attack, a penetration of the container. Joseph says that as there is no notion of what it is to be understood by another person, these patients seem not to have a concept of mind, a way of being with another person that is of understanding and being understood by two separate individuals.

Non-resonance stands out in a group as an inability to take part in dialogue or exchange. This can be observed in the psychosomatic patient, the emotionally illiterate person for whom the language of the emotions is utterly alien. It is fascinating to witness the changes that can occur: the growth of the capacity to listen and to be listened to with understanding; to develop a language that can grasp recurrent and subtle states of feelings; and to see and hear such a patient begin to tune in to the emotional life of others. In the group, non-resonance can progress to resonance and to mirroring in a way that may well not be possible in dyadic therapy. The patient eventually manages to become part of and contribute to the emotional life of others, thereby entering into an intersubjective world.

I now return to the distinction between resonance and echo. The Jungian analyst Patricia Berry (2008) has given subtle attention to the meaning of Echo in the Narcissus myth. Echo does not have an identity: to speak she needs another's words and surroundings that will echo her. Before becoming involved with Narcissus, with whom she falls passionately in love, she had dallied with the demigod Pan, that desirous animal force that claims to be everything: we still use the prefix 'pan-' to express that all-encompassing attitude. Pan desires loving and sexual echoing, but Echo flees him, rejecting his demand to echo everything. Echo's own desire is for Narcissus, Pan's opposite – singular, self-contained and self-enclosed by his own image. He stands for the particular, and Echo will not unite with Pan the general. In a fascinating footnote to his chapter on narcissism, Havelock Ellis says that when Pan was rejected by Echo, he was taught the art of masturbation by his father, the god Hermes, so as to be able to console and comfort himself (Ellis 1915/2018). Thus, Pan also stands for the auto-erotic, the seeking of bodily satisfaction in oneself as a consolation for the loss of the other.

Now, why has Echo lost her voice? It is because she deceived Hera, queen of Olympus; by her chattering, she had allowed Zeus to go on sexually dallying with her sister nymphs. As punishment for this distracting chattering, Hera deprives her of her own powers of speech, restricting her ever after to be the echo of others. Now, Hera the queen is a stickler for facts, forms and order. She is a literaliser; for her, the real is the actual. Zeus is always escaping from her to propagate the world, for if she were to retain control over him, there would be no development, no unexpected strange occurrences. The relationship between Hera and Zeus brings to my mind the relationship between Margaret Dumont and Groucho Marx!

Echo's very presence and chattering threatens Hera by showing up the emptiness in formal order. Echo finds the gaps, the holes, the hollows, the echoing possibilities; her actions show up the gaps in Hera's concept of faithfulness in marriage. It is Echo who makes possible the acts of covert fertility. It is her words that allow Zeus to procreate and allow new forms to be born. But through Hera's curse, Echo is condemned to be repetitive and find a new form for herself. Her attention and her passion now centre on Narcissus, who exemplifies self-absorption, the search for beauty in a self-mirroring image but who also directs his longing downwards, seeking depth. This depth is what Echo longs to find for herself through attracting the love of Narcissus.

In the verbal interplay between them, the words circle within themselves autogeneratively. The words are not direct; they are not object-related; they are not a dialogue; they lack depth. Narcissus calls out for the company of others, but all he finds is Echo. Every occurrence between them is a reoccurrence. Echo pursues Narcissus and he flees from her, for what he seeks is his own identity based on separateness and sameness, whereas Echo is totally dependent on her surroundings. Echo's painful passion, her longing for the unrealisable, kept at an agonised distance, represents an intrapsychic distance, an imaginative distancing. Narcissus repudiates Echo, who symbolises dependency on surroundings, and he returns to his own self-entrapped world. Berry writes that to develop the echo in one's narcissism, one must achieve a certain painful distance in and by which this echo can sound.

In therapy we maintain and protect a distant nearness that is in touch with the intrapsychic, but we preserve Echo's longing and suffering for the work of the analysis. Echoing distance creates space for beauty, a painful beauty that has no happy ending but ends in transformation. Echo's body wastes away, consumed by love and grief, and she becomes etiolated, transformed into a body of stone and air. Through this transformation we can hear echoes and transform them, in turn, into resonance. We train our ears to hear and transform what we hear into meaningful form. This kind of resonance is central to the proto-conversation between the mother and her infant. It involves a fine coordination between the facial expressions, vocalisations and body movements of mother and child, such that they can be conceived as a single system made up of two people.

Meares (2000: 70) writes that the pleasure that generates value comes from events in the environment that match or are concordant with models of the individual's ongoing personal experience. This matching, or concordance, is of a very particular kind. It involves a resonance with what is known of oneself, however dim or tenuously formed this knowing may be. Pleasure arises when the responses of the other show a re-cognition of personal reality. This may not be the 'reality' as shown to the world. The concordance, resonance or re-presentation is with that complex of feelings, imaginings and memories that can be sensed as the core of individual experience. There is a feeling of well-being that arises when the responses of the other resonate with what is sensed as being the most personal of one's own experiences. The feeling of well-being creates a sense of personal value, which enables us to have a core of sense of self-worth.

Non-resonance can slowly give way to more harmonious ways of relating to both oneself and the selves of others. I have seen this happen in group analysis, though the process is pain-giving and painstaking. Some patients who have come to an impasse in dyadic therapies are able to make more progress in group analysis through the presence of other resonating persons, resonating others whose inner processes are made both visible and audible through mirroring and resonance. I found much to confirm this thesis in the important paper by the Boston group for the study of change who find that, in the process of psychotherapy, there is something more than interpretation (Stern et al. 1998).

Conclusion: Group mothering

I replace the noun for the group as mother with the active mothering that an analytic group can give, by listening attentively and by responding both sympathetically and empathically. Perhaps in the session described above, the mothering was enhanced by the absence of men, but I have witnessed occasions when the men also provided such caring and understanding responses.

What I hope to have illustrated above is the growth of intersubjectivity, the sense of one person entering into the experiences of the other, exchanging with them, having access to their own self at the same time as the self of the other. Thus, both intrapsychic and interpersonal processes take place simultaneously. In the group-analytic group, all the members participate in this gradual deepening of the exchanges between peers, fellow members who are not constrained by their roles as are therapists with their patients in a dyadic situation. After many years of experience, I am convinced that these are the processes that bring about therapeutic change and that the therapist's principal and basic function is to provide the group's psychic envelope and maintain the medium in which the group matrix slowly evolves. To do this adequately, the therapist must genuinely value the group experience and see it as something that s/he is privileged to be able to offer and also to be part of.

In the sessions described above, there was a sense of deep engagement with varied experiences, with mothers who do not give back to their children the sense that their tyrannical, angry feelings can be accepted, understood and converted into meaningful communications and experiences, ones that can lead to growth in relationships rather than disruption and pain. There can be a failure of dialogue, a failure of sonorous exchanges, but now this can be looked at, recognised and grieved over together. I understand that this is the group as mother and the group as *mothering*.

Members can generate the experience between themselves and for each other. In this medium, quite profound regressions can safely be experienced and held, often feared previously as threats of disintegration, madness or the fear of breakdown. Being heard, held and understood through the fear of regression can allow recognition of the need to re-experience early relationships and their disruptive effects on the developing self. The self that unfolds is also the self that can be held; the mirroring, echoing, resonance and understanding that the group offers does not lead to the fate that Ovid described in his legend but more to that which Milton (2003) wrote about in *Paradise Lost*. Milton writes of how Eve, never having seen herself before, is entranced by her reflection in a pool where she might have suffered the same fate as Narcissus. When a voice speaks to her to tell her of the danger she is in, she is able to leave and seek Adam, her human counterpart and companion. This is the voice of knowledge and understanding, a voice that urges on the self, entranced with its own reflection, that the fate of the human being is to be found in relationship with others.

> I thither went
> With unexperienced thought, and laid me down
> On the green bank, to look into the clear
> Smooth lake, that to me seem'd another sky.
> As I bent down to look, just opposite
> A shape within the wat'ry gleam appear'd,
> Bending to look on me: I started back,
> It started back; but pleased I soon return'd;
> Pleased it return'd as soon with answ'ring looks
> Of sympathy and love: there I had fix'd

Mine eyes till now, and pined with *vain desire*,
Had not a voice thus warn'd me. What thou seest,
What there though seest, fair Creature, is thyself.
(Milton 2003: 98)

Note

1 This chapter is an edited version of a paper published as Chapter 5 in *Desire, Passion and Gender: Clinical Implications*, edited by L. Navaro, R. Friedman, and S. L. Schwartzberg (2011), pp. 65–80.

Grateful thanks are extended to the editors for their consent to the publication of this paper here and to the publishers, Nova Science Publishers. (Ed.)

Section VI

End matter

Appendix 1: Malcolm Pines, author: Books and papers published in journals and books

The twelve previously published papers in Malcolm Pines's earlier collection, *Circular Reflections: Selected Papers on Group Analysis and Psychoanalysis* (1998), are marked *.

The present collection, *The Journey from Psychoanalysis to Group Analysis: Further Papers of Malcolm Pines*, contains twenty papers, nine of which were previously published. They are all marked **.

An earlier catalogue of Pines's writings is available in 'Malcolm Pines Bibliography', *Circular Reflections* (1998), pp. 227–234.

A. Biographical

Journal title	Subject	Author(s)	Vol.	Issue	Pages	Date	Year
Group Analysis	Interview with Malcolm Pines	Malcolm Pines, Martin Weegmann	43	3	372–401	Aug 27	2010
Group Analysis	Malcolm Pines et al.: The Art of Teaching Group Analysis	Harold Behr	43	3	241–252	Sep	2010
Group Analysis	A Conversation with Malcolm Pines: Part One	Juan Tubert-Oklander, Reyna Hernández-Tubert	43	4	476–495	Dec	2010
Group Analysis	A Conversation with Malcolm Pines: Part Two	Juan Tubert-Oklander, Reyna Hernández-Tubert	44	1	3–26	Mar	2011
Group Analysis	Reminiscences and Reflections on My Life in Psychiatry and Psychotherapy	Malcolm Pines	48	2	13–24	May 26	2015
Group Analysis	Malcolm Pines as I Knew Him	Harold Behr	55	1	118–120	Mar	2022
Group Analysis	Malcolm Pines (1925–2021). A Personal Reflection	Sue Einhorn	55	1	129–132	Mar	2022
Group Analysis	Malcolm Pines Obituary	John Schlapobersky	55	1	121–128	Mar	2022

B. Book reviews by Malcolm Pines

Journal	Book reviewed	Vol.	Issue	Page(s)	Date	Year
Group Analysis	*The Interpretation of Language Volume I: Understanding the Symbolic Meaning of Language Volume II: Understanding the Unconscious Meaning of Language* by Theodore Thass Thienemann	7	2	126–129	Jul 1	1974
Group Analysis	*Quotation from The Discovery of the Individual 1050–1200* by Colin Morris	8	2	120	May 1	1975
Group Analysis	*Psychodrama: Theory and Therapy* by Ira A. Greenberg	9	1	47	Mar 1	1976
Group Analysis	*The Art and Technique of Analytic Group Therapy* by Martin Grotjahn	11	1	68–70	Apr 1	1978
Group Analysis	*The Borderline Patient* by Roy Grinker and Beatrice Werble	11	2	168–169	Aug 1	1978
Group Analysis	*Structuring the Therapeutic Process: Compromise with Chaos* by Murray Cox	11	3	281–282	Dec 1	1978
Group Analysis	*Group Approaches in Psychiatry* by J. Stuart Whiteley and John Gordon	12	2	171	Aug 1	1979
Group Analysis	*Psychoanalytic Psychology: The Development of Freud's Thought* by Raymond E. Fancher	12	2	173–174	Aug 1	1979
Group Analysis	*The Psychoanalysis of Organisations* by Robert de Board	12	2	177–179	Aug 1	1979
Group Analysis	*The Therapeutic Self* by John G. Watkins	12	2	179–180	Aug 1	1979
Group Analysis	*Ego-Psychology 2* by Gertrude Blank and Reuben Blank	12	3	271–273	Dec 1	1979
Group Analysis	*Intensive Psychotherapy of the Borderline Patient* by Richard D. Chessick	12	3	273–274	Dec 1	1979
Group Analysis	*The Therapeutic Interaction* by Robert Langs	12	3	274–275	Dec 1	1979
Group Analysis	*From Group Dynamics to Group Psychoanalysis* by Morton Kissen	13	1	77–78	Apr 1	1980
Group Analysis	*Faces in a Cloud – Subjectivity in Personality Theory* by Robert Stollerow and George Attwood	13	1	82–83	Apr 1	1980

Group Analysis	*The Psychoanalytic Study of Society* by W. Muensterberger, L. Boyer Bryce and S. A. Grolnick	17	3	265–266	Dec 1	1984
Group Analysis	*The Quiet Profession: Supervisors of Psychotherapy* by Anne Alonso	20	4	381	Dec 1	1987
Group Analysis	*In Defense of Narcissism: The Creative Self in Search of Meaning* by Carl Goldberg	21	1	90	Mar 1	1988
Group Analysis	*Descent into Conflict, 1945: A Doctor's War* by David H. Clark	29	3	414–415	Sep 1	1996
Group Analysis	*W. R. Bion. War Memoirs 1917–19*	31	1	124	Mar 1	1998
Group Analysis	*Love in a Time of Loneliness* by Paul Verhaeghe	33	2	305–306	Jun 1	2000
Group Analysis	*The Neuroscience of Human Relationships, Attachment and the Developing Social Brain* by Louis Cozolino	40	4	562–563	Dec 1	2007
Group Analysis	*The French Revolution: A Tale of Terror and Hope for Our Times* by Harold Behr	48	3	394–396	Aug 27	2015

C. Editorials by Malcolm Pines et al.

Journal	Title		Vol.	Issue	Page(s)	Date	Year
Group Analysis	Editorial	Malcolm Pines	19	1	3–4	Mar 1	1986
Group Analysis	Editorial	Malcolm Pines	19	2	99	Jun 1	1986
Group Analysis	Editor's Note	Malcolm Pines	21	3	210	Sep 1	1988
Group Analysis	Editorial Note	Malcolm Pines	22	2	130	Jun 1	1989
Group Analysis	Editorial	Malcolm Pines	24	1	5	Mar 1	1991
International Review of Psychoanalysis	Guest Editorial	Malcolm Pines, R. Wisbey	18		321–324		1991
Group Analysis	Editorial	Malcolm Pines	31	4	387–388	Dec 1	1998
Group Analysis	Editorial Introduction	Malcolm Pines	32	3	291–292	Sep 1	1999
Group Analysis	Editorial	Malcolm Pines	33	3	315	Sep 1	2000
Group Analysis	Editor's Note	Malcolm Pines	34	1	4	Mar 1	2001
Group Analysis	Editor's Response to 'The Social Unconscious: A Post-Foulkesian Perspective' by Farhad Dalal	Malcolm Pines	34	4	557–559	Dec 1	2001
Group Analysis	Editor's Introduction	Malcolm Pines	35	1	4	Mar 1	2002
Group Analysis	Editorial Introduction	Malcolm Pines, Luisa Brunori	36	4	503–506	Dec 1	2003

D. Papers in *Group Analysis*

Article	Author(s)	Vol.	Issue	Page(s)	Date	Year
Therapeutic Community	Helle Munro, Malcolm Pines, David Clark	3	1	15–23	May 1	1970
Discussion on Relationship between Psychoanalysis and Group Analysis	Martin Grotjahn, Malcolm Pines, S. H. Foulkes, Werner W. Kemper	3	1	42–56	May 1	1970
Section II: Second European Symposium on Group Analysis	Malcolm Pines, Earl Hopper, A. C. Robin Skynner, Ilse Seglow, M. M. Berger, Minnie L. J. Abercrombie	5	2	77–102	Aug 1	1972
Section V Diverse Communications, Reports	Helle Munro, Malcolm Pines	6	3	185–193	Nov 1	1973
II (c) Therapeutic Community	Malcolm Pines	7	1	46–49	Apr 1	1974
Section IV Group-Analytic Commentary	Malcolm Pines	7	2	112–116	Jul 1	1974
The Group-Analytic Practice	Lionel Kreeger, Malcolm Pines	7	3	146–147	Nov 1	1974
A Prospect of Group Analysis	Malcolm Pines	10	1	49–55	Apr 1	1977
Group-analytic psychotherapy of the Borderline Patient*	Malcolm Pines	11	2	115–126	Aug 1	1978
Framework Patients	Malcolm Pines	11	3	245–247	Dec 1	1978
Group Psychotherapy: Frame of Reference for Training	Malcolm Pines	12	3	210–218	Dec 1	1979
Articles: How a Group Develops over Time	Malcolm Pines	12	2	109–113	Aug	1979
The Frame of Reference of Group Psychotherapy	Malcolm Pines	13	1	16–21	Apr 1	1980
Correspondence	Malcolm Pines, Louis Zinkin, Gregory van der Kleij, Meg Sharpe, Josephine Lomax-Simpson	13	3	157–160	Dec 1	1980

What to Expect in the Psychotherapy of the Borderline Patient	Malcolm Pines	13	3	168–177	Dec 1	1980
From: Malcolm Pines	Malcolm Pines	13	3	204–205	Dec 1	1980
On 'Group Analysis: Taking the Non-problem Seriously' by Caroline Garland XV/1, pp. 4–14	Dennis Brown, Malcolm Pines, Robin Skynner	15	1	53–55	Apr 1	1982
Reflections on Mirroring*	Malcolm Pines	15	Supp.	1–26	May 10	1982
Group Psychotherapy for Students and Teachers – A Selected Bibliography 1946–1979	Malcolm Pines	15	2	198–199	Aug 1	1982
The Group-Analytic View of Culture and Civilization: Response to Yiannis Gabriel	Malcolm Pines	16	2	145–151	Aug 1	1983
Psychoanalysis, Psychodrama and Group Psychotherapy: Step-Children of Vienna	Malcolm Pines	19	2	101–112	Jun	1986
Shame – What Psychoanalysis Does and Does Not Say	Malcolm Pines	20	1	16–31	Mar 1	1987
Bion: A Group-Analytic Appreciation	Malcolm Pines	20	3	251–262	Sep 1	1987
Mediation Papers: A Group-Analytic Response	Malcolm Pines	21	1	57–59	Mar 1	1988
Group Analysis and Healing*	Malcolm Pines	22	4	417–429	Dec 1	1989
The Matrix of Group Analysis: An Historical Perspective**	Malcolm Pines	24	2	99–109	Jun 1	1991
'Elaboration of the Negative' and Other Concepts: A Tribute to Eduardo Cortesão	Malcolm Pines	25	2	151–167	Jun 1	1992
The Self as a Group: The Group as a Self**	Malcolm Pines	29	2	183–190	Jun 1	1996
The Contributions of Ernest Hutten to Group Analysis	Malcolm Pines	29	2	277	Jun 1	1996

Dialogue and Selfhood: Discovering Connections**	Malcolm Pines	29	3	327–341	Sep 1	1996
Centennial Celebration to Commemorate the Birth and Work of Norbert Elias	Malcolm Pines	30	4	475–476	Dec 1	1997
Alfreda Galt, Collaborator of Trigant Burrow, 1910–1998	Malcolm Pines	32	1	156	Mar 1	1999
Patrick de Maré: A Man Ahead of His Time	Malcolm Pines	33	1	8–10	Mar 1	2000
The Coherency of Group Analysis**	Malcolm Pines	35	1	13–26	Mar 1	2002
Falling in and out of Class Structures	Malcolm Pines	35	3	406–410	Sep 1	2002
The Time Unlimited Group	Malcolm Pines	36	2	224–227	Jun 1	2003
Social Brain and Social Group: How Mirroring Connects People**	Malcolm Pines	36	4	507–513	Dec 1	2003
Foreword	Malcolm Pines	38	2	179–180	Jun 1	2005
Response to Lecture by Ralph Stacey	Malcolm Pines	38	4	495–498	Dec 1	2005
How Can Group Analysis Become an Academic Discipline?	Malcolm Pines	39	2	273–280	Jun 1	2006
Ave Atque Vale	Malcolm Pines	39	2	281–282	Jun 1	2006
Special Section: Papers Presented at the GAS 2005 Symposium, Molde: Editorial	Malcolm Pines, Tom Ormay	39	3	291	Sep 1	2006
Group Analysis and the Affective Disorders**	Malcolm Pines	40	3	357–365	Sep 1	2007
Minding the Gap: Commentary on 'The Body of Shame in the Circle of the Group'	Malcolm Pines	41	2	180–181	Jun 1	2008
The Matrix of Group Analysis: An Historical Perspective**	Malcolm Pines	42	1	5–15	Mar 1	2009
A Commentary on Ernest Wolf's 'Group Helplessness and Rage'	Malcolm Pines	42	2	197–198	May 20	2009

Introduction: A Celebration of the Life and Work of Patrick de Maré	Malcolm Pines	42	3	278–279	Aug 19	2009
Clinical Work in Small Groups	Malcolm Pines	42	3	280–281	Aug 19	2009
A Commentary on Nielsen, Luggin, Thygesen and Aagaard's 'The Use of Substitutes—Continuity and the Group-as-a-Whole'	Malcolm Pines	42	4	376–377	Dec	2009
Comment on Taha et al.'s 'Power of Love and Love of Power'	Malcolm Pines	43	2	190–191	Jun 1	2010
On Narcissism, Evolution and Group Dynamics: A Tribute to Malcolm Pines	Sigmund Karterud	43	3	301–310	Aug 27	2010
Malcolm Pines' Contribution to Group Analysis	Rocco Antonio Pisani	43	3	328–336	Aug 27	2010
End Note	Malcolm Pines	43	3	402	Aug 27	2010
Learning Peace: Here and Now – The Intercultural Competence of Groups	Malcolm Pines	43	4	465–475	Dec 17	2010
Postscript: To Articles Published to Honour Malcolm Pines at His 85th Birthday	Kevin Power	43	4	559–561	Dec 17	2010
Comment on 'The Median Group and Psychiatry: Reclaiming Mind' by Roberto Schöllberger	Malcolm Pines	44	2	236–238	Jun 13	2011
Introduction	Malcolm Pines	46	2	120–122	May 28	2013
Introduction to a New Book Dedicated to Anneliese Heigl-Evers	Malcolm Pines	46	3_suppl	37–39	Aug 27	2013
Steps towards a Basic Theory of Groups	Malcolm Pines	48	2	120–125	May 26	2015
Preface to Correspondence between R. A. Pisani and E. J. Anthony	Malcolm Pines	52	2	242–243	Feb 9	2019

E. Papers published in other journals

Journal title	Paper	Author(s)	Vol.	Issue	Page(s)	Date	Year
Psychotherapy and Psychosomatics	Borderline Personality Organisation	Malcolm Pines	25	1/6	58–62		1975
Postgraduate Medical Journal	A Psychoanalytic View of Sleep	Malcolm Pines	52	603	26–31	Jan	1976
International Journal of Group Psychotherapy	The Frame of Reference of Group Psychotherapy	Malcolm Pines	31	3	275–285		1981
British Journal of Psychiatry	Reading about Psychoanalysis	Malcolm Pines	138		164–167		1981
International Journal of Group Psychotherapy	Psychoanalysis and Group Analysis	Malcolm Pines	33	2	155–170		1983
Analytic Psychotherapy & Psychopathology	Group-analytic psychotherapy and the Borderline Patient*	Malcolm Pines	1	1	57–70		1984
The International Review of Psycho-Analysis	Reflections on Mirroring*	Malcolm Pines	11	1	27–42		1984
Group	Psychic Development and the Group Analytic Situation*	Malcolm Pines	9	1	24–37		1985
Psychoanalytic Inquiry	Mirroring and Child Development*	Malcolm Pines	5	2	211–231		1985
Clínica y Análisis Grupal	Coherency and Disruption in the Sense of Self*	Malcolm Pines	10	41	425–443	Jul–Sep	1986
Neurologia et Psychiatrica	The Borderline Personality: Concepts and Criteria	M. Jackson, M. Pines	9		54–67		1986
Neurologia et Psychiatrica	The Borderline Personality: Psychodynamics and Treatment	M. Jackson, Mal-colm Pines, B. Stevens	9		66–68		1986
British Journal of Psychotherapy	Coherency and Disruption in the Development of the Self	Malcolm Pines	2	3	180–185	Mar	1986

British Journal of Psychotherapy	Change and Innovation, Decay and Renewal in Psychotherapy*	Malcolm Pines	4	1	76–85		1987
Psychoanalytic Psychology	On History and Psychoanalysis*	Malcolm Pines	6	2	121–135		1989
Current Opinion in Psychiatry	Borderline Personality Disorder and Its Treatment	Malcolm Pines	2	3	362–367		1989
Psychoanalytic Psychotherapy	An English Freud?	Malcolm Pines	5	1	1–9		1990
Holistic Medicine	Psychological Aspects of Energy	Malcolm Pines	5		5–15		1990
Psychoanalytic Inquiry	Group Analysis and the Corrective Emotional Experience: Is It Relevant?	Malcolm Pines	10	3	389–408		1990
International Review of Psychoanalysis	Once More the Question of Revising the Standard Edition	Malcolm Pines	18		325–330		1991
International Journal of Group Psychotherapy	Group-Analytic Psychotherapy	Jeff Roberts, Malcolm Pines	42	4	469–494		1992
British Journal of Psychotherapy	The Universality of Shame: A Psychoanalytic Approach	Malcolm Pines	11	3	346–357	Mar	1995
Mind and Human Interaction	Psychoanalysis and Group Analysis: The Jews and the Germans	Malcolm Pines	7	1	20–30	Feb	1996
International Journal of Therapeutic Communities	Forgotten Pioneers: An Unwritten History of the Therapeutic Community**	Malcolm Pines	20	1	23–42	Spring	1999
Group	Shepherding Group Analysis: Shepherds Past, Present and Future	Malcolm Pines	24	1	49–57	Feb	2000
Funzione Gamma University 'Sapienza' Rome	Bion, Foulkes and Empathy	Malcolm Pines	https://www.funzione-gamma.it/wp-content/uploads/2022/11/bion-foulkes-empathy3e.pdf				2012

F. Lectures and responses by Malcolm Pines

Occasion/Publication	Title	Vol	Issue	Page	Date	Year
Sixth Annual Foulkes Lecture, London 1982	Reflections on Mirroring: Sixth Annual Foulkes Lecture. *Group Analysis 15, Supplement**	15	2	S: 1–S26	Aug 1	1982
	Circular Reflections (1998)			17–39		
Keynote address, Canadian Association of Group Psychotherapy, Banff 1983	Psychic Development and the Group Analytic Situation. *Group* (1983)*	9	1	24–37	Oct 29	1983
	Circular Reflections (1998)			59–76		
The Arbours Lecture, London 1986	Change and Innovation, Decay and Renewal in Psychotherapy. *British Journal of Psychotherapy* (1987)*	4	1	76–85	Feb 11	1986
	Circular Reflections (1998)			117–129		
Freud Memorial Lecture, University College London 1986	On History and Psychoanalysis. *Psychoanalytic Psychology* (1989)*	6	2	121–135		1986
	Circular Reflections (1998)			167–181		1998
Keynote Lecture, International Conference of Psychodrama and Analytic Group Psychotherapy, Buenos Aires 1986	Psychoanalysis, Psychodrama and Group Psychotherapy: Step-Children of Vienna. *Group Analysis* (1986)	19	2	101–112		August 1985
Association for Psychoanalytic Psychotherapy Lecture, London 1989	What Should a Psychotherapist Know – Dedicated to Tom Main. *Circular Reflections* (1998)*			131–149		1989

Keynote Lecture, Eighth European Symposium in Group Analysis, Oxford 1990	The Historical Matrix of Group Analysis: A Perspective from the History of Ideas. *Group Analysis* (1991)**	24	2	99–109	Sept	1990
Keynote Lecture, Regional Meeting of the International Association of Group Psychotherapy, Taipei, Taiwan 1993	The 'In-Between'**					1993
Keynote Lecture, Ninth European Symposium on Group Analysis 'Boundaries and Barriers', Heidelberg 1993	Psychoanalysis and Group Analysis: The Jews and The Germans. Figure-Ground Relationships. Circular Reflections (1998)*			153–165	Sept	1993
Opening Paper, Congress of the International Association for the History of Psychoanalysis, Berlin 1994	Dissent in Context Schisms in the Psychoanalytic Movement*				Jul 21	1994
	Circular Reflections (1998)			103–116		
Paper given at the Third National Congress of the Italian Group Analytic Society, Rome	Ideology and Tolerance in Clinical Group Analysis					1995
Group Analysis	Response to Lecture by Lise Rafaelsen	29	2	158–159	Jun 1	1996
Keynote Lecture, Meeting of the Israeli Association for Group Psychotherapy, Jerusalem 1996	Group Analysis and Its Surrounding and Supporting Network. *Group Analysis* (1996)**	35	1	13–26		1996
	'Die Kohärenz der Gruppenanalyse.' Gropenpsychotherapie und Gruppendynamik: Psychosozial.'Symboltheorie in Psychoanalyse und Gruppenanalyse'. Pines, M. (2013)	26	H1	9–18		2013

Maxwell Jones Lecture, Henderson Hospital, Sutton, 1998	Forgotten Pioneers: An Unwritten History of the Therapeutic Community.				Jun 26	1998
	Journal of Therapeutic Communities 20 (1): 23–42**	20	1	23–42		
Keynote Lecture EGATIN, Study Day: European Group Analytic Training Institutions Network, Copenhagen, Denmark	Training in Group Analysis: Where We Have Come From**			Unpublished		2000
Keynote Lecture, European Symposium in Group Analysis, Bologna	Changing Times, Changing Realities: A Group-Analytic Perspective on the History of Psychotherapy**			Unpublished	Aug	2001
Group Analysis	Response to Lecture by Ralph Stacey	38	4	495–498	Dec 1	2005
Group Analysis	Response to Harold Lecture by Harold Behr	44	4	470–471	Oct 28	2011

G. Papers published in books

Title	Author	Book title	Year	Publisher
Psychotherapy outside the National Health Service: Training in Dynamic Aspects of Psychotherapy, pp. 274–295	Malcolm Pines	Varma, V. (Ed.), *Psychotherapy Today*	1974	London, Constable
The Large Group – An Overview, pp. 291–311	Malcolm Pines	Kreeger, L. (Ed.), *The Large Group: Dynamics and Therapy*	1975	London, Constable
Group Psychotherapy with Difficult Patients, pp. 102–119	Malcolm Pines	Wolberg, L. R., and Aronson, M. L., *Group Psychotherapy*	1976	New York, Stratton Intercontinental Medical Books
The Doctor Patient Relationship, pp. 102–119	Malcolm Pines	Krauss, S., *Encyclopaedic Handbook of Medical Psychology*	1976	London, Butterworths
The Contributions of S. H. Foulkes to Group-analytic psychotherapy	Malcolm Pines	Wolberg, L. R., Aronson, M. L., and Wolberg, A. R. (Eds.), *Group Therapy: An Overview*	1978	New York, Stratton Intercontinental Medical Books
Therapeutic Communities in Teaching Hospitals, pp. 23–30	Malcolm Pines	Hinshelwood, R. D., and Manning, N., *Therapeutic Communities: Reflections and Progress*	1979	London, Routledge & Kegan Paul
The Frame of Reference of Group Psychotherapy TNH	Malcolm Pines	De Moor, W., and Windgarden, H. R. (Eds.), *Psychotherapy Research & Training*	1980	Elsevier/N. Holland Bio Medical Press
Group Analysis (Group-Analytic Psychotherapy), 3rd ed., 1985, pp. 132–177**	Malcolm Pines, L. E. Hearst, H. L. Behr	Gazda, G. M. (Ed.), *Basic Approaches to Group Psychotherapy and Group Counseling*	1982	Springfield, IL, Charles C. Thomas
Mirroring and Child Development: Psychodynamic and Psychological Interpretations* TNH	Malcolm Pines	Honess, T., and Yardley, K. (Eds.), *Self and Identity: Perspectives across the Lifespan*	1987	London, Routledge & Kegan Paul

Mirroring and Group Therapy in Borderline and Narcissistic Patients TNH	Malcolm Pines	Slavinska-Holy, N. (Ed.), *Borderline & Narcissistic Patients in Therapy*	1988	New York, International Universities Press
Group Analysis ISW [KUT]	Malcolm Pines, M. Marrone	Kutash, I., and Wolf, A. (Eds.), *Group Psychotherapist's Handbook: Contemporary Theory and Technique*	1990	New York, Columbia University Press
Group-analytic psychotherapy and the Borderline Patient, pp. 31–44*	Malcolm Pines	Roth, B. E., Stone, W. N., and Kibel, H. D. (Eds.), *The Difficult Patient in Group: Group Psychotherapy with Borderline and Narcissistic Disorders*	1990	American Group Psychotherapy Association, Monograph Series, Madison, CT, International Universities Press
The Development of the Psychodynamic Movement, pp. 206–231	Malcolm Pines	Berrios, G., and Freeman, H. (Eds.), *150 Years of British Psychiatry 1841–1991*	1991	London, Gaskell
The Borderline Patient, pp. 97–106 Interminable Patients, pp. 112–114	Malcolm Pines	Roberts, J., and Pines, M., *The Practice of Group Analysis*	1991	London, Routledge, Chapman and Hall
A History of Psychodynamic Psychiatry in Britain, pp. 183–208*	Malcolm Pines	Holmes, J. (Ed.), *Textbook of Psychotherapy and Psychiatric Practice*	1991	London, Churchill Livingstone
'Group Analysis', pp. 29–47	Malcolm Pines, Sylvia Hutchinson	Alonso, A., and Swiller, H. I. (Eds.), *Group Therapy in Clinical Practice*	1993	American Psychiatric Press
Borderline Phenomena in Analytic Groups, pp. 128–148	Malcolm Pines	Pines, M., and Schermer, V. L., *Ring of Fire. Primitive Affects and Object Relations in Group Psychotherapy*	1994	London, Routledge

The Self as a Group: The Group as a Self, pp. 24–29**	Malcolm Pines	Harwood, I. N. H., and Pines, M. (Eds.), *Self Experiences in Group: Intersubjective and Self Psychological Pathways to Human Understanding*	1998	London, Jessica Kingsley Publishers
The Illumination of Dreams, pp. 25–36	Malcolm Pines	Neri, C., Pines, M., and Friedman, R., *Dreams in Group Psychotherapy: Theory and Technique*	2002	London, Jessica Kingsley Publishers
Bion and Foulkes on Empathy				
Group Methods in Adult Psychiatry, pp. 1350–1368	John Schlapobersky, Malcolm Pines	Gelder, M., et al. (Eds.), *New Oxford Textbook of Psychiatry. Second edition*	2009	Oxford, Oxford University Press
Group Analysis and Group Analytic Psychotherapy, pp. 264–268	John Schlapobersky, Malcolm Pines	Tschuschke, V. (Ed.), *Gruppenpsychotherapie und Gruppendynamik*	2010	Stuttgart, Thieme
Narcissus and Echo: Vision and Hearing in Early Development and Some Applications to Individual and Group Psychotherapy**	Malcolm Pines	Navaro, L., Friedman, R., and Schwartzberg, S. L. (Eds.), *Desire, Passion and Gender: Clinical Implications*	2011	New York, Nova Publishers
Afterword, p. 245	Malcolm Pines	Harwood, I., Stone, W., and Pines, M., *Self-Experiences in Group, Revisited: Affective Attachments, Intersubjective Regulations, and Human Understanding*	2012	London, Routledge

H. Books written and edited by Malcolm Pines

The Evolution of Group Analysis	M. Pines, Ed.	International Library of Group Analysis	Routledge	1984 Reissued Jessica Kingsley Publishers 2000
Bion and Group Psychotherapy	M. Pines, Ed.	International Library of Group Analysis	Routledge	1985 Reissued Jessica Kingsley Publishers 2000
The Practice of Group Analysis	M. Pines and J. Roberts, Eds.	International Library of Group Analysis	Routledge	1991
Ring of Fire – Primitive Affects and Object Relations in Group Psychotherapy	M. Pines and V. Schermer, Eds.	International Library of Group Analysis	Routledge	1994
Circular Reflections: Selected Papers on Group Analysis and Psychoanalysis	M. Pines	International Library of Group Analysis	Routledge	1998
Self Experiences in Group: Intersubjective and Self Psychological Pathways to Human Understanding	M. Pines and I. Harwood, Eds.	International Library of Group Analysis	Routledge	1998
Group Psychotherapy of the Psychoses – Concepts, Interventions and Contexts	M. Pines and V. Schermer, Eds.	International Library of Group Analysis	Routledge	1999
Building on Bion: Roots – Origins and Context of Bion's Contributions to Theory and Practice	M. Pines and R. Lipgar, Eds.	International Library of Group Analysis	Jessica Kingsley Publishers	2002
Building on Bion: Branches – Contemporary Developments and Applications of Bion's Contributions to Theory and Practice	M. Pines and R. Lipgar, Eds.	International Library of Group Analysis	Jessica Kingsley Publishers	2002
Dreams in Group Psychotherapy	M. Pines, C. Neri, and R. Friedman, Eds.	International Library of Group Analysis	Jessica Kingsley Publishers	2002
Self Experiences in Group Revisited: Affective Attachments, Intersubjective Regulations, and Human Understanding	M. Pines, I. Harwood, and W. Stone, Eds.	International Library of Group Analysis	Jessica Kingsley Publishers	2012

I. Obituaries in *Group Analysis* by Malcolm Pines

Obituary	Vol.	Issue	Page(s)	Date	Year
T. F. Main (1911–1990)	23	4	431–432	Dec 1	1990
Martin Grotjahn (1904–1990): A Personal Tribute	25	3	317–318	Sep 1	1992
Romano Fiumara	25	4	498	Dec 1	1992
Eric Trist (1909–1993)	27	1	118	Mar 1	1994
Louis Zinkin (1925–1993)	27	1	119	Mar 1	1994
Dennis Brown (1928–2004)	37	4	562–563	Dec 1	2004
Maureen Spurgeon (1941–2007)	41	1	116	Mar 1	2008
Patrick de Maré (1916–2008)	41	2	210–211	Jun 1	2008
Colin James (1937–2008)	41	3	308–309	Sep 1	2008
Elinor Field (née Nathan) (1926–2006)	41	3	310–311	Sep 1	2008
Juan Campos (1928–2009)	42	1	96–98	Mar 1	2009
Introduction: A Celebration of the Life and Work of Patrick de Maré (1916–2008)	42	3	278–279	Sep	2009
Adele Mittwoch (1926–2011)	44	2	243–244	Jun 13	2011
Stuart Whiteley (1926–2012)	46	1	104	June	2013
E. James Anthony (1916–2014)	48	2	222–225	June	2015

Appendix 2: Malcolm Pines, editor: International Library of Group Analysis

In 1981, Malcolm Pines established the International Library of Group Psychotherapy and Group Process. In 1998, with the publication of *Circular Reflections*, he changed the name of the series to the International Library of Group Analysis (ILGA). The library was first published by Routledge (1981–1995) and then by Jessica Kingsley Press (JKP, 1997–2003), where the newly named series was numbered. Some titles were first published by Routledge and reissued by JKP. Some are still available; many are out of print.[1]

In 2009, the concept was revived as the New International Library of Group Analysis, edited by Earl Hopper.

Series editor: Malcolm Pines Author/editor of title	Title	Year of publication	Publisher
Agazarian, Y. M., and Peters, R.	*The Visible and Invisible Group – Two Perspectives on Group Psychotherapy and Group Process*	1981	Routledge
Caine, T. M., Wijesinghe, O. B. A, and Winter, D. A.	*Personal Styles in Neurosis – Implications for Small Group Psychotherapy and Behaviour Therapy*	1981	Routledge
Kutter, P.	*Basic Aspects of Psychoanalytic Group Therapy*	1982	Routledge
Jones, M.	*The Process of Change*	1982	Routledge
Gabriel, Y.	*Freud and Society*	1983	Routledge
Anzieu, D.	*The Group and the Unconscious*	1984	Routledge
Pines, M. (Ed.)	*The Evolution of Group Analysis* [reissued as ILGA:16]	1983	Routledge
Pines, M. (Ed.)	*Bion and Group Psychotherapy*	1985	Routledge
Whitaker, D. S.	*Using Groups to Help People*	1985	Routledge
Roberts, J., and Pines, M. (Eds.)	*The Practice of Group Analysis*	1991	Routledge
Wardi, D.	*Memorial Candles – Children of the Holocaust*	1992	Routledge
Kennard, D., Roberts, J., and Winter, D. A.	*A Workbook of Group-Analytic Interventions* [reissued as ILGA, 2000]	1993	Routledge
Ashbach, C., and Schermer V. L. (Eds.)	*Object Relations, the Self and the Group*	1994	Routledge
Boyd, R. D.	*Personal Transformations in Small Groups – A Jungian Perspective*	1994	Routledge
Schermer, V. L., and Pines, M. (Eds.)	*Ring of Fire – Primitive Affects and Object Relations in Group Psychotherapy*	1994	Routledge
Sharpe, M. (Ed.)	*The Third Eye – Supervision of Analytic Groups*	1995	Routledge
Pines, M. [ILGA:1]	*Circular Reflections – Selected Papers on Group Analysis and Psychoanalysis*	1998	JKP
Schermer, V. L., and Pines, M. (Eds.) [ILGA:2]	*Group Psychotherapy of the Psychoses – Concepts, Interventions and Contexts*	1999	JKP

Marrone, M., and Diamond, N. [ILGA:3]	*Attachment and Interaction*	1998	JKP
Harwood, I. N. H., and Pines, M. (Eds.) [ILGA:4]	*Self Experiences in Group: Intersubjective and Self Psychological Pathways to Human Understanding* [separately issued in 'Psychoanalytic Inquiry Book Series', 2012]	1998	JKP
Dalal, F. [ILGA:5]	*Taking the Group Seriously – Towards a Post-Foulkesian Group Analytic Therapy*	1998	JKP
Evans, J. [ILGA:6]	*Active Analytic Group Therapy for Adolescents*	1998	JKP
Thompson, S. [ILGA:7]	*The Group Context*	1998	JKP
Neri, C. [ILGA:8]	*Group*	1998	JKP
Edelson, M., and Berg, D. N. [ILGA:9]	*Rediscovering Groups – A Psychoanalyst's Journey Beyond Individual Psychology*	1999	JKP
Ettin, M. F. [ILGA:10]	*Foundations and Applications of Group Psychotherapy – A Sphere of Influence*	1999	JKP
Agazarian, Y. M., and Gantt, S. P. [ILGA:11]	*Autobiography of a Theory – Developing a Theory of Living Human Systems and Its Systems-Centered Practice*	2000	JKP
Pines, M. (Ed.) [ILGA:16]	*The Evolution of Group Analysis* [reprint of 1983]	2000	JKP
Pines, M. (Ed.)	*Bion and Group Psychotherapy* [paperback edition of 1985 text]	2000	JKP
Kennard, D., Roberts, J., and Winter, D. A. [ILGA:13]	*A Workbook of Group-Analytic Interventions*	2000	JKP
Brown, D., and Zinkin, L. (Eds.)	*The Psyche and the Social World – Developments in Group-Analytic Theory* [cited as 1994 ILGP&GP]	2000	JKP
Chazan, R. [ILGA:14]	*The Group as Therapist*	2001	JKP
Sandison, R. [ILGA:12]	*A Century of Psychiatry, Psychotherapy and Group Analysis – A Search for Integration*	2001	JKP
Neri, C., Pines, M., and Friedman, R. [ILGA:18]	*Dreams in Group Psychotherapy: Theory and Technique*	2002	JKP

Ringer, T. M. [TNH]	*Group Action: The Dynamics of Groups in Therapeutic, Educational and Corporate Settings* [not an ILGA title: Malcolm Pines contributed foreword, pp. 13–14]	2002	JKP
Lipgar, R. M., and Pines, M. (Eds.) [ILGA:20]	*Building on Bion: Roots – Origins and Context of Bion's Contributions to Theory and Practice*	2002	JKP
Lipgar, R. M., and Pines, M. (Eds.) [ILGA:21]	*Building on Bion: Branches – Contemporary Developments and Applications of Bion's Contributions to Theory and Practice*	2002	JKP
Hopper, E. [ILGA:22]	*The Social Unconscious – Selected Papers*	2003	JKP
Hopper, E. [ILGA:23]	*Traumatic Experience in the Unconscious Life of Groups – The Fourth Basic Assumption: Incohesion: Aggregation/Massification or (ba) I:A/M*	2003	JKP
Tubert-Oklander, J., and Hernández de Tubert, R. [ILGA:24]	*Operative Groups – The Latin-American Approach to Group Analysis*	2003	JKP
Schneider, S., and Weinberg, H. (Eds.) [ILGA:25]	*The Large Group Re-Visited – The Herd, Primal Horde, Crowds and Masses*	2003	JKP
Billow, R. M. [ILGA:26]	*Relational Group Psychotherapy – From Basic Assumptions to Passion*	2003	JKP

Note

1 We believe these titles represent a comprehensive list, but would welcome additions or amendments from readers who may know of other books in the series that we could not trace. (Ed.)

Bibliography

Abelin, E. L. (1980). Triangulation, the Role of the Father, and the Origins of Core Gender Identity During the Rapprochement Subphase. In R. F. Lax, S. Bach, and J. A. Burland (Eds.), *Rapprochement: The Critical Subphase of Separation-Individuation*. New York, Jason Aronson.

Abercrombie, M. L. J. (1963). *The Anatomy of Judgement*. London, Hutchinson.

Abercrombie, M. L. J. (1969). *Group Methods in Education*. Society for Research in Higher Education. Monograph.

Abraham, A. (1973a). Group Tensions as Measured by Configurations of Different Self and Transself Aspects. *Group Process* 5: 71–89.

Abraham, A. (1973b). More about Individual and Group Matrix. *Group Analysis* 6 (2): 105–110.

Abraham, A. (1973c). A Model for Exploring Intra- and Interindividual Process in Groups. *International Journal of Group Psychotherapy* 23 (1): 3–22.

Abraham, A. (1991). Beyond Transference: The Relationship Between Freud and Rolland. *Group Analysis* 24 (2): 171–183.

Abse, D. W. (1974). *Clinical Notes on Group-Analytic Psychotherapy*. Bristol, John Wright & Sons.

Abse, D. W. (1979). Trigant Burrow and the Inauguration of Group Analysis in the U.S.A. *Group Analysis* 12 (3): 218–229.

Adler, A. (1925/2011). *The Practice and Theory of Individual Psychology*. Mansfield Centre, CT, Martino Publishing.

Aichhorn, A. (1925/1955). *Wayward Youth: A Psychoanalytic Study of Delinquent Children, Illustrated by Actual Case Histories*. New York, Meridian Books. First published in 1925 as *Verwahrloste Jugend*.

Alexander, F., Eisenstein, S., and Grotjahn, M. (1966). *Psychoanalytic Pioneers*. New York, Basic Books.

Alexander, F., and French, T. M. (1946). *Psychoanalytic Therapy: Principles and Application*. New York, Ronald Press.

Andersen, H. C. (1983). *The Complete Fairy Tales and Stories*. New York, Anchor Books.

Ansermet, F., and Magistretti, P. (2007). *Biology of Freedom: Neural Plasticity, Experience, and the Unconscious*. London, Handsel.

Anthony, E. J. (1965). Age and Syndrome in Group Psychotherapy. *Topical Problems in Psychotherapy* 5: 80–89.

Anthony, E. J. (1978). The Group-Analytic Circle and Its Ambient Network: 2nd Foulkes Lecture. *Group Analysis* 11 (Supplement 1): 1–18. Also in Pines, M. (Ed.). (1983). *The Evolution of Group Analysis*. London, Routledge. Reissued 2000, London, Jessica Kingsley, pp. 29–53.

Anzieu, D. (1989). *The Skin Ego: A Psychoanalytic Approach to the Self*. New Haven, CT, Yale University Press.

Arendt, H. (1978). *The Life of the Mind. Volume One: Thinking and Volume Two: Willing*. New York, Harcourt Brace Jovanovich.

Arroyave, F., and Pangbourne, J. (1976). Group Methods in the Treatment of Alcoholics. *Group Analysis* 9 (1): 32–33.

Auden, W. H. (1936/2018). *Letters From Iceland*. London, Faber.

Aunger, R. (2000). Memes. In R. I. M. Dunbar and L. Barrett (Eds.), *The Oxford Handbook of Evolutionary Psychology*. Oxford, Oxford University Press, pp. 599–603.

Bachelard, G. (1992). *The Poetics of Space*. London, Beacon.

Bakhtin, M. (1981). *The Dialogic Imagination: Four Essays*. Ed. Michael Holquist. Trans. Caryl Emerson and Michael Holquist. Austin, University of Texas Press.

Balint, M. (1959). *Thrills and Regressions*. New York, International Universities Press.

Balint, M. (1968). *The Basic Fault: Therapeutic Aspects of Regression*. London, Tavistock Publishers.

Barker, P. (2008) *The Regeneration Trilogy: Regeneration, The Ghost Road, The Eye in the Door*. London, Penguin.

Barnes, B., Ernst, S., and Hyde, K. (1999). *An Introduction to Groupwork: A Group-Analytic Perspective*. London, Macmillan.

Barton, R. A., and Dunbar, R. I. M. (1997). Evolution of the Social Brain. In A. Whiten and R. W. Byrne (Eds.), *Machiavellian Intelligence*. Cambridge, Cambridge University Press, pp. 240–263.

Barwick, N., and Weegmann, M. (2017). *Group Therapy: A Group-Analytic Approach*. London, Routledge.

Bateman, A. W., and Fonagy, P. (1999). Effectiveness of Partial Hospitalization in the Treatment of Borderline Personality Disorder: A Randomized Controlled Trial. *American Journal of Psychiatry* 156 (10): 1563–1569.

Bateman, A. W., and Fonagy, P. (2000). Effectiveness of Psychotherapeutic Treatment of Personality Disorder. *British Journal of Psychiatry* 177: 138–143.

Beebe, B., and Lachmann, F. M. (1992). The Contributions of Mother-Infant Mutual Influence to the Origins of Self- and Object Representations. In N. J. Skolnick and S. C. Warshaw (Eds.), *Relational Perspectives in Psychoanalysis*. Hillsdale, NJ, Analytic Press, pp. 83–118.

Beebe, B., and Lachmann, F. M. (2012). *The Origins of Attachment: Infant Research and Adult Treatment*. London, Routledge.

Behr, H. L., and Hearst, L. E. (1977). Group Analysis Goes into Napsbury. *Group Analysis* 10 (3): 264–266.

Behr, H. L., and Hearst, L. E. (2005). *Group-Analytic Psychotherapy: A Meeting of Minds*. London, Whurr Publishers.

Benjamin, J. (1992). Recognition and Destruction: An Outline of Intersubjectivity. In N. J. Skolnick and S. C. Warshaw (Eds.), *Relational Perspectives in Psychoanalysis*. Hillsdale, NJ, Analytic Press, pp. 43–60.

Bergin, A. E., and Garfield, S. L. (Eds.) (1994). *Handbook of Psychotherapy and Behavior Change*. Fourth edition. New York, Wiley.

Berlin, I. (1976). *Vico and Herder: Two Studies in the History of Ideas*. London, Hogarth Press.

Berry, P. (1992). Echo and Beauty. In R. K. Papadopoulos (Ed.), *Carl Gustav Jung: Critical Assessments. Volume II: The Structure and Dynamics of the Psyche*. London, Routledge.

Berry, P. (2008). *Echo's Subtle Body: Contributions to an Archetypal Psychology*. Dallas, Spring Publications.

Bion, W. R. (1962). *Learning from Experience*. London, Heinemann.

Bion, W. R. (1968/1998). *Experiences in Groups and Other Papers*. London, Tavistock Publications.

Bion, W. R. (1990). *Memoir of the Future*. London, Karnac.

Bion, W. R. (1992). *Cogitations*. London, Karnac.

Bion, W. R., and Rickman, J. (1943). Intra-group Tensions in Therapy. *Lancet* 242 (6274): 678–681.

Bion Talamo, P., Borgogno, F., and Merciai, S. A. (Eds.) (2000). *W. R. Bion: Between Past and Future*. London, Routledge.

Blaffer Hrdy, S. (2009). *Mothers and Others: The Evolutionary Origins of Mutual Understanding*. Cambridge, MA, Harvard University Press.

Blake, R. (1980). The Group Matrix. *Group Analysis* 13 (3): 177–183.

Bolognini, S. (1999/2006). *Like Wind, Like Wave: Fables from the Land of the Repressed*. New York, Other Press.

Bowlby, J. (1965). *Child Care and the Growth of Love*. London, Pelican.

Bowlby, J. (1969). *Attachment and Loss. Vol. 1: Attachment*. London, Hogarth Press.

Bowlby, J. (1973). *Attachment and Loss. Vol. 2: Separation Anxiety and Anger*. London, Hogarth Press.

Bowlby, J. (1980). *Attachment and Loss. Vol. 3: Sadness and Depression*. London, Hogarth Press.

Bramley, W. (1979). *Group Tutoring: Concepts and Case Studies*. New York, Nichols Publishing.

Bramley, W., and Andry, R. G. (1977). A Group Analytic Approach to Training. *Group Analysis* 10 (1): 32–39.

Brazelton, T. B., Yogman, M. W., Als, H., and Tronick, E. (1979). The Infant as a Focus for Family Reciprocity. In M. Lewis and L. A. Rosenblum (Eds.), *The Child and Its Family, Vol. 2*. New York, Plenum, pp. 29–43.

Bridgeland, M. (1971). *Pioneer Work with Maladjusted Children: A Study of the Development of Therapeutic Education*. London, Staples Press.

Bridger, H. (1946). The Northfield Experiment. *Bulletin of the Menninger Clinic* 10 (3): 81–86.

Brierly, M. (1951). *Trends in Psycho-analysis*. London, Hogarth Press and Institute of Psychoanalysis.

Britvić, D., Radelić, N., and Urlić, I. (2006). Long-Term Dynamic-Oriented Group Psychotherapy of Posttraumatic Stress Disorder in War Veterans: Prospective Study of Five-Year Treatment. *Croatian Medical Journal* 47 (1): 76–84.

Brody, S. (1956). *Patterns of Mothering: A Study of Maternal Influence During Infancy*. Introduction by René A. Spitz. New York, International Universities Press.

Bromberg, P. M. (1993). Shadow and Substance: A Relational Perspective on Clinical Process. *Psychoanalytic Psychology* 10: 147–168.

Brothers, L. (1997). *Friday's Footprint: How Society Shapes the Human Mind*. Oxford, Oxford University Press.

Broucek, F. J. (1982). Shame and Its Relation to Early Narcissistic Developments. *International Journal of Psychoanalysis* 63: 369–378.

Brown, D. (1979). Some Reflections on Bion's Basic Assumptions From a Group-Analytic Viewpoint. *Group Analysis* 12 (3): 204–210.

Brown, D. (1985). Bion and Foulkes: Basic Assumptions and Beyond. In M. Pines (Ed.), *Bion and Group Psychotherapy*. London, Routledge, pp. 192–219.

Brown, D. G. (1988). Confrontation in the Group Analytic Matrix: Toward a Classification. *Group* 12: 191–197.

Brown, D. (1994/2000). Self Development Through Subjective Interaction: A Fresh Look at 'Ego Training in Action'. In D. Brown and L. Zinkin (Eds.), *The Psyche and the Social World: Developments in Group-Analytic Theory*. London, Routledge, pp. 80–89. Republished in Maratos, J. (Ed.). (2006). *Resonance and Reciprocity: Selected Papers by Dennis Brown*. London, Routledge, pp. 107–123.

Brown, D., and Zinkin, L. (Eds.) (1994/2000). *The Psyche and the Social World: Developments in Group-Analytic Theory*. London, Routledge. Reissued 2000, London, Jessica Kingsley.

Brüne, M., Ribbert, H., and Schiefenhövel, W. (Eds.). (2003). *The Social Brain: Evolution and Pathology*. Chichester, Wiley.

Buber, M. (1958/2000). *I and Thou*. Trans. Ronald Gregor Smith. New York, Scribner.

Burke, E. (2007). *A Letter From Mr. Burke, to a Member of the National Assembly: In Answer to Some Objections to His Book on French Affairs*. Ann Arbor, MI, University of Michigan Library.

Burlingame, G. M., Fuhriman, A., and Mosier, J. (2003). The Differential Effectiveness of Group Psychotherapy: A Meta-analytic Perspective. *Group Dynamics: Theory, Research, and Practice* 7 (1): 3–12.

Burrow, T. (1924–1927). *To Freud. Sigmund Freud Papers: General Correspondence, 1871–1996*. Library of Congress, https://www.loc.gov/item/mss3999000493. Accessed 12 February 2024.

Burrow, T. (1926). Psychoanalytic Improvisations and the Personal Equation. *Psychoanalytic Review* 13: 173–186.

Burrow, T. (1927). *The Social Basis of Consciousness: A Study in Organic Psychology Based Upon a Synthetic and Societal Concept of the Neuroses*. New York, Harcourt, Brace.

Burrow, T. (1927a) The Problem of Transference. *British Journal of Medical Psychology*, 1827, Vol 7, pp. 193–202.

Burrow, T. (1958). *The Search for Man's Sanity: The Selected Letters of Trigant Burrow*. Ed. W. E. Galt. New York, Oxford University Press.

Burrow, T. (1984). *Toward Social Sanity and Human Survival*. New York, Horizon House Books.

Burrow, T. (1992). *The Basis of Group-Analysis or the Analysis of the Reactions of Normal and Neurotic Individuals*. Classics in Group Psychotherapy, Ed. K. Roy MacKenzie. New York, Guilford Press.

Burrows, S. (1981). *Distorting Mirrors: Visions of the Crowd in Late Nineteenth-Century France*. New Haven, CT, Yale University Press.

Butler, S. (1903). *The Way of All Flesh*. London, Grant Richards.

Cacioppo, J. T., and Patrick, W. (2009). *Loneliness: Human Nature and the Need for Social Connection*. London, Norton.

Canetti, E. (1984). *Crowds and Power*. New York, Farrar, Straus and Giroux.

Cannon, W. B. (1932). *The Wisdom of the Body*. New York, Norton.

Castaneda, C. (1968/1998). *The Teachings of Don Juan. A Yaqui Way of Knowledge*. Berkeley, University of California Press. Thirtieth anniversary edition 1998, New York, Washington Square Press.

Champernowne, I. (1975). *The One and Only Me*. Niles, IL, Argus Communications.

Chance, M. R. A. (1980). *Group Cohesion and Intellectual Coherence. The Ethological Basis of Intelligence and Its Integration of the Personality*. Paper presented at the VII International Congress of Group Psychotherapy, Copenhagen, August 1980. In *Congress Proceedings*. New York, Plenum Press.

Cheney, D. L., and Seyfarth, R. M. (2007). *Baboon Metaphysics: The Evolution of a Social Mind*. Chicago, University of Chicago Press.

Chiesa, M. (1997). A Combined In-Patient/Out-Patient Programme for Severe Personality Disorders. *Therapeutic Communities* 18 (4): 297–309.

Cilasun, J., Schlapobersky, J. R., Papanastassiou, M., and Thomas, A. (2022). The Large Group in Training Parts I and II. *Group Analysis* 55 (3): 407–440.

Cooley, C. H. (1902). *Human Nature and the Social Order*. New York, Charles Scribner's Sons. Revised edition 1922.

Corbella, S. (2003). *Storie e luoghi del gruppo*. Milan, Raffaello Cortina Editore.

Cordess, C., and Cox, M. (Eds.) (1996). *Forensic Psychotherapy: Crime, Psychodynamics and the Offender Patient*. London, Jessica Kingsley.

Cortesão, E. L. (1974). Transference Neurosis and the Group-Analytic Process. *Group Analysis* 7 (3): 4–10.

Cox, M. (1978/1995). *Structuring the Therapeutic Process: Compromise with Chaos – the Therapist's Response to the Individual and the Group*. London, Jessica Kingsley.

Cox, M. (1990). The Group as Poetic Play-Ground: From Metaphor to Metamorphosis. Foulkes Lecture to the Group Analytic Society, London. Unpublished.

Cox, M. (1998). *Remorse and Reparation*. London, Jessica Kingsley.

Cox, M., and Theilgaard, A. (1987/1994). *Mutative Metaphors in Psychotherapy: The Aeolian Mode*. London, Jessica Kingsley.

Cox, M., and Theilgaard, A. (1994). *Shakespeare as Prompter: The Amending Imagination and the Therapeutic Process*. London, Jessica Kingsley.

Cozolino, L. (2002). *The Neuroscience of Psychotherapy: Building and Rebuilding the Human Brain*. New York, Norton.

Cozolino, L. (2006). *The Neuroscience of Human Relationships: Attachment and the Developing Social Brain*. New York, Norton.

Cozolino, L. (2010). *The Neuroscience of Psychotherapy: Healing the Social Brain*. Second edition. London, Norton.

Craparo, G. (2019). *Rediscovering Pierre Janet: Trauma, Dissociation, and a New Context for Psychoanalysis*. London, Routledge.

Critchley, M., and Critchley, E. A. (1998). *John Hughlings Jackson: Father of English Neurology*. Oxford, Oxford University Press.

Crook, J. H. (1980). *The Evolution of Human Consciousness*. Oxford, Oxford University Press.

Daelemans, S., and Maranhão, T. (1990). Psychoanalytic Dialogue and the Dialogic Principle. In T. Maranhão (Ed.), *The Interpretation of Dialogue*. Chicago, University of Chicago Press, pp. 219–241.

Dalal, F. (1998; 1981). *Taking the Group Seriously: Towards a Post-Foulkesian Group-Analytic Theory*. London, Jessica Kingsley.

Damasio, A. (1994). *Descartes' Error: Emotion, Reason, and the Human Brain*. London, Putnam Publishing.

Darwin, C. R. (1838). *Notebook M: [Metaphysics on Morals and Speculations on Expression*]. CUL-DAR125.- Edited by Paul Barrett and John van Wyhe (Darwin Online), http://darwin-online.org.uk. Accessed 12 February 2024.
De Maré, P. B. (1972). *Perspectives in Group Psychotherapy: A Theoretical Background*. London, George Allen and Unwin.
De Maré, P. B. (1975). The Politics of Large Groups. In L. Kreeger (Ed.), *The Large Group: Dynamics and Therapy*. London, Constable.
De Maré, P. B. (1977). Group Analytic Principles in Natural and Stranger Groups. *Group Analysis* 10 (1): 16–21.
De Maré, P. B. (1980). *The Median Group Method*. Paper presented at the VII International Congress of Group Psychotherapy, Copenhagen, August 1980. In *Congress Proceedings*. New York, Plenum Press.
Dewey, J. (1954). *The Public and Its Problems*. London, Swallow.
Dick, B. M. (1975/1983). A Ten-Year Study of Out-Patient Analytic Group Therapy. *British Journal of Psychiatry* 127 (4): 365–375. Reissued in Pines, M. (Ed.). (1983). *The Evolution of Group Analysis*. London, Routledge.
Diel, P. (1980). *Symbolism in Greek Mythology: Human Desire and Its Transformations*. London, Shambhala.
Dilthey, W. (1914/1988). *Introduction to the Human Sciences: An Attempt to Lay a Foundation for the Study of Society and History*. London, Harvester Wheatsheaf.
Doidge, N. (2007). *The Brain That Changes Itself: Stories of Personal Triumph From the Frontiers of Brain Science*. London, Viking.
Donald, M. (1991). *Origins of the Modern Mind: Three Stages in the Evolution of Culture and Cognition*. Cambridge, MA, Harvard University Press.
Donald, M. (2007). Evolutionary Origins of the Social Brain. In O. Vilarroya and F. Forn i Argimon (Eds.), *Social Brain Matters*. New York, Rodopi, pp. 216–222.
Dowrick, S. (1992). *Intimacy & Solitude*. London, Women's Press.
Dunbar, R. I. (2009). The Social Brain Hypothesis and Its Implications for Social Evolution. *Annual of Human Biology* 36 (5): 562–572.
Edelman, G. M. (1987). *Neural Darwinism: The Theory of Neuronal Group Selection*. London, Basic Books.
Eissler, K. R. (Ed.). (1948). *Searchlights on Delinquency: New Psychoanalytic Studies*. New York, International Universities Press.
Elias, N. (1968/2000). Homo clausus. In P. du Gay, J. Evans, and P. Redman (Eds.), *Identity: A Reader*. London, Sage.
Elias, N. (1978) *What Is Sociology? Vol. 5 of Collected Works*. Eds. R. Kilminster and S. Mennell. Dublin, University College Press.
Elias, N. (1991/2001). *The Society of Individuals*. Third edition. New York, Continuum International.
Elias, N. (2000). *The Civilizing Process*. London, Wiley-Blackwell.
Ellis, Havelock (1915/2018). *Sexual Inversion*. London, Adeptio's Vintage Edition.
Emde, R. N. (Ed.). (1980). Editor's Introduction: The Developmental Orientation. *Psychoanalysis and Contemporary Thought* 3 (2): 123–129.
Emde, R. N. (1981). Changing Models of Infancy and the Nature of Early Development: Remodeling the Foundations. *Journal of the American Psychoanalytic Association* 29 (1): 179–218.
Emde, R. N. (1983). The Prerepresentational Self and Its Affective Core. *Psychoanalytic Study of the Child* 38 (1): 165–192.

Emde, R. N. (1988). Development Terminable and Interminable. I. Innate and Motivational Factors From Infancy. *International Journal of Psychoanalysis* 69 (Pt 1): 23–42.

Emde, R. N. (1990). Mobilizing Fundamental Modes of Development: Empathic Availability and Therapeutic Action. *Journal of the American Psychoanalytic Association* 38 (4): 881–913.

Emde, R. N. (1992a). Positive Emotions for Psychoanalytic Theory: Surprises From Infancy Research and New Directions. In T. Shapiro and R. N. Emde (Eds.), *Affect: Psychoanalytic Perspectives*. Madison, CT, International Universities Press, pp. 5–44.

Emde, R. N. (1992b). Amae, Intimacy, and the Early Moral Self. *Infant Mental Health Journal* 13 (1): 34–42.

Emde, R. N., Biringen, Z., Clyman, R. B., and Oppenheim, D. (1991). The Moral Self of Infancy: Affective Core and Procedural Knowledge. *Developmental Review* 11 (3): 251–270.

Erdman, D. V. (Ed.). (1988). *The Complete Poetry & Prose of William Blake*. Berkeley, University of California Press.

Erikson, E. H. (1950/1995). *Childhood and Society*. New York, Norton; Vintage, 2009.

Ezriel, H. (1973). Psychoanalytic Group Therapy. In L. R. Wolberg and E. K. Schwartz (Eds.), *Group Therapy: An Overview*. New York, International Medical Books, pp. 183–210.

Fairbairn, W. R. D. (1949). Steps in the Development of an Object-Relations Theory of the Personality. *British Journal of Medical Psychology* 22 (1–2): 26–31.

Fairbairn, W. R. D. (1994). *Psychoanalytic Studies of the Personality*. London, Routledge.

Federn, P. (1952). *Ego Psychology and the Psychoses*. London, Basic Books.

Feldman, M., and Spillius, E. B. (1999). *Psychic Equilibrium and Psychic Change: Selected Papers of Betty Joseph*. London, Routledge.

Fenichel, O., and Rangell, L. (1996). *The Psychoanalytic Theory of Neurosis*. New York, Norton.

Fiumara, G. C. (1990). *The Other Side of Language: A Philosophy of Listening*. London, Routledge.

Fiumara, R. (1991). Brain, Mind and Matrix from an Evolutionary Viewpoint. *Group Analysis* 24 (4): 409–418.

Fiumara, R., and Zanasi, M. (1989). Depression of the Group and Depression in the Group. *Group Analysis* 22 (1): 49–57.

Fogel, A. (1993). *Developing Through Relationships*. Chicago, University of Chicago Press.

Fonagy, P., and Bateman, A. (2004). *Psychotherapy for Borderline Personality Disorder: Mentalization-Based Treatment*. Oxford, Oxford University Press.

Fonagy, P., Gergely, G., Jurist, E. L., and Target, M. (2002). *Affect Regulation, Mentalization, and the Development of the Self*. New York, Other Press.

Fonagy, P., and Target, M. (1996–2000). 'Playing With Reality' Papers. *International Journal of Psycho-Analysis* 77 (1996): 217–233; 77 (1996): 459–470; 81 (2000): 853–874.

Foulkes, S. H. (1938). On Introjection. *International Journal of Psychoanalysis* 18: 269–290. Reissued in Foulkes (1990a), pp. 57–78.

Foulkes, S. H. (1948). *Introduction to Group-Analytic Psychotherapy: Studies in the Social Integration of Individuals and Groups*. London, William Heinemann. Reissued in 1983, London, Karnac Classics.

Foulkes, S. H. (1964/1984). *Therapeutic Group Analysis*. London, George Allen and Unwin. Reissued in 1984, London, Karnac.

Foulkes, S. H. (1971). Access to Unconscious Processes in the Group Analytic Group. *Group Analysis* 4 (1): 4–14.

Foulkes, S. H. (1973). Address to the First European Workshop. *Group Analysis* 6 (2): 72–77.

Foulkes, S. H. (1975/1986). *Group-analytic psychotherapy: Method and Principles*. London, Gordon and Breach. Reprinted 1986, London, Karnac.

Foulkes, S. H. (1975). Qualification as a Psychoanalyst as an Asset as Well as a Hindrance for the Future Group Analyst. *Group Analysis* 8 (3): 180–182.

Foulkes, S. H. (1977). On the Concept of Resonance. In L. Wolberg and M. Aronson (Eds.), *Group Therapy: An Overview*. New York, Stratton International Books, pp. 52–58. Reissued in Foulkes, S. H. (1990). *Selected Papers: Psychoanalysis and Group Analysis*. London, Karnac, pp. 297–305.

Foulkes, S. H. (1990a). *Selected Papers: Psychoanalysis and Group Analysis*. Ed. E. Foulkes. London, Karnac.

Foulkes, S. H. (1990b). Book Review of Norbert Elias's *The Civilizing Process*. In *Selected Papers: Psychoanalysis and Group Analysis*, ed. E. Foulkes. London, Karnac, pp. 79–82.

Foulkes, S. H., and Anthony, E. J. (1981; 1988; 1991) *Group Psychotherapy: The Psychoanalytic Approach*. London, Penguin. Second edition 1965. Reissued 1983, London, Karnac.

Foulkes, S. H., and Stewart Prince, G. (1972). *Psychiatry in a Changing Society*. London, Tavistock Publications.

Freeman, W. J. (1995). *Societies of Brains: A Study in the Neuroscience of Love and Hate*. New York, Psychology Press.

Freeman, W. J. (2001). *How Brains Make Up Their Minds*. New York, Columbia University Press.

Freud, A. (1989). *Normality and Pathology in Childhood*. London, Routledge.

Freud, S. (1900, 1901). *The Interpretation of Dreams (I, II)*. In J. Strachey (Ed.), Standard Edition. London, Hogarth Press, Vols. IV, V.

Freud, S. (1905). *Fragment of an Analysis of a Case of Hysteria*. In J. Strachey (Ed.), Standard Edition. London, Hogarth Press, Vol. VII, pp. 1–122.

Freud, S. (1910). *Five Lectures on Psycho-analysis*. In J. Strachey (Ed.), Standard Edition. London, Hogarth Press, Vol. XI, pp. 1–56.

Freud, S. (1913). *Totem and Taboo*. In J. Strachey (Ed.), Standard Edition. London, Hogarth Press, Vol. XIII, pp. 1–163.

Freud, S. (1917). *On Narcissism: An Introduction*. In J. Strachey (Ed.), Standard Edition, London, Hogarth Press, Vol. XIV, pp. 73–102.

Freud, S. (1921). *Group Psychology and the Analysis of the Ego*. In J. Strachey (Ed.), Standard Edition. London, Hogarth Press, Vol. XVIII, pp. 67–144.

Freud, S. (1923). *The Ego and the Id*. In J. Strachey (Ed.), Standard Edition. London, Hogarth Press, Vol. XIX, pp. 1–66.

Freud, S. (1927). *The Future of an Illusion*. In J. Strachey (Ed.), Standard Edition. London, Hogarth Press, Vol. XXI, pp. 3–56.

Freud, S. (1930). *Civilization and Its Discontents*. In J. Strachey (Ed.), Standard Edition. London, Hogarth Press, Vol. XXI, pp. 59–145.

Freud, S. (1933). *Why War?* In J. Strachey (Ed.), Standard Edition, London, Hogarth Press, Vol. XXII, pp. 197–215.

Freud, S. (1939). *Moses and Monotheism*. In J. Strachey (Ed.), Standard Edition. London, Hogarth Press, Vol. XXIII, pp. 3–137.
Garland, C. (Ed.). (1980). The Survivor Syndrome Workshop. *Group Analysis* (November special issue).
Garland, C. (1982). Group-Analysis: Taking the Non-Problem Seriously. *Group Analysis* 15 (1): 4–14. doi:10.1177/053331648201500102.
Gay, P. (1989). *Freud: A Life for Our Time*. London, Macmillan.
Gazzaniga, M. S. (1985). *The Social Brain: Discovering the Networks of the Mind*. London, Basic Books.
Gazzaniga, M. S. (2009). *Human: The Science Behind What Makes Us Unique*. New York, Harper Perennial.
Geertz, C. (1973). *The Interpretation of Cultures: Selected Essays*. New York, Basic Books.
Gergely, G., and Watson, J. S. (1996). The Social Biofeedback Theory of Parental Affect-Mirroring: The Development of Emotional Self-Awareness and Self-Control in Infancy. *International Journal of Psychoanalysis* 77 (Pt 6): 1181–1212.
Ginsburg, L. M. (1985). The Imprint of Sigmund Freud's Interest in Porcupines Upon the Psychoanalytic Study of Group Constructs. *Psychoanalysis and Contemporary Thought* 8 (4): 515–528.
Glover, E. (1931). The Therapeutic Effect of Inexact Interpretation: A Contribution to the Theory of Suggestion. *International Journal of Psychoanalysis* 12: 397–411.
Goethe, J. W. von (1890). *Faust*. Third edition. Trans. B. Taylor. London, Ward, Lock.
Goethe, J. W. von (2005). *Selected Poetry*. London, Penguin.
Goldberg, A. (Ed.). (1983). *The Future of Psychoanalysis: Essays in Honor of Heinz Kohut*. New York, International Universities Press.
Goldstein, K. (1939/2000). *The Organism: A Holistic Approach to Biology Derived From Pathological Data in Man*. New York, Zone Books. Reissued Cambridge, MA, Zone Books, introduced by Oliver Sachs.
Goldstein, K. (1940). *Human Nature in the Light of Psychopathology*. Cambridge, MA, Harvard University Press.
Goldstein, K., and Gelb, A. (1918). Psychologische Analysen hirnpathologischer Fälle auf Grund von Untersuchungen Hirnverletzter [Psychological analysis of cases of brain disease]. *Zeitschrift für die gesamte Neurologie und Psychiatrie* 41: 1–142.
Gosling, R. H. (1981). A Study of Very Small Groups. In J. S. Grotstein (Ed.), *Do I Dare Disturb the Universe? A Memorial to W. R. Bion*. Beverly Hills, Caesura Press.
Green, A. (1975). The Analyst, Symbolization and Absence in the Analytic Setting. *International Journal of Psychoanalysis* 56: 1–22.
Gregory, R. L. (1997). Knowledge in Perception and Illusion. *Philosophical Transactions of the Royal Society* 352: 1121–1128.
Griffiths, P., and Pringle, P. (1997). *Psychosocial Practice Within a Residential Setting*. London, Karnac.
Groddeck, G. (1977). *The Meaning of Illness: Selected Psycho-analytic Writings*. New York, International Universities Press.
Grotjahn, M. (1993). *The Art and Technique of Analytic Group Therapy*. Northvale, NJ, Jason Aronson.
Grotstein, J. (1985). Some Perspectives on Empathy From Others and Toward One-Self. In J. Lichtenberg (Ed.), *Empathy, Vol. 1*. Hillsdale, NJ, Analytic Press, pp. 201–215.
Grotstein, J. (1993). *Splitting and Projective Identification*. London, Jason Aronson.

Guimón, J., Atienza, J. L., Duro, P., Trojaola, B., Ehrensperger, S., and Ayerra, J. M. (2004). The Role of Groups in a Changing Mental Health Scenario. *European Journal of Psychiatry* 18: 9–19.

Hakeem, A. (2009). Forensic Group Psychotherapy: Estela Welldon's Contribution to Working with Groups at the Portman Clinic. *British Journal of Psychotherapy* 25 (2): 230–238.

Haldane, J. B. S. (1932). *The Causes of Evolution*. London, Longmans, Green.

Harris, A. (1992). Dialogues as Transitional Space: A Rapprochement of Psychoanalysis and Developmental Psycholinguistics. In N. J. Skolnick and S. C. Warshaw (Eds.), *Relational Perspectives in Psychoanalysis*. Hillsdale, NJ, Analytic Press, pp. 119–146.

Harrison, T. (2000). *Bion, Rickman, Foulkes and the Northfield Experiments: Advancing on a Different Front*. London, Jessica Kingsley.

Hartmann, H. (1958). *Ego Psychology and the Problem of Adaptation*. New York, International Universities Press.

Hayward, J. E. S. (1959). Solidarity: The Social History of an Idea in Nineteenth Century France. *International Review of Social History* 4 (2): 261–284.

Hayward, J. E. S. (1961). The Official Social Philosophy of the French Third Republic: Léon Bourgeois and Solidarism. *International Review of Social History* 6 (1): 19–48.

Hearst, L. E. (1980). *Restoring the Impaired Self as an Essential Corrective Experience in Group Analysis*. Paper presented at the VII International Congress on Group Psychotherapy, Copenhagen, August. In *Congress Proceedings*. New York, Plenum Press.

Hedges, L. E. (1983). *Listening Perspectives in Psychotherapy*. New York, Jason Aronson.

Heinzel, R., Beyer, F., and Klein, T. (2000). Outpatient Psychoanalytic Individual and Group Psychotherapy in a Nationwide Catamnestic Study in Germany. *Group Analysis* 33 (3): 353–372.

Hess, E. H. (1958). 'Imprinting' in Animals. *Scientific American* 198 (3): 81–93.

Hobson, R. F. (1979). 'The Messianic Community'. In R. D. Hinshelwood and N. Manning (Eds.), *Therapeutic Communities: Reflections and Progress*. London, Routledge and Kegan Paul.

Hobson, R. P., and Lee, A. (1999). Imitation and Identification in Autism. *Journal of Child Psychology and Psychiatry* 40 (4): 649–659.

Hobson, R. P., Wimpory, D. C., Williams, J. M., and Nash, S. (2000). Are Infants With Autism Socially Engaged? A Study of Retrospective Parental Reports. *Journal of Autism and Developmental Disorders* 30 (6): 525–536.

Hoffman, E. (2001). *The Secret*. London, Secker & Warburg.

Holman, C. (1999). Social Mind, Social Brain: What Changes in Group Therapy? *Group Analysis* 32 (1): 157–164.

Holmes, J. (2004). Disorganized Attachment and Borderline Personality Disorder: A Clinical Perspective. *Attachment & Human Development* 6: 181–190.

Holquist, M. (1981). Introduction. In M. Bakhtin, *The Dialogic Imagination*. Austin, University of Texas Press, pp. xii–xiii.

Holquist, M. (1990). *Dialogism: Bakhtin and His World*. London, Routledge.

Hopper, E. (1981). A Comment on Professor M. Jahoda's 'Individual and Group'. In M. Pines and L. Rafaelsen (Eds.), *The Proceedings of the VII International Congress of Group Psychotherapy*. London, Plenum.

Horowitz, M., Fridhandler, B., and Stinson, C. (1992). Person Schemas and Emotion. In T. Shapiro and R. N. Emde (Eds.), *Affect: Psychoanalytic Perspectives*. Madison, CT, International Universities Press, pp. 173–208.

Hughes, H. S. (1979). *Consciousness and Society: The Reorientation of European Social Thought 1890–1930*. Brighton, Harvester.

Hutchinson, S. (1986). Styles in Group Analysis. Unpublished paper.

Hutten, E. H. (1983). Meaning and Information in the Group Process. In M. Pines (Ed.), *The Evolution of Group Analysis*. London, Routledge and Kegan Paul, pp. 151–166.

Hutten, E. H. (1984). The Self in the Group. *Group Analysis* 17 (2): 122–133.

Huxley, J. (1992). *Evolutionary Humanism*. London, Prometheus Books.

Huxley, J., *et al.* (Eds.). (2010). *Evolution: The Modern Synthesis*. Cambridge, MA, MIT Press.

James, D. C. (1980). W. R. Bion's Contribution to the Field of Group Therapy: An Appreciation. In L. R. Wolberg and M. L. Aronson (Eds.), *Group and Family Therapy: An Overview*. New York, Brunner/Mazel.

James, D. C. (1985). Bion's 'Containing' and Winnicott's 'Holding' in the Context of the Group Matrix. *International Journal of Group Psychotherapy* 34 (2): 201–213.

James, W. (1890/2017). *The Principles of Psychology*. Pantianos Classics.

James, W. (1978). *The Writings of William James: A Comprehensive Edition*. Chicago, University of Chicago Press.

James, W. (2013). *Principles of Psychology*. Fifth edition. London, Cosimo.

Jay, M. (1973). *The Dialectic Imagination – A History of the Frankfurt School and the Institute of Social Research, 1923–1950*. London, William Heinemann Medical Books.

Jennings, H. (1947). Sociometric Differentiation of the Psychegroup and the Sociogroup. *Sociometry* 10 (1): 71–79.

Jones, J. M. (1995). *Affects as Process: An Inquiry into the Centrality of Affect in Psychological Life*. Hillsdale, NJ, Analytic Press.

Jones, M. (1968/2013). *Social Psychiatry: A Study of Therapeutic Communities*. Second edition. London, Routledge.

Jung, K. G. (1991). *The Archetypes and the Collective Unconscious*. London, Routledge.

Kadis, A. L., Krasner, J. D., Weiner, M. F., Winick, C., and Foulkes, S. H. (1974). *Practicum of Group Psychotherapy*. Second edition. New York, Harper & Row.

Kanas, N. (1996). *Group Therapy for Schizophrenic Patients*. New York, American Psychiatric Press.

Kegan, R. (1983). *The Evolving Self: Problem and Process in Human Development*. Cambridge, MA, Harvard University Press.

Kern, S. (1992). *The Culture of Love: Victorians to Moderns*. Cambridge, MA, Harvard University Press.

Kernberg, O. F. (1975). *Borderline Conditions and Pathological Narcissism*. New York, Jason Aronson.

Kernberg, O. F. (1981/2012). *The Inseparable Nature of Love and Aggression: Clinical and Theoretical Perspectives*. Washington, DC, American Psychiatric Publishing.

Kernberg, P. (2006). *Beyond the Reflection: The Role of the Mirror Paradigm in Clinical Practice*. New York, Other Press.

King, P. (Ed.). (2003). *No Ordinary Psychoanalyst: The Exceptional Contributions of John Rickman*. London, Karnac.

King, P., and Steiner, R. (Eds.). (1992). *The Freud-Klein Controversies 1941–45*. London, Routledge.
Kitayama, S., Duffy, S., Kawamura, T., and Larsen, J. T. (2003). Perceiving an Object and Its Context in Different Cultures: A Cultural Look at New Look. *Psychological Science* 14 (3): 201–206.
Klein, G. S. (1976). *Psychoanalytic Theory: An Exploration of Essentials*. New York, International Universities Press.
Kohut, H. (1966). Forms and Transformations of Narcissism. *Journal of the American Psychoanalytic Association* 14 (2): 243–272.
Kohut, H. (1971). *The Analysis of the Self*. Chicago, University of Chicago Press.
Kohut, H. (1977). *The Restoration of the Self*. New York, International Universities Press.
Kohut, H. (1984). *How Does Analysis Cure?* Chicago, University of Chicago Press.
Kohut, H. (1985). *Self Psychology and the Humanities: Reflections on a New Psychoanalytic Approach*. New York, Norton.
Kosseff, J. W. (1975). The Leader Using Object-Relations Theory. In Z. A. Liff and J. Aronson (Eds.), *The Leader in the Group*. New York, Jason Aronson.
Kreeger, L. (Ed.). (1975). *The Large Group*. London, Constable.
Kris, E. (1977). *The Selected Papers of Ernst Kris*. New Haven, CT, Yale University Press.
Kropotkin, P. (1902/2008). *Mutual Aid: A Factor of Evolution*. Second edition. London, Forgotten Books.
Kumin, I. (1996). *Pre-object Relatedness: Early Attachment and the Psychoanalytic Situation*. New York, Guilford Press.
Lacan, J. (1977). *Écrits. A Selection*. London, Tavistock Publications.
Landauer, K. (1914). Spontanheilung einer Katatonie. *Zeitschrift für ärztliche Psychoanalyse* 2: 441–459.
Landauer, K. (1924). Passive Technik: Zur Analyse narzißtischer Erkrankungen. *Internationale Zeitschrift für Psychoanalyse* 10: 415–422.
Landauer, K. (1936). Die Affekte und ihre Entwicklung. *Imago* 22, 275–291.
Landauer, K. (1991). *Theorie der Affekte und andere Schriften zur Ich-Organisation*. Ed. H.-J. Rothe. Frankfurt am Main, Fischer.
Langs, R. (1977). *Classics in Psychoanalytic Technique*. New York, Jason Aronson.
Leal, M. R. M. (1968). Transference Neurosis in Group-Analytic Treatment. *Group Analysis* 1 (2): 99–109.
Leal, R. (1983). Why Group Analysis Works. In M. Pines (Ed.), *The Evolution of Group Analysis*. London, Routledge and Kegan Paul, pp. 183–196.
Le Bon, G. (1895/2019). *The Crowd: A Study of the Popular Mind*. Independent Publishers. Digireads B0831TJ1J3.
LeBlanc, A. (2001). The Origins of the Concept of Dissociation: Pierre Janet, His Nephew Paul, and the Problem of Post-hypnotic Suggestion. *History of Science* 39 (1): 57–69.
Lecourt, E. (1990). The Musical Envelope. In D. Anzieu, *Psychic Envelopes*. London, Karnac, pp. 211–235.
Lenn, R., and Stefano, K. (2012). *Small, Large, and Median Groups: The Work of Patrick de Maré*. London, Karnac.
Levin, D. M. (1989). *The Listening Self: Personal Growth, Social Change and the Closure of Metaphysics*. London, Routledge.

Lewin, K. (1951). *Field Theory in Social Science: Selected Theoretical Papers*. Ed. D. Cartwright. New York, Harper.

Lewin, K. (1977). *Resolving Social Conflicts & Field Theory in Social Science*. Joint Edition. Washington, DC, American Psychological Association.

Lewis, M., and Brooks-Gunn, J. (1979). *Social Cognition and the Acquisition of Self*. New York, Plenum.

Lichtenberg, J. D. (1991). *Psychoanalysis and Infant Research*. Hillsdale, NJ, Analytic Press.

Lichtenstein, H. (1977). *The Dilemma of Human Identity*. New York, Jason Aronson.

Lipgar, R. (2003). Re-discovering Bion's Experiences in Groups: Notes and Commentary on Theory and Practice. In R. Lipgar and M. Pines (Eds.), *Building on Bion. Roots. Origins and Context of Bion's Contributions to Theory and Practice*. London, Jessica Kingsley, pp. 29–58.

Lipgar, R., and Pines, M. (2003a). *Building on Bion: Roots. Origins and Context of Bion's Contributions to Theory and Practice*. London, Jessica Kingsley.

Lipgar, R., and Pines, M. (2003b). *Building on Bion: Branches. Contemporary Developments and Applications of Bion's Contributions to Theory and Practice*. London, Jessica Kingsley.

Loewald, H. W. (1988). On the Mode of Therapeutic Action of Psychoanalytic Psychotherapy. In A. Rothstein (Ed.), *How Does Treatment Help?* Madison, CT, International Universities Press, pp. 51–59.

Loewald, H. W. (1989). *Papers on Psychoanalysis*. New Haven, CT, Yale University Press.

Loewenstein, R. (1966). *Psychoanalysis: A General Psychology*. Ed. R. M. Loewenstein. New York, International Universities Press.

Lucie-Smith, E., Arell, B., Fuchs, A., and Karjalainen, T. (1995). *Desire: Borealis 7* [Catalogue of a photo exhibition, 17 August – 1 October 1995]. Helsinki, Nordic Arts Center.

Lyons-Ruth, K. (1999). The Two-Person Unconscious: Intersubjective Dialogue, Enactive Relational Representation, and the Emergence of New Forms of Relational Organization. *Psychoanalytic Inquiry* 19 (4): 576–617.

Mahler, M. S. (1968). *On Human Symbiosis and the Vicissitudes of Individuation*. New York, International Universities Press.

Mahler, M. S., Pine, F., and Bergman, A. (1975). *The Psychological Birth of the Human Infant: Symbiosis and Individuation*. New York, Basic Books.

Main, T. F. (1946). The Hospital as a Therapeutic Institution. *Bulletin of the Menninger Clinic* 10 (3): 66–70.

Main, T. F. (1977). The Concept of the Therapeutic Community: Variations and Vicissitudes. *Group Analysis* 10 (2): 2–16.

Main, T. (2001). *The Ailment and Other Psychoanalytic Essays*. Ed. J. Johns. London, Routledge Classics.

Malan, D. H. (1963). *A Study of Brief Psychotherapy*. London, Tavistock.

Malan, D. H. (1999). *Individual Psychotherapy and the Science of Psychodynamics*. Second edition. Oxford, Butterworth-Heinemann.

Malan. D. H., Balfour, F. H., Hood, V. G., and Shooter, A. M. (1976). Group Psychotherapy: A Long-Term Follow-Up Study. *Archives of General Psychiatry* 33 (1): 1303–1315.

Malloch, S., and Trevarthen, C. (2010). *Communicative Musicality: Exploring the Basis of Human Companionship*. Oxford, Oxford University Press.

Maranhão, T. (1990). *The Interpretation of Dialogue*. Chicago, University of Chicago Press.

Maratos, J. (Ed.). (2006). *Resonance and Reciprocity: Selected Papers by Dennis Brown*. London, Routledge.

Maratos, J. (Ed.). (2015). *Foundations of Group Analysis for the Twenty-First Century*. London, Routledge.

Margalit, A. (1996). *The Decent Society*. Cambridge, MA, Harvard University Press.

Margulies, A. (1989). *The Empathic Imagination*. New York, Norton.

Martin, E. S. (1882). *Sly Ballads in Harvard China*. Boston, A. Williams.

Maslow, A. H. (1943). A Theory of Human Motivation. *Psychological Review* 50 (4): 370–396.

Maslow, A. H. (1954). *Motivation and Personality*. New York, Wiley.

Maslow, A. H. (1962). *Toward a Psychology of Being*. New York, Wiley.

Masuda, T., and Nisbett, R. E. (2001). Attending Holistically Versus Analytically: Comparing the Context Sensitivity of Japanese and Americans. *Journal of Personality and Social Psychology* 81 (5): 922–934.

McDougall, J. (1989). *Theaters of the Body: A Psychoanalytic Approach to Psychosomatic Illness*. London, Norton.

McLaurin, A. (1981). Virginia Woolf and Unanism. *Journal of Modern Literature* 9: 115–122.

McLaurin, A. (1984). Consciousness and Group Consciousness in Virginia Woolf. In E. Warner (Ed.), *Virginia Woolf: A Centenary Perspective*. London, Macmillan, pp. 28–40.

Mead, G. H. (1934/2015). *Mind, Self, & Society*. Ed. Charles W. Morris. Chicago, University of Chicago Press.

Mead, G. H. (1964). *Selected Writings*. Chicago, University of Chicago Press.

Meares, R. (2000). *Intimacy and Alienation*. London, Brunner-Routledge.

Medoff, D. (2009). Freud's Reply to Einstein on Delivering Mankind From War. *Peace Review* 21 (4): 437–441.

Meissner, W. W. (1996). Empathy in the Therapeutic Alliance. *Psychoanalytic Inquiry* 16 (1): 39–53.

Meltzoff, A. (1997). Explaining Facial Imitation: A Theoretical Model. *Early Development and Parenting* 6 (3–4):179–192.

Mennell, S. (2001). The Other Side of the Coin: Decivilizing Processes. In T. Salumets (Ed.), *Norbert Elias and Human Interdependencies*. Montreal, McGill-Queen's University Press, pp. 32–49.

Menninger, K. A. (1946). Foreword. *Bulletin of the Menninger Clinic* 10 (3): 65.

Menninger, K. A., and Holzman, P. S. (1973). *Theory of Psychoanalytic Technique*. New York, Basic Books.

Menzies Lyth, I. E. P. (1960). A Case-Study in the Functioning of Social Systems as a Defence Against Anxiety: A Report on a Study of the Nursing Service of a General Hospital. *Human Relations* 13 (2): 95–121.

Merleau-Ponty, M. (1968). *The Visible and the Invisible*. Trans. A. Lingis. Evanston, IL, Northwestern University Press.

Midgley, N. (2007). Anna Freud: The Hampstead War Nurseries and the Role of the Direct Observation of Children for Psychoanalysis. *The International Journal of Psychoanalysis* 88 (4): 939–959.

Milton, J. (2003). *Paradise Lost*. London, Penguin Classics: Kindle edition.

Mitchell, J. (2000). *Psychoanalysis and Feminism: A Radical Reassessment of Freudian Psychoanalysis*. New York, Basic Books.

Mohr, G. J. (1966). August Aichhorn. Friend of the Wayward Youth. In F. Alexander *et al.* (Eds.), *Psychoanalytic Pioneers*. New York, Basic Books.

Montessori, M. (1948/1986). *The Discovery of the Child*. New York, Ballantine Books.

Moreno, J. L. (1932). *The First Book on Group Psychotherapy*. Beacon, NY, Beacon House.

Moreno, J. L. (1934). *Who Shall Survive? A New Approach to the Problem of Human Interrelations*. Beacon, NY, Beacon House.

Morson, G. S. (Ed.). (1986). *Bakhtin: Essays and Dialogues on His Work*. Chicago, University of Chicago Press.

Morson, G. S., and Emerson, C. (1990). *Mikhail Bakhtin: Creation of a Prosaics*. San Francisco, Stanford University Press.

Moscovici, S. (1985). *The Age of the Crowd: A Historical Treatise on Mass Psychology*. Cambridge, Cambridge University Press.

Mulgan, J. (1997). *Connnexity: How to Live in a Connected World*. London, Chatto & Windus.

Müller-Freienfels, R. (1935). The Evolution of Modern Psychology. In *The Psychology of Super-Individual Psychic Life*. Trans. W. B. Wolfe. New Haven, CT, Yale University Press, pp. 400–458.

Napolitani, D. (1980). *Beyond the Individual: The Relationship Between Subject and Group in a Group-Analytic Perspective*. Paper presented at the VII International Congress of Group Psychotherapy, Copenhagen, August. In *Congress Proceedings*. New York, Plenum.

Navaro, L., Friedman, R., and Schwartzberg, S. L. (Eds.). (2011). *Desire, Passion and Gender: Clinical Implications*. New York, Nova Science.

Neri, C., Pines, M., and Friedman, R. (2002). *Dreams in Group Psychotherapy: Theory and Technique*. London, Jessica Kingsley.

Nitsun, M. (1996). *The Anti-Group: Destructive Forces in the Group and Their Creative Potential*. London, Routledge.

Nye, R. A. (1975). *The Origins of Crowd Psychology: Gustave LeBon and the Crisis of Mass Democracy in the Third Republic*. London, Sage.

Oliner, P. M., Oliner, S. P., Baron, L., Blum, L. A., Krebs, D., and Smolenska, M. Z. (1992). *Embracing the Other: Philosophical, Psychological, and Historical Perspectives on Altruism*. New York, New York University Press.

Ornstein, P. H. (Ed.). (1978). *The Search for the Self: Selected Writings of Heinz Kohut*. Four volumes. New York, International Universities Press.

Ornstein, P. (1988). Multiple Curative Factors and Processes in the Psychoanalytic Psychotherapies. In A. Rothstein (Ed.), *How Does Treatment Help? On the Modes of Therapeutic Action of Psychoanalytic Psychotherapy*. Madison, CT, International Universities Press, pp. 105–128.

Ortega y Gasset, J. (1963). *Meditations on Quixote*. London, Norton.

Ovid. (1993). *Metamorphoses of Ovid. Book 3: Narcissus and Echo*. Trans. A. Mandelbaum. New York, Harcourt Brace.

Oxford University Press. (2018). *Oxford Dictionaries*. https://premium.oxforddictionaries.com. Accessed 12 February 2024.

Panksepp, J. (1998). *Affective Neuroscience: The Foundations of Human and Animal Emotions*. New York, Oxford University Press.

Papoušek, H., Jürgens, U., and Papoušek, M. (Eds.). (1992). *Nonverbal Vocal Communication: Comparative & Developmental Approaches*. Cambridge, Cambridge University Press.

Paskauskas, R. A. (Ed.). (1993). *The Complete Correspondence of Sigmund Freud and Ernest Jones 1908–1939*. Cambridge, MA, Belknap Press.

Person, E. S. (1991). Romantic Love: At the Intersection of the Psyche and the Cultural Unconscious. *Journal of the American Psychoanalytic Association* 39 (Supplement): 383–411.

Pertegato, E. G. (2014). Foulkes' Roots in Trigant Burrow's Writings. *Group Analysis* 47 (3): 312–328.

Pertegato, E. G., and Pertegato, G. O. (2019). *From Psychoanalysis to Group Analysis: The Pioneering Work of Trigant Burrow*. London, New International Library of Group Analysis.

Piaget, J., and Inhelder, B. (1967). *The Child's Conception of Space*. London, Norton.

Pichon-Rivière, E. (1971). *El proceso grupal: Del psicoanálisis a la psicología social (I)* [*The group process: From psychoanalysis to social psychology (I)*]. Buenos Aires, Nueva Visión.

Pichon-Rivière, E. (1995). *Diccionario de psicología social: Thematic Compilation of Writings by Pichon-Rivière, Joaquín, and Cols*. Buenos Aires, Nueva Visión.

Pines, D. (1994). *A Woman's Unconscious Use of Her Body*. London, Routledge.

Pines, M. (1975). Group Psychotherapy With Difficult Patients. In L. R. Wolberg, M. L. Aronson, and A. R. Wolberg (Eds.), *Group Therapy: An Overview*. New York, Stratton Intercontinental Books.

Pines, M. (1978a). Psycho-Analysis and Group Analysis. *Group Analysis* 11 (1): 8–20.

Pines, M. (1978b). The Contributions of S. H. Foulkes to Group Analytic Psychotherapy. In L. R. Wolberg, M. L. Aronson, and A. R. Wolberg (Eds.), *Group Therapy 1978 – An Overview*. New York, Stratton Intercontinental Medical Book.

Pines, M. (1978c). Group-analytic psychotherapy of the Borderline Patient. *Group Analysis* 11 (2): 115–126.

Pines, M. (1980). Group Psychotherapy: Frame of Reference for Training. In W. de Moor and H. R. Wijngaarden (Eds.), *Psychotherapy: Research and Training*. New York, Elsevier North-Holland Biomedical Press, pp. 233–244.

Pines, M. (1982/1997). Reflections on Mirroring: Sixth Annual Foulkes Lecture. *Group Analysis* 15 (Supplement); and in *Circular Reflections: Selected Papers on Group Analysis and Psychoanalysis*. London, Jessica Kingsley, pp. 17–39.

Pines, M. (Ed.). (1983a). *The Evolution of Group Analysis*. London, Routledge.

Pines, M. (1983b). The Contribution of S. H. Foulkes to Group Therapy. In M. Pines (Ed.), *The Evolution of Group Analysis*. London, Routledge, pp. 265–285.

Pines, M. (1983c). The Fundamentals of Group-Analytic Therapy. In M. Pines (Ed.), *The Evolution of Group Analysis*. London, Routledge.

Pines, M. (1984a). Reflections on Mirroring. *International Review of Psychoanalysis* 11: 27–42.

Pines, M. (1984b). The Frame of Reference of Group-Analytic Psychotherapy. In T. E. Lear (Ed.), *Spheres of Group Analysis*. London, Group-Analytic Society Publications, pp. 20–28.

Pines, M. (1984c). Mirroring in Group Analysis as a Developmental and Therapeutic Process. In T. E. Lear (Ed.), *Spheres of Group Analysis*. London, Group-Analytic Society Publications, pp. 118–136.

Pines, M. (1984d). Group-analytic psychotherapy and the Borderline Patient. *Analytic Psychotherapy & Psychopathology* 1 (1): 57–70.

Pines, M. (1985a). Psychic Development and the Group Analytic Situation. *Group Analysis* 9: 24–37.

Pines, M. (Ed.). (1985b). *Bion and Group Psychotherapy*. London, Routledge.

Pines, M. (1986). Psychoanalysis, Psychodrama and Group Psychotherapy: Step-Children of Vienna. *Group Analysis* 19 (2): 101–112.

Pines, M. (1987a). Shame – What Psychoanalysis Does and Does Not Say. *Group Analysis* 20 (1): 16–31.

Pines, M. (1987b). Mirroring and Child Development: Psychodynamic and Psychological Interpretations. In T. Honess and K. Yardley (Eds.), *Self and Identity: Perspectives Across the Lifespan*. London, Routledge and Kegan Paul, pp. 19–37.

Pines, M. (1988a). Mirroring and Group Analysis. In N. Slavinska-Holy (Ed.), *Borderline and Narcissistic Patients in Therapy*. New York, International Universities Press, pp. 143–171.

Pines, M. (1988b). Mediation Papers: A Group-Analytic Response. *Group Analysis* 21 (1): 57–59.

Pines, M. (1989). Group Analysis and Healing. *Group Analysis* 22 (4): 417–429.

Pines, M. (1990). Group Analysis and the Corrective Emotional Experience: Is It Relevant? *Psychoanalytic Inquiry* 10: 389–408.

Pines, M. (1991a) The Matrix of Group Analysis: An Historical Perspective. *Group Analysis* 24 (2): 99–109.

Pines, M. (1991b). A History of Psychodynamic Psychiatry in Britain. In J. Holmes (Ed.), *Textbook of Psychotherapy and Psychiatric Practice*. London, Churchill Livingstone.

Pines, M. (1995). The Universality of Shame: A Psychoanalytic Approach. *British Journal of Psychotherapy* 11 (3): 346–357.

Pines, M. (1998). *Circular Reflections: Selected Papers on Group Analysis and Psychoanalysis*. London, Jessica Kingsley.

Pines, M. (2000). Shepherding Group Analysis: Shepherds Past, Present and Future. In *Group*. 24(1): 49–57.

Pines, M. (2002). The Illumination of Dreams. In C. Neri, M. Pines, and R. Friedman (Eds.), *Dreams in Group Psychotherapy: Theory and Technique*. London, Jessica Kingsley, pp. 25–36.

Pines, M. (2003a). Social Brain and Social Group: How Mirroring Connects People. *Group Analysis* 36 (4): 507–513.

Pines, M. (2003b). Bion and Foulkes on Empathy. In R. M. Lipgar and M. Pines (Eds.), *Building on Bion: Roots. Origins and Context of Bion's Contributions to Theory and Practice*. London, Jessica Kingsley.

Pines, M. (2007). The Group-as-a-Whole Approach in Foulkesian Group-analytic psychotherapy. In G. M. Saiger, S. Rubenfeld, and M. D. Dluhy (Eds.), *Windows into Today's Group Therapy*. London, Routledge.

Pines, M. (2012). Bion, Foulkes and Empathy. In: *Funzione Gamma, University 'Sapienza', Rome*. https://www.funzionegamma.it/en/bion-foulkes-and-empathy

Pines, M., Hearst, L. E., and Behr, H. L. (1982). Group Analysis (Group-Analytic Psychotherapy). In G. M. Gazda (Ed.), *Basic Approaches to Group Psychotherapy and Group Counselling*. Springfield, IL, Charles C. Thomas, pp. 132–178.

Pines, M., and Roberts, J. (1991). *The Practice of Group Analysis*. London, Routledge.

Pines, M., and Schermer, V. L. (1994). *Ring of Fire. Primitive Affects and Object Relations in Group Psychotherapy*. London, Routledge.

Pines, M., and Schermer, V. L. (1999). *Group Psychotherapy of the Psychoses: Concepts, Interventions and Contexts*. London, Jessica Kingsley.
Pirandello, L. (1922/1995). *Six Characters in Search of an Author*. London, Penguin.
Poland, W. S. (1975). Tact as a Psychoanalytic Function. *International Journal of Psychoanalysis* 56 (2): 155–162.
Powell, A. (1991). Matrix, Mind and Matter: From the Internal to the Eternal. *Group Analysis* 24 (3): 299–315.
Powles, W. E. (1989). Group Therapy With Affective Disorders: Critical Impression of Trends and Strategies. *Group Analysis* 22 (1): 7–17.
Rafaelsen, L., and Linnemann, E. (1980). *Training Programme in Group Analysis*. Paper presented at the VII International Congress of Group Psychotherapy, Copenhagen, August. In *Congress Proceedings*. New York, Plenum.
Ramachandran, V. S., and Blakeslea, S. (1999). *Phantoms in the Brain: Human Nature and the Architecture of Mind*. London, Fourth Estate Publishers.
Rangell, L. (1980). *The Mind of Watergate: An Exploration of the Compromise of Integrity*. New York, Norton.
Rangell, L. (2006). *The Road to Unity in Psychoanalytic Theory*. New York, Jason Aronson.
Rapaport, D. (1960). The Structure of Psycho-analytic Theory: A Systematizing Attempt. *Psychological Issues 6. Monograph*.
Rawls, J. (2005). *A Theory of Justice*. Cambridge, MA, Harvard University Press.
Redl, F. (1966). *When We Deal With Children: Selected Writings*. New York, Free Press.
Redl, F., and Wineman, D. (1965). *Children Who Hate: A Sensitive Analysis of the Antisocial Behavior of Children in Their Response to the Adult World*. New York, Macmillan.
Reich, W. (1945a). *Character Analysis*. New York, Orgone Institute Press.
Reich, W. (1945b). *The Sexual Revolution: Toward a Self-Governing Character Structure*. New York, Orgone Institute Press.
Reich, W. (1946). *The Mass Psychology of Fascism*. New York, Orgone Institute Press.
Renier, O. (1976). Groups as Part of an In-Service Day Release Course for Residential Social Workers. *Group Analysis* 9 (1): 41–42.
Reppen, J. (1980). Symposium: George Klein's Psychoanalytic Theory in Perspective. *Psychoanalytic Review* 67 (2): 159–160.
Resnik, S. (1995). *Mental Space*. London, Karnac.
Rey, H. (1994). *Universals of Psychoanalysis in the Treatment of Psychotic and Borderline States*. London, Free Association Books.
Rickman, J. (1957a). *Selected Contributions to Psycho-Analysis*. Ed. W. C. M. Scott. London, Hogarth Press and The Institute of Psycho-Analysis. Reissued 2003, London, Karnac, with a new preface.
Rickman, J. (1957b). *Number and the Human Sciences, Psycho-analysis and Culture*. Reprinted in *Selected Contributions to Psycho-Analysis*. Ed. W. C. M. Scott. London, Hogarth Press and The Institute of Psycho-analysis.
Rickman, J. (2003). *No Ordinary Psychoanalyst: The Extraordinary Contributions of John Rickman*. Ed. Pearl King. London, Karnac.
Ridley, M. (1996). *The Origins of Virtue*. London, Viking.
Rieber, R. W. (Ed.). (1987–1999). *The Collected Works of L. S. Vygotsky*. Six volumes. London, Springer.
Rizzolatti, G., and Craighero, L. (2004). The Mirror-Neuron System. *Annual Review of Neuroscience* 27: 69–192.
Rizzolatti, G., and Sinigaglia, C. (2008). *Mirrors in the Brain: How Our Minds Share Actions and Emotions*. New York, Oxford University Press.

Robbins, M. (1996). *Conceiving of Personality*. New Haven, CT, Yale University Press.

Roberts, J. P. (1982). Foulkes' Concept of the Matrix. *Group Analysis* 15 (2): 111–126.

Rogers, C. R. (1951). *Client-Centered Therapy: Its Current Practice, Implications, and Theory*. London, Constable.

Rose, N. (1985). *The Psychological Complex: Psychology, Politics and Society in England, 1869–1939*. London, Routledge and Kegan Paul.

Rosenfeld, H. (1965). *Psychotic States: A Psychoanalytical Approach*. London, Routledge. Reissued 1982, London, Karnac.

Rösing, W., and Barthel-Rösing, M. (2017). *Pioneers of Group Analysis*. Wilhelm Rösing Film, https://www.roesingfilm.de/filme/pioneers-of-group-analysis. Accessed 12 February 2024.

Rothschild, E. (2001). *Economic Sentiments: Adam Smith, Condorcet and the Enlightenment*. Cambridge, MA, Harvard University Press.

Rothstein, A. (Ed.). (1988). *How Does Treatment Help? On the Modes of Therapeutic Action of Psychoanalytic Psychotherapy*. Madison, CT, International Universities Press, pp. 51–59.

Ruesch, J., and Bateson, G. (1951). *Communication: The Social Matrix of Psychiatry*. New York, Norton.

Rycroft, C. (1968). *A Critical Dictionary of Psychoanalysis*. New York, Basic Books.

Sander, L. (2008). *Living Systems, Evolving Consciousness, and the Emerging Person*. New York, Analytic Press.

Sandler, J. (1987). *From Safety to Superego: Selected Papers of Joseph Sandler*. London, Karnac.

Schilder, P. (1938/1999). *Psychotherapy*. Vol. 27 of the 38-volume series. New York, General Psychology.

Schilder, P. (1999). *The Image and Appearance of the Human Body: Studies in the Constructive Energies of the Psyche*. London, Routledge.

Schindler, W. (1951). Family Pattern in Group Formation and Therapy. *International Journal of Group Psychotherapy* 1 (2): 100–105.

Schindler, W. (1966). The Role of the Mother in Group Psychotherapy. *International Journal of Group Psychotherapy* 16 (2): 198–202.

Schlapobersky, J. R. (Ed.). (1987). *Selected Papers of Robin Skynner. Vol. 1. Explorations With Families: Group Analysis and Family Therapy*. London, Methuen. Reissued 1988, London, Routledge.

Schlapobersky, J. R. (Ed.). (1989). *Selected Papers of Robin Skynner. Vol. 2. Institutes and How to Survive Them*. London, Methuen. Reissued 1990, London, Routledge.

Schlapobersky, J. R. (1995/2000). The Language of the Group: Monologue, Dialogue and Discourse in Group Analysis. In D. Brown and L. Zinkin (Eds.), *The Psyche and the Social World*. London, Routledge. Reissued London, Jessica Kingsley, pp. 211–231; and in J. Schlapobersky (2016), *From the Couch to the Circle: Group-Analytic Psychotherapy In Practice*. Hove, UK, Routledge, pp. 112–113.

Schlapobersky, J. R. (1996). Forensic Psychotherapy: A Group-Analytic Perspective – From the Speech of Hands to the Language of Words. In C. Cordess and M. Cox (Eds.), *Forensic Psychotherapy: Crime, Psychodynamics and the Offender Patient*. London, Jessica Kingsley, pp. 227–244.

Schlapobersky, J. R. (2001). The Social World of the Forsaken Psyche: The Fall of Icarus. *Group Analysis* 34 (4): 485–500.

Schlapobersky, J. R. (2015a). On Making a Home Amongst Strangers: The Paradox of Group Psychotherapy. 39th Foulkes Memorial Lecture, London, May 2015. *Group Analysis* 48 (4): 406–432.

Schlapobersky, J. R. (2015b). Group Psychotherapy in the United Kingdom: Report for Special Edition. *International Journal of Group Psychotherapy* 65 (4): 565–576.

Schlapobersky, J. R. (2016). *From the Couch to the Circle: Group-Analytic Psychotherapy in Practice*. Hove, UK, Routledge.

Schlapobersky, J. R. (2021). *When They Came for Me: The Hidden Diary of an Apartheid Prisoner*. London, Berghahn Books and Cape Town, Jonathan Ball.

Schlapobersky, J. R. (2022). Finding a Voice; Bearing Witness to the Voices of Others; Coming Out of the Shadows Together: Basic Principles of Group Psychotherapy. In P. Verhagen and A. ter Haar (Eds.), *Leerboek Groepspsychotherapie*. Amsterdam, Boom de Tijdstroom, pp. 179–191.

Schlapobersky, J. R. (2024). From Toxic Bonds to Healing Relationships. A Journey through Group Analytic Theory and Practice. *Group Analysis* 57 (2): 129–160. doi:10.1177/05333164241245904.

Schlapobersky, J. R., and Bamber, H. (1988), Rehabilitation Work With Victims of Torture in London: The Reclamation of Time and Space. In D. Miserez (Ed.), *Refugees – The Trauma of Exile. The Humanitarian Role of Red Cross and Red Crescent*. Dordrecht, Martinus Nijhoff, pp. 206–222.

Schlapobersky, J. R., and Pines, M. (2009). Group Methods in Adult Psychiatry. In M. Gelder *et al.* (Eds.), *New Oxford Textbook of Psychiatry*. Second edition. Oxford, Oxford University Press, pp. 1350–1368.

Schlapobersky, J. R., and Pines, M. (2010). Group Analysis and Group Analytic Psychotherapy. In V. Tschuschke (Ed.), *Gruppenpsychotherapie und Gruppendynamik*. Stuttgart, Thieme, pp. 264–268.

Schlesinger, H. J. (1988). Historical Overview of the Mode of Therapeutic Action of Psychoanalytic Psychotherapy. In A. Rothstein (Ed.), *How Does Treatment Help? On the Modes of Therapeutic Action of Psychoanalytic Psychotherapy*. Madison, CT, International Universities Press, pp. 7–27.

Schore, A. N. (1994). *Affect Regulation and the Origin of Self: The Neurobiology of Emotional Development*. Hillsdale, NJ, Lawrence Erlbaum.

Searles, H. (1986/2018). *Collected Papers on Schizophrenia and Related Subjects*. London, Routledge.

Shapiro, T., and Emde, R. N. (1992) (Eds.). *Affect: Psychoanalytic Perspectives*. Madison, CT, International Universities Press.

Sharpe, M. (1977). Group Themes in a District General Hospital Psychiatric Unit – Shrodells, Watford, England. *Group Analysis* 10 (3): 266–273.

Shweder, R. A. (2003). *Why Do Men Barbecue? Recipes for Cultural Psychology*. Cambridge, MA, Harvard University Press.

Sigrell, B. (1979). An Evaluation of an Educational Programme in Group Psychotherapy. *Group Analysis* 12 (1): 55–56.

Sinason, V. (2010). *Mental Handicap and the Human Condition: An Analytic Approach to Intellectual Disability*. London, Free Association Books.

Skynner, A. C. R. (1969). A Group-Analytic Approach to Conjoint Family Therapy. *Journal of Child Psychology and Psychiatry* 10 (2): 81–106.

Skynner, A. C. R. (1983). Group Analysis and Family Therapy. In M. Pines (Ed.), *The Evolution of Group Analysis*. London, Routledge, pp. 326–343.

Skynner, A. C. R. (1986). What Is Effective in Group Psychotherapy? *Group Analysis* 19 (1): 5–22.

Skynner, A. C. R. (1987). *Explorations With Families: Group Analysis and Family Therapy*. Ed. J. R. Schlapobersky. London, Methuen. Reissued London, Routledge, 1990.

Skynner, A. C. R. (1989a). *Institutes and How to Survive Them: Mental Health Training and Consultation*. Ed. J. R. Schlapobersky. London, Methuen. Reissued London, Routledge, 1991.

Skynner, A. C. R. (1989b). Be Sure to Feed the Goose That Lays the Golden Eggs: A Discussion on the Myth of Altruism. In J. R. Schlapobersky (Ed.), *Institutes and How to Survive Them: Mental Health Training and Consultation*. London, Methuen. Reissued London, Routledge, 1991.

Slater, P. E. (1966). *Microcosm: Structural, Psychological and Religious Evolution in Groups*. New York, Wiley.

Slavin, M. O., and Kriegman, D. (1992). *The Adaptive Design of the Human Psyche: Psychoanalysis, Evolutionary Biology, and the Therapeutic Process*. London, Guilford Press.

Smart, N. (1994). *Worldviews: Crosscultural Explorations of Human Beliefs*. New York, Prentice Hall.

Smith, A. (1759/2010). *The Theory of Moral Sentiments*. London, Penguin.

Smith, A. (1776/2003). *The Wealth of Nations*. London, Bantam Classics.

Smith, J. M. (1975). Survival Through Suicide [Book Review of E. O. Wilson's Sociobiology: The New Synthesis]. *New Scientist*, 28 August.

Sofer, R. N. (1978). *Ethics and Society in England: The Revolution in the Social Sciences 1870–1914*. Berkeley, University of California Press.

Spaas, L. (2000). *Echoes of Narcissus*. New York, Berghahn.

Spencer, H. (2000). *First Principles of a New System of Philosophy*. London, Admant.

Sroufe, L. A., and Waters, E. (1977). Attachment as an Organizational Construct. *Child Development* 48: 1184–1199.

Stacey, R. (2003). *Complexity and Group Processes: A Radically Social Understanding of Individuals*. London, Routledge.

Stern, D. (1998). *The Interpersonal World of the Infant*. London, Karnac.

Stern, D. N., Sander, L. W., Nahum, J. P., Harrison, A. M., Lyons-Ruth, K., Morgan, A. C., Bruschweilerstern, N., and Tronick, E. Z. (1998). Non-interpretive Mechanisms in Psychoanalytic Therapy: The 'Something More' Than Interpretation. *International Journal of Psycho-analysis* 79: 903–921.

Sternberg, T. (1982). Defence Mechanisms and the Working Through of Resistances in Group Therapy. *Group Analysis* 15 (3): 261–277.

Stevens, A. (1993). *Withymead: A Jungian Community for the Healing Arts*. London, Coventure.

Stolorow, R. D., Brandchaft, B., and Atwood, G. E. (1988). *Psychoanalytic Treatment: An Intersubjective Approach*. New York, Routledge.

Stone, W. (1996). *Group Psychotherapy for People With Chronic Mental Illness*. New York, Guilford Press.

Storr, A. (1986). *The Essential Jung: Selected Writings*. London, Fontana Press.

Sullivan, H. S. (1964). *The Fusion of Psychiatry and Social Science*. New York, Norton.

Sutherland, J. D. (1952). Notes on Psychoanalytic Group Therapy: I. Therapy and Training. *Psychiatry* 15: 111–117.

Suttie, I. D. (1935/1988). *The Origins of Love and Hate*. London, Free Association Books.

Tarde, G. (1903). *The Laws of Imitation*. New York, Henry Holt.

Taylor, James (Ed.). (1985). *Selected Writings of John Hughlings Jackson*. Two volumes. Birmingham, AL, Classics of Neurology & Neurosurgery Library.

Tolpin, M. (1983). Corrective Emotional Experience: A Self Psychological Revelation. In A. Goldberg (Ed.), *The Future of Psychoanalysis*. New York, International Universities Press, pp. 363–379.

Torres, N. (2003). Gregariousness and the Mind: Wilfred Trotter and Wilfred Bion. In R. Lipgar and M. Pines (Eds.), *Building on Bion: Roots. Origins and Context of Bion's Contributions to Theory and Practice*. London, Jessica Kingsley, pp. 85–117.

Trevarthen, C. (1979). Communication and Cooperation in Early Infancy: A Description of Primary Intersubjectivity. In M. Bullowa (Ed.), *Before Speech: The Beginning of Human Communication*. London, Cambridge University Press, pp. 321–347.

Trevarthen, C. (1993a). The Self Born in Intersubjectivity: The Psychology of an Infant Communicating. In U. Neisser (Ed.), *The Perceived Self: Ecological and Interpersonal Sources of Self-Knowledge*. New York, Cambridge University Press, pp. 121–173.

Trevarthen, C. (1993b). The Function of Emotions in Early Infant Communication and Development. In J. Nadel and L. Camaioni (Eds.), *New Perspectives In Early Communicative Development*. London, Routledge, pp. 48–81.

Trotter, W. (1916/2005). *Instincts of the Herd in Peace and War*. London, Cosimo Classics.

Trotter, W. (1941). *The Collected Papers of Wilfred Trotter F.R.S.* Oxford, Oxford University Press.

Tubert-Oklander, J. (2009). El museo y el taller. Algunas reflexiones sobre la vitalidad de los textos [The museum and the workshop: Some reflections on the vitality of texts]. In *Hermenéutica analógica y condición humana* [*Analogical hermeneutics and the human condition*]. Analogía Filosófica, special number 24.

Tubert-Oklander, J. (2010). A Gentle Revolutionary: The Influence of Malcolm Pines on My Thinking and Practice. *Group Analysis* 43 (3): 228–240.

Tyson, P., and Tyson, R. (1990). *Psychoanalytic Theories of Development*. New Haven, CT, Yale University Press.

Urlić, I. (2004). Trauma and Reparation, Mourning and Forgiveness: The Healing Potential of the Group. *Group Analysis* 37 (4): 453–471.

Usandivaras, R. J. (1986). Foulkes' Primordial Level in Clinical Practice. *Group Analysis* 19 (2): 113–124.

Valsiner, J., and Van der Veer, R. (2000). *The Social Mind: Construction of the Idea*. London, Cambridge University Press.

Verhaeghe, P. (1999). *Love in a Time of Loneliness*. London, Rebus Press.

Voloshinov, V. N. (1986). *Marxism and the Philosophy of Language*. Cambridge, MA, Harvard University Press.

Vonofakos, D., and Hinshelwood, B. (2012). Wilfred Bion's Letters to John Rickman (1939–1951). *Psychoanalysis and History* 14 (1): 53–94.

Vygotsky, L. S. (1962/2012). *Thought and Language*. Cambridge, MA, MIT Press.

Vygotsky, L. S. (1978). *Mind in Society: The Development of Higher Psychological Processes*. Cambridge, MA, Harvard University Press.

Vygotsky, L. S. (1981). The Genesis of Higher Mental Functions. In J. V. Wertsch (Ed.), *The Concept of Activity in Soviet Psychology*. Armonk, NY, M. E. Sharpe, pp. 144–188.

Waal, F. de (1982). *Chimpanzee Politics: Power and Sex Among Apes*. Baltimore, Johns Hopkins University Press.
Waal, F. de (1996). *Good Natured: The Origins of Right and Wrong in Humans and Other Animals*. Cambridge, MA, Harvard University Press.
Waal, F. de (2009). *The Age of Empathy: Nature's Lessons for a Kinder Society*. New York, Harmony Books.
Wallas, G. (1908/1961). *Human Nature in Politics*. London, Archibald Constable.
Watkins, J. G. (1978). *The Therapeutic Self: Developing Resonance – Key to Effective Relationships*. London, Human Sciences Press.
Weinshel, E. M. (1975). 'The Analyst as the Conscience of the Analysis', Written with Victor Calef. In Robert S. Wallerstein (Ed.), *Commitment and Compassion in Psychoanalysis: Selected Papers of Edward M. Weinshel*. London, Analytic Press, pp. 245–265.
Weiss, J., Sampson, H., and Mount Zion Psychotherapy Research Group. (1986). *The Psychoanalytic Process: Theory, Clinical Observation & Empirical Research*. New York, Guilford Press.
Welldon, E. V. (1992). *Mother, Madonna, Whore: The Idealization and Denigration of Motherhood*. London, Karnac.
Welldon, E. V. (1997). Let the Treatment Fit the Crime: Forensic Group Psychotherapy. 20th Foulkes Lecture. *Group Analysis* 30 (1): 9–26.
Welldon, E. V. (2012). *Playing With Dynamite: A Personal Approach to the Psychoanalytic Understanding of Perversions, Violence, and Criminality*. London, Karnac.
Wender, L. (1936). The Dynamics of Group Psychotherapy and Its Application. *Journal of Nervous and Mental Disease* 84 (1): 54–60.
Wertheimer, M. (1959). *Productive Thinking*. New York, Harper Collins.
Wertsch, J. V. (1985). *Vygotsky and the Social Formation of Mind*. Cambridge, MA, Harvard University Press.
Wertsch, J. V. (1991). *Voices of the Mind: A Sociocultural Approach to Mediated Action*. London, Harvester Wheatsheaf.
Wexler, B. E. (2008). *Brain and Culture: Neurobiology, Ideology, and Social Change*. Cambridge, MA, MIT Press.
Whitaker, D. S. (2001). *Using Groups to Help People*. London, Routledge.
Whitehead, C. (Ed.). (2008). *The Origin of Consciousness in the Social World*. Exeter, Imprint Academic.
Whiteley, S. (2004). The Evolution of the Therapeutic Community. *Psychiatric Quarterly* 75 (3).
Whiten, A., and Byrne, R. W. (Eds.). (1997). *Machiavellian Intelligence*. Cambridge, Cambridge University Press.
Wickström, G., and Bendix, T. (2000). The 'Hawthorne Effect' – What Did the Original Hawthorne Studies Actually Show? *Scandinavian Journal of Work, Environment & Health* 26 (4): 363–367.
Widener, A. (1979). *Gustave Le Bon: The Man and His Works*. Indianapolis, Liberty Press.
Wilke, G. (2003). The Large Group and Its Conductor. In R. Lipgar and M. Pines (Eds.), *Building on Bion: Branches. Contemporary Developments and Applications of Bion's Contributions to Theory and Practice*. London, Jessica Kingsley, pp. 70–105.
Williams, B. (1969). The Idea of Equality. In J. Feinberg (Ed.), *Moral Concepts*. Oxford, Oxford University Press.

Winnicott, D. W. (1945). *Getting to Know Your Baby*. London, Heinemann Medical Books.

Winnicott, D. W. (1951). Transitional Objects and Transitional Phenomena. *International Journal of Psychoanalysis* 35. Also in *Through Paediatrics to Psycho-analysis*, London, Hogarth Press, pp. 229–242, and *Playing and Reality*, London, Routledge Classics, pp. 1–34.

Winnicott, D. W. (1957). Further Thoughts on Babies as Persons. In J. Hardenberg (Ed.), *The Child and the Outside World: Studies in Developing Relationships*. London, Tavistock, pp. 134–140.

Winnicott, D. W. (1958a). The Capacity to Be Alone. *International Journal of Psychoanalysis* 39: 146–420.

Winnicott, D. W. (1958b). The Observation of Children in a Set Situation. In *Through Paediatrics to Psychoanalysis*. London, Hogarth Press, p. 58.

Winnicott, D. W. (1960). The Theory of the Parent-Infant Relationship. *International Journal of Psychoanalysis* 41: 585–595.

Winnicott, D. W. (1965/1985). *The Maturational Process and the Facilitating Environment*. London, Hogarth Press.

Winnicott, D. W. (1967/1971). *Playing and Reality*. London, Tavistock.

Winnicott, D. W. (1968). The Use of an Object and Relating Through Identification. *International Journal of Psycho-Analysis* 50: 711–716.

Winnicott, D. W. (1973). *The Child, the Family, and the Outside World*. Harmondsworth, UK, Penguin.

Winnicott, D. W. (1975). *Through Paediatrics to Psycho-analysis*. London, Hogarth Press.

Wolf, E. S. (2002). *Treating the Self: Elements of Clinical Self Psychology*. New York, Guilford Press.

Wolff, H. H., and Solomon, E. B. (1973). Individual and Group Psychotherapy: Complementary Growth Experiences. *International Journal of Group Psychotherapy* 23 (2): 177–184.

Wrangham, R., and Peterson, D. (1977/1996). *Demonic Males: Apes and the Origin of Human Violence*. London, Bloomsbury.

Wright, K. (2009). *Mirroring and Attunement: Self-Realization in Psychoanalysis and Art*. London, Routledge.

Wundt, W. (1911/2019). *Principles of Physiological Psychology Vols. I, II, III*. London, Forgotten Books.

Wundt, W. (1994). *Elements of Folk Psychology*. London, Gryphon Editions. Second edition, 2009, London, Biblioba.

Wurmser, L. (1981). *The Mask of Shame*. Baltimore, Johns Hopkins University Press.

Yalom, I. D., and Leszcz, M. (2005). *The Theory and Practice of Group Psychotherapy*. Fifth edition. New York, Basic Books.

Zeldin, I. (1979). *France 1948–1945: Politics and Anger*. Oxford, Oxford University Press.

Zinkin, L. (1983). Malignant Mirroring. *Group Analysis* 16 (2): 113–126.

Zinkin, L. (1989). The Group as Container and Contained. *Group Analysis* 22 (3): 227–234.

Index